VIRAL PATHOGENESIS
AND IMMUNOLOGY

Viral Pathogenesis
and Immunology

Cedric A. Mims

Professor of Microbiology
Guy's Hospital Medical School
London

AND

David O. White

Professor of Microbiology
University of Melbourne

BLACKWELL

SCIENTIFIC PUBLICATIONS

Oxford London Edinburgh
Boston Palo Alto Melbourne

© 1984 by
Blackwell Scientific Publications
Editorial offices:
Osney Mead, Oxford OX2 0EL
8 John Street, London WC1N 2ES
9 Forrest Road, Edinburgh EH1 2QH
52 Beacon Street, Boston
   Massachusetts 02108, USA
706 Cowper Street, Palo Alto
   California 94301, USA
99 Barry Street, Carlton
   Victoria 3053, Australia

First published 1984

Typeset by Acorn Bookwork
Salisbury, Wilts.
Printed in Great Britain
at the University Press, Cambridge

DISTRIBUTORS

USA
   Blackwell Mosby Book Distributors
   11830 Westline Industrial Drive
   St Louis, Missouri 63141

Canada
   Blackwell Mosby Book Distributors
   120 Melford Drive, Scarborough
   Ontario M1B 2X4

Australia
   Blackwell Scientific Book Distributors
   31 Advantage Road, Highett
   Victoria 3190

British Library
Cataloguing in Publication Data

Mims, Cedric A.
   Viral pathogenesis and immunology.
   1. Virus diseases—Immunological
   aspects
   I. Title   II. White, David O.
   616.9'25079   RC114.5

   ISBN 0-632-00193-9

Dedication

Both authors trained in Frank Fenner's department at the Australian National University in Canberra and were inescapably influenced by Sir Macfarlane Burnet. This book is dedicated to Burnet and Fenner—the former stands as no less than the father of modern virology and immunology, and the latter, among many other things, a classic contributor in viral pathogenesis. The book may not be as good as the one they would have written, but it reflects both the interests and the influence of these great men.

Contents

Introduction

Pathogenesis was for many years, and perhaps justifiably, regarded as a messy, unsatisfactory area for virus research—a sad state of affairs that was lamented by early enthusiasts (Mims, 1964). That view has been transformed. People now want to find out just how viruses cause diseases. In the first place, the extraordinary flowering of immunology is giving a much clearer understanding of host defence mechanisms, susceptibility to disease, and immunopathology. At the same time, research progress in virology itself has paved the way for better studies of pathogenesis; viral genes and their products can be identified and it is not unreasonable to hope that, before long, certain virus diseases will be described at the molecular level.

Burnet pointed out in 1955 that '. . . since most virus diseases are non-lethal, the termination of the disease and the elimination of virus from the body are at least as important as the initiation and development of infection' (Burnet, 1955, p. 204). Pathogenesis cannot be studied without also considering immunology and host defences.

This book surveys the pathogenesis of virus infection and gives to immunological phenomena the attention they deserve. It ends with a chapter on viral vaccines, an area of applied immunovirology in which exciting developments are taking place. Except for the briefest mention of RNA tumour viruses under persistent infections, we have not dealt with viruses and tumours. It is as up to date as a book can be, and fully referenced. We have given recent references where possible because they refer to earlier work, and we apologise to the many scientists whose papers have not been cited because of constraints of space.

This is the first book to deal centrally with viral pathogenesis and immunology. It is now a fast moving, fascinating subject and new work will soon alter the details, but we hope that the general principles outlined here will continue to be useful.

Chapter One
Basic Characteristics of Viruses

DEFINITION OF VIRUS

We tend to think of viruses as the smallest of the microorganisms responsible for infectious disease. Yet, strictly speaking, they are not microorganisms, for they are not cells. Unlike bacteria, they contain no organelles and have no metabolism. Consisting basically of a nucleic acid genome enclosed within a protective coat of protein, they are metabolically inert until they enter the host cell upon which they are absolutely dependent for their replication. It is true that most viruses do carry a nucleic acid polymerase which can under certain experimental situations transcribe messenger RNA from the viral genome in a test-tube, and that certain additional steps involved in viral replication have been successfully accomplished *in vitro*; however, under natural circumstances, viruses are capable of multiplying only inside living cells. They are thus obligate intracellular parasites, which utilise the organelles and metabolic pathways of the host cell for their own reproduction.

1

Viruses parasitise all of God's creatures. There are viruses of all vertebrates—not only mammals (see Fenner *et al.*, 1974), but also birds, reptiles, fish and amphibia (Andrewes *et al.*, 1978). There are viruses of invertebrates, especially insects (Gibbs, 1973; Tinsley and Harrap, 1978) but also protozoa (Diamond and Mattern, 1976). There are viruses of plants (Matthews, 1981), even of algae (Sherman and Brown, 1978) and fungi (Hollings, 1978). Even the smallest free-living creatures, the bacteria, are parasitised by viruses (Luria *et al.*, 1978). Indeed, there is reason to believe that the number of distinct species of viruses on earth far exceeds the number of species of all other living things. Every species that has been studied, e.g. man, monkey, mouse, *E. coli*, has yielded dozens of different viruses. By no means all of them produce disease, though many do under certain circumstances. This book is concerned only with mammalian viruses, and in particular with those responsible for disease in man.

STRUCTURE OF VIRUSES

Nucleic acid

The genome of a virus consists of either DNA or RNA. The latter is unique in biology—no other living creature employs RNA as its repository of genetic information. Furthermore, viral nucleic acid (NA), whether DNA or RNA, may be single- or double-stranded. It may be linear or circular. It may consist of a single 'polycistronic' molecule, analogous to a chromosome comprised of a string of genes; alternatively, the genome may be 'segmented', occurring as a number of distinct molecules, each being a separate gene. Moreover, single-stranded viral nucleic acid may be of positive or negative 'polarity'. If positive it represents meaningful information and the viral RNA acts as messenger RNA; if negative, i.e. complementary RNA, messenger RNA must first be transcribed from it by a transcriptase carried in the virion (Bishop, 1977). The nature of the viral nucleic acid dictates the strategy of viral replication. It also forms the basis of viral classification (Baltimore, 1971).

Protein

The nucleic acid (NA) is enclosed within a protein coat, which presumably serves to protect the genome from degradation, to package at least one copy of each essential NA molecule, to hold the NA in the correct conformation with respect to its transcriptase, and to repress the transcription of certain 'early' genes. The more complex viruses may have an inner core of protein in close apposition with the NA, which in turn is surrounded by one (or sometimes two) concentric shells of protein, which display a particular type of symmetry, described below.

Isometric viruses

The introduction of negative staining to electron microscopy (see Brenner and Horne, 1959) revealed, quite unexpectedly, that the outer protein coat of most viruses is in fact a thing of beauty as well as practicality (review: Horne and Wildy, 1979). The protein molecules are arranged symmetrically to form an isometric structure, in the shape of an icosahedron, i.e. a 20-sided solid, each face being an equilateral triangle (review: Caspar, 1965). As first pointed out by Caspar and Klug (1962), one would expect that, for reasons of genetic economy (Crick and Watson, 1956), the shell of a virus particle would ideally consist of a number of repeating units of the same protein molecule, and that the optimal arrangement of such units to produce a stable tightly-packed array with minimum stress on the bonds between them would be that particular type of polyhedron known as an icosahedron. In fact, although the shells of some small viruses are constructed entirely of such identical units, most use at least one additional type of polypeptide, e.g. at the vertices of the icosahedron, to stabilise the structure. To use the terminology first introduced by Lwoff *et al.* (1959) and now widely adopted, the virus particle ('virion') has an outer shell ('capsid') composed of morphological units ('capsomers') arranged with 'icosahedral symmetry'. Each capsomer consists of one or a small number of protein molecules. There are, however, some viruses of known icosahedral symmetry (e.g. picornaviruses), the capsomers of which are not clearly visible by electron microscopy.

Enveloped viruses with tubular nucleocapsids

In a second form of symmetry, 'helical symmetry', the capsomers surround the viral NA in the form of a helix or spiral to form a 'tubular nucleocapsid'. Most mammalian RNA viruses have this form, the tube being flexible, wound into a coil, and enclosed within a lipoprotein envelope. Many plant and bacterial viruses consist of rod-shaped tubular nucleocapsids, but they are 'naked', having no envelope. The envelope is acquired by the virion during release by 'budding' from the infected cell; it consists therefore of plasma membrane from which cellular proteins have been displaced by viral glycoproteins that project from the envelope as 'peplomers', or 'spikes' (Compans and Klenk, 1979). Hence, although the viral envelope contains no cellular proteins, its lipids are cellular, and the oligosaccharide side-chains on the virus-coded glycoproteins as well as on the cellular glycolipids are determined in part by the cell's glycosyl transferases. While all vertebrate viruses with nucleocapsids of helical symmetry are enveloped, only a minority of those with isometric nucleocapsids also have an envelope (e.g. the Herpesviridae). A few families of viruses, notably the retroviruses and poxviruses, have more complex structures still.

The relative sizes and shapes of viruses of the major families of animal viruses are depicted diagrammatically in Fig. 1.1.

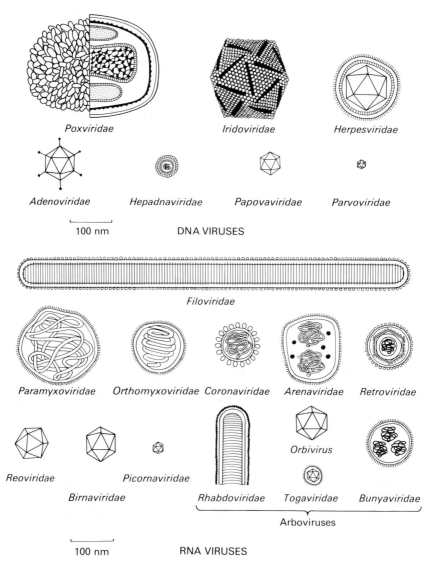

Fig. 1.1. Diagram illustrating the shapes and relative sizes of animal viruses of the major families (bar = 100 nm). Courtesy of Fenner *et al.* (1985) *Veterinary Virology*. Academic Press, New York.

CLASSIFICATION OF VIRUSES

At the conclusion of World War II we knew of only a handful of human viruses, but hundreds more have been discovered subsequently, largely as a result of the exploitation of cell culture (Enders *et al.*, 1949). Systematic attempts to develop taxonomic criteria for classifying viruses began only in the 1960s and have since that time been under the control of the International Committee on Taxonomy of Viruses (ICTV) (see Fenner *et al.*, 1974; Matthews, 1983).

Vertebrate viruses are currently classified into about 20 families (for review and comprehensive listing, see Matthews, 1982) on the basis of a number of parameters which may be grouped under two main headings: (1) the nature of the genome and (2) the structure of the virion. More specifically, the information considered most fundamental is:

Nucleic acid
   DNA or RNA
   Molecular weight (MW)
   Single-stranded (SS) or double-stranded (DS)
   Linear or circular
   Polycistronic or segmented
   Polarity + or − (if SS)
Virion
   Size
   Shape
   Symmetry of capsid (icosahedral or helical)
   Transcriptase in virion?
   Envelope?

Pathogenetic and epidemiological properties determining such crucial matters as host range and mode of transmission, which have been incorporated into useful cryptograms (Fenner and Gibbs, 1983), are not generally regarded as crucial taxonomic criteria for assigning viruses to families. A single family may accommodate viruses with comparable genomes and morphology which nevertheless have totally distinct host ranges and modes of transmission. For instance, the Rhabdoviridae and Reoviridae families contain viruses of plants and insects as well as of vertebrates, including man.

Classification within families, into genera, then species, types and strains is currently based mainly on serology (review: Schmidt, 1979). In general, internal proteins tend to be relatively conserved through recent evolution and are often common to a number of viruses, whereas antigenic drift in surface proteins has led to the emergence of different serotypes. Though rather more complicated, methods are now available for assessing the degree of similarity between the genomes of viruses. Genetic homology can be determined by molecular hybridisation, or the precise nucleotide sequence of the viral nucleic acid can be determined chemically (see Laver and Air, 1980; Nayak, 1981). Such procedures for characterising the genome have been used not only to construct dendrograms, tracing the recent evolution of influenza viruses by antigenic drift and shift (Air *et al.*, 1981), but also to estimate the antiquity of herpesviruses (Nahmias *et al.*, 1981) and retroviruses (Weiss *et al.*, 1982) indigenous to, or integrated into the genome of, particular host species believed, from the fossil records, to have evolved hundreds of millions of years ago.

The physicochemical properties of the genome and structural features of the virion which characterise the known families of DNA and RNA viruses are summarised in Tables 1.1 and 1.2.

THE FAMILIES OF MAMMALIAN VIRUSES: PEN PORTRAITS

Papovaviruses

Small icosahedral DNA viruses noted for capacity to produce tumours *in vivo* and to transform cultured cells (review: Sambrook, 1981). Circular molecule of ds DNA. Nuclear replication.

Papillomavirus genus (virion: 55 nm; DNA 5×10^6 daltons) contains numerous host-specific viruses, including many human serotypes, causing benign skin papillomas (warts) in animals. Polyomavirus genus (virion 45 nm; DNA 3×10^6 daltons) contains the famous polyoma virus (of mice) and SV40 (of monkeys) used as experimental models for the study of carcinogenesis. The human polyomaviruses, BK & JC, commonly produce inapparent infection and may be reactivated by immunosuppression.

Adenoviruses

Medium-sized icosahedral DNA viruses distributed widely in animals and birds (review: Wigand *et al.*, 1982; Ginsberg, 1984). Nuclear multiplication, basophilic inclusions. Some haemagglutinate rat or monkey RBC. Some are oncogenic in baby rodents.

Now 39 known human species (previously designated 'types') recovered from throat or faeces. Infections usually asymptomatic, e.g. persistent infections of tonsils and adenoids, but some types responsible for conjunctivitis, pharyngitis and other respiratory infections. Role in gastroenteritis unknown but uncultivable virions often visualised by EM in faeces.

Table 1.1 Properties of the virions of the recognised families of DNA animal viruses.

Family	Genome[a] Mol. wt. ($\times 10^6$)	Genome[a] Nature[b]	Shape[c]	Virion Size (nm)	Transcriptase
Papovaviridae	3–5	D, circular	Icosahedral (72)	45–55	–
Adenoviridae	20–30	D, linear	Icosahedral (252)	70–90	–
Herpesviridae	80–150	D, linear	Icosahedral (162), enveloped	Envelope 120–150; capsid 100–110	–
Iridoviridae	130–140	D, linear	Icosahedral (~1500) enveloped	Capsid, 190	+
Poxviridae	120–200	D, linear	Brick-shaped, sometimes enveloped	$300 \times 240 \times 100$	+
Parvoviridae	1.5–2.2	S, linear	Icosahedral (32)	18–26	–
Hepadnavirus group	1.8	D(S), circular[d]	Spherical	42	–

[a]Genome invariably a single molecule.
[b]D, double-stranded; S, single-stranded.
[c]Figure in parentheses indicates number of capsomers in icosahedral capsids.
[d]Circular molecule is double-stranded for most of its length but contains a single-stranded region of variable length.

Courtesy of White & Fenner (in press). *Medical Virology*, 3rd edn. Academic Press, New York.

Table 1.2 Properties of the virions of the recognised families of RNA animal viruses.

Family	Genome		Virion				
	Mol. wt. ($\times 10^6$)	Nature[a]	Envelope	Shape[b]	Size (nm)	Transcriptase	Symmetry of nucleocapsid[c]
Picornaviridae	2.6	S, 1	–	Icosahedral	20–30	–	Icosahedral (20–30)
Caliciviridae	2.8	S, 1	–	Icosahedral	35–39	–	Icosahedral (35–39)
Togaviridae	4	S, 1	+	Spherical	40–70	–	Icosahedral (25–35)
Orthomyxoviridae	5	S, 8	+	Spherical	80–120	+	Helical (9–15)
Paramyxoviridae	5.7	S, 1	+	Spherical	100–300	+	Helical (12–17)
Coronaviridae	6	S, 1	+	Spherical	75–160	–	Helical (11–13)
Arenaviridae	5	S, 2	+	Spherical	110–130	+	Helical (?)
Bunyaviridae	5.5	S, 3	+	Spherical	90–100	+	Helical (2–2.5)
Retroviridae	2×3[d]	S, 1	+	Spherical	80–100	+(Reverse)	Helical (?)
Rhabdoviridae	4	S, 1	+	Bullet-shaped	170×70	+	Helical (5)
Filovirus group	4.2	S, 1	+	Filamentous	800×80	?+	Helical
Reoviridae	12–15	D, 10–12	–	Icosahedral	60–80	+	Icosahedral (45–60)
Birnavirus group	4.8	D, 2	–	Icosahedral	60	+	Icosahedral (45)

[a] All molecules linear; S, single-stranded; D, double-stranded; number, number of molecules in genome.
[b] Some enveloped viruses are very pleomorphic (sometimes filamentous).
[c] Figure in brackets indicates diameter (nm) of nucleocapsids.
[d] Inverted dimer.

Courtesy of White & Fenner (in press). *Medical Virology*, 3rd edn. Academic Press, New York.

Herpesviruses

Large icosahedral enveloped DNA viruses (review: Roizman *et al.*, 1981; Roizman, 1982–4), noted for tendency to establish persistent (often latent) infections and to be reactivated by immunosuppression. DNA ds, linear, containing reiterated sequences, wrapped around a protein core; enclosed within an icosahedral capsid which is in turn surrounded by a bilayered membrane. Nuclear replication. Produce intranuclear inclusions and often giant cells in culture and *in vivo*. Spread usually by mucosal secretions, e.g. saliva, otherwise respiratory or urinary.

The family contains over 80 viruses, widely spread throughout vertebrates and invertebrates. Many species, e.g. different monkeys carry their own unique herpesvirus. Well-known examples in animals and birds include pseudorabies (swine), malignant catarrhal fever (wildebeest), infectious rhinotracheitis (cattle, cats), equine rhinopneumonitis (equine abortion) and infectious laryngotracheitis (chickens). Many animal species have unique cytomegaloviruses. Several herpesviruses are oncogenic, e.g. Lucké virus of frogs, Marek's disease virus of chickens, *Herpesvirus saimiri* and *Herpesvirus ateles* in monkeys.

All four human herpesviruses are common and important (review: Nahmias *et al.*, 1981; Roizman, 1982). Herpes simplex, type 1: primary—pharyngitis; recurrent—'cold sores'. Also kerato-conjunctivitis, meningo-encephalitis, etc. Type 2: herpes genitalis, neonatal herpes. Varicella-zoster: primary—chickenpox; recurrent—herpes zoster ('shingles'). Cytomegalovirus (review: Ho, 1982): inapparent, persistent, with shedding into saliva, urine; severe congenital abnormalities (cytomegalic inclusion disease) in newborn; lethal pneumonitis, hepatitis in immunocompromised. EB virus (review: Epstein and Achong, 1979; Kieff *et al.*, 1982): infectious mononucleosis (glandular fever) in adolescents; persists in B lymphocytes; associated with nasopharyngeal carcinoma in Chinese, and Burkitt lymphoma.

Iridoviruses

Very large complex icosahedral double-stranded DNA viruses many of which infect insects, others amphibia or fish (review: Goorha and Granoff, 1979). African swine fever virus is the most important agent affecting mammals. No known human iridoviruses.

Poxviruses

The largest viruses (review: Fenner *et al.*, 1985), just visible by light microscopy. Complex brick-shaped virion containing very long linear molecule of cross-linked ds DNA and transcriptase plus several other enzymes in a protein core surrounded by a complex series of membranes. Cytoplasmic multiplication. Dermatotrophic—characteristic skin lesions. Transmission by contact, airborne, or mechanically by arthropods (e.g. myxomatosis of rabbits).

Host-specific poxviruses infect numerous animals and birds. Man occasionally acquires zoonotic infections, e.g. cowpox, milker's nodes and orf. Molluscum contagiosum unique to man. Smallpox eradicated by vaccination in 1980.

Parvoviruses

Tiny icosahedral viruses with unique genome of single-stranded DNA (review: Berns, 1983). Nuclear replication. Infect insects and mammals, e.g. rat virus (Kilham), feline panleukopenia virus, Aleutian mink disease virus, and a probable human parvovirus that infects blood-forming cells in the bone marrow. The four serotypes of human adeno-associated virus (AAV) are defective, requiring concurrent infection with 'helper' adenovirus or herpesvirus. Found in human throat but not known to cause disease.

Hepadnaviruses

Small spherical DNA viruses causing hepatitis and persistent infections (review: Tiollais *et al.*, 1981; Marion and Robinson, 1983). Very short circular double-stranded DNA molecule containing a single-stranded region of variable length, associated with DNA polymerase inside an icosahedral protein 'core' (HB_cAg) which is in turn enclosed within a closely adherent 'envelope' containing cellular lipids, glycoproteins and 'surface' antigen (HB_sAg). The 42 nm virion ('Dane particle') is usually accompanied by excess 22 nm HB_sAg particles. Nuclear replication in hepatocytes. Yet to be grown conventionally *in vitro*, but cultured cells can be transfected with viral DNA.

Tentative Hepadnaviridae family contains the hepatitis viruses of woodchuck, ground squirrel and duck. Human hepatitis B virus (review: Szmuness *et al.*, 1982), of which there are several subtypes, is transmitted principally by blood, but also saliva, semen, perinatally, especially from chronic carriers. May progress to chronic hepatitis, cirrhosis, hepatocellular carcinoma.

Picornaviruses

The smallest RNA viruses (review: Cooper *et al.*, 1978; Perez-Bercoff, 1979). Icosahedral, non-enveloped virion contains polycistronic linear ss RNA of positive polarity (positive sense, i.e. infectious) which is poly-adenylated at its 3'-end and has a small protein, VP_g attached to its

5'-end. Cytoplasmic multiplication, cytocidal for cultured cells. Generally host-specific and spread by alimentary or respiratory routes.

A large and important family, divided into four major genera: *Enterovirus*, *Rhinovirus*, *Cardiovirus* and *Aphthovirus*.

Enteroviruses are acid-stable (at pH 3) and infect the enteric tract of animals such as pigs, cattle, rodents and monkeys as well as man. Human enteroviruses (review: Grist *et al.*, 1978) were originally divided into the polioviruses (three serotypes, producing paralytic poliomyelitis), echoviruses (32 types) and coxsackieviruses (23 types of coxsackie A, six types of B), the latter being distinguished by their pathogenicity for infant mice. Following recognition that this distinction is rather artificial, more recently discovered enteroviruses have been simply numbered sequentially from 68 onwards. The latest, enterovirus 72, is the agent of hepatitis A (review: Szmuness *et al.*, 1982). The other enteroviruses habitually multiply asymptomatically in the gut but may also cause diseases ranging from mild undifferentiated 'summer febrile illnesses', rashes, respiratory infections, and vesicular pharyngitis (coxsackie A), through moderately debilitating episodes of 'aseptic' meningitis or myalgia (Bornholm disease—coxsackie B), to more serious diseases including carditis (often lethal in the newborn—coxsackie B), pancreatitis or haemolytic uraemia (coxsackie B), pneumonia (enterovirus 68), pandemic acute haemorrhagic conjunctivitis, sometimes with radiculomyelitis (enterovirus 70), or encephalitis (enterovirus 71). The *Rhinoviruses* (review: Macnaughton, 1982) are acid-labile and are the major aetiological agent of the common cold; there were 113 distinct serotypes at the last count. The rodent viruses known as EMC, ME and Mengo constitute the *Cardiovirus* genus, while genus *Aphthovirus* accommodates the seven serotypes (and numerous subtypes) of the virus causing foot-and-mouth disease in cloven-hooved animals (review: Brooksby, 1982). Certain unclassified insect viruses also appear to belong to the Picornaviridae family.

Caliciviruses

Small icosahedral RNA viruses resembling picornaviruses, but somewhat larger with distinct capsid morphology and genome strategy (review: Schaffer, 1979). This new family now accommodates the feline calicivirus, vesicular exanthema of swine virus, and the human caliciviruses causing gastroenteritis, the prototype of which was originally designated Norwalk virus (Greenberg *et al.*, 1981).

Astroviruses

Small isometric non-enveloped viruses somewhat resembling picornaviruses or caliciviruses but displaying a characteristic star-shaped outline (review: Holmes, 1979). Recovered from faeces of lambs, calves and human neonates, and may cause diarrhoea. Uncultured; genome undefined; unclassified taxonomically.

Togaviruses

Small icosahedral enveloped RNA viruses (review: Porterfield *et al.*, 1978; Schlesinger, 1980). RNA, single-stranded, linear, non-segmented, positive polarity. Haemagglutinate at defined pHs. Cytoplasmic multiplication.

Most togaviruses belong to the genera *Alphavirus* and *Flavivirus*, and are arboviruses, i.e. multiply in a blood-sucking arthropod and are transmitted by bite to a vertebrate (but not all togaviruses are arboviruses and not all arboviruses are togaviruses). The vector is usually a mosquito, less commonly a tick, sandfly, or gnat, in which the togavirus may be maintained indefinitely by transovarial infection. The natural vertebrate reservoir is a bird, mammal or reptile in which the infection is often inapparent. Infection of man normally produces subclinical infection or a syndrome characterised by fever, arthralgia, with or without a rash (e.g. the viruses of dengue, chikungunya, o'nyong-nyong, Ross River). However, togaviruses can also give rise to several of the most lethal human diseases. These fall into two main clinical entities: encephalitis (e.g. Japanese, St Louis, Eastern equine, Western equine, Venezuelan equine, and Australian encephalitis viruses) and haemorrhagic fever (e.g. yellow fever—in which hepatitis is a conspicuous feature; dengue—usually reinfection with a different serotype, often leading to death from dengue shock syndrome (Halstead, 1981a); Kyasanur Forest disease—India; Omsk haemorrhagic fever—U.S.S.R.). There are dozens of such togaviruses, each with its own characteristic ecological niche in some corner of the world (review: Theiler and Downs, 1973; Berge, 1975).

Some togaviruses are not arthropod-borne but spread in more conventional ways. Members of the genus *Pestivirus* include the viruses of mucosal disease (bovine virus diarrhoea), hog cholera (European swine fever), and possibly equine arteritis and lactic dehydrogenase viruses. The *Rubivirus* genus accommodates the virus causing rubella in man (and the congenital rubella syndrome in the foetus).

Orthomyxoviruses

Quite large enveloped RNA viruses with nucleocapsid of helical symmetry. The genome consists of eight separate molecules of single-stranded RNA of negative polarity, each comprising a separate gene, with its own transcriptase. Two types of glycoprotein project from the envelope: haemagglutinin (agglutinates erythrocytes) and neuraminidase (cleaves sialic acid from glycoproteins) (review: Laver and Air, 1980).

Influenza A viruses are widespread in birds (e.g. ducks, turkeys, chickens, pelagic birds) and mammals (horses, pigs, man). Genetic reassortment produces subtypes with novel HA genes which precipitate pandemics of human influenza ('antigenic shift'). Point mutations in the HA gene generate new strains ('antigenic drift') (review: Webster *et al.*, 1982).

Paramyxoviruses

Large pleomorphic enveloped RNA viruses (review: Choppin and Compans, 1975). Nucleocapsid has helical symmetry. Non-segmented single-stranded RNA of negative polarity, plus transcriptase. Envelope contains two glycoproteins: haemagglutinin (often carrying neuraminidase activity also = HN) and fusion (F) protein. Cytoplasmic inclusions, syncytia, haemadsorption (usually). Respiratory spread.

Important pathogens in animals include the viruses of canine distemper, rinderpest (cattle), Newcastle disease (birds), and parainfluenza viruses affecting various animals.

The family contains four human pathogens, all common and important: measles, mumps, parainfluenza (types 1–4) and respiratory syncytial (RS) virus. Parainfluenza viruses are a common cause of croup (laryngotracheobronchitis) while RS virus causes regular winter epidemics of bronchiolitis/pneumonitis in infants (review: Jackson and Muldoon, 1973).

Coronaviruses

Quite large pleomorphic RNA viruses of helical symmetry with large club-shaped projections from the envelope (review: Siddell *et al.*, 1983). RNA linear, single-stranded, non-segmented, of positive polarity. Cytoplasmic multiplication.

The family includes the viruses of infectious bronchitis of chickens and transmissible gastroenteritis of pigs, among others. Murine hepatitis and feline infectious peritonitis viruses establish persistent infections.

Several human serotypes cause common colds, especially in adults during winter, and perhaps recurrent wheezing in asthmatic children and chronic bronchitis in adults. Coronavirus-like particles are often seen in faeces but their role in human gastroenteritis is uncertain.

Arenaviruses

Quite large pleomorphic enveloped RNA viruses with a protein core of currently unknown structure, club-shaped peplomers and, uniquely, non-functional ribosomes (review: Rawls and Leung, 1979). RNA, single-stranded, segmented (two species of 'viral' RNA of negative polarity, two of cellular ribosomal RNA, and one of ? cellular transfer RNA), plus transcriptase. Cytoplasmic multiplication.

Most arenaviruses cause persistent inapparent infections in their natural rodent host (e.g. lymphocytic choriomeningitis (LCM) virus in mice), being transmitted vertically, including congenitally. Horizontal spread via excreta, especially urine, to man can produce lethal disease, e.g. Junin and Machupo viruses, producing Argentine and Bolivian haemorrhagic fevers respectively, and the virus of (West African) Lassa fever (review: Buckley and Casals, 1978).

Bunyaviruses

Large spherical enveloped RNA arboviruses of helical symmetry (review: Bishop and Shope, 1979). RNA single-stranded, segmented into three circular (end hydrogen-bonded) molecules, of negative-polarity, plus transcriptase. Genetic reassortment between bunyaviruses is readily demonstrable in the laboratory. Though only recently defined, the family already contains well over 100 species, virtually all of them arthropod-borne. Transovarial, transstadial and venereal transmission have been demonstrated in some arthropods.

The *Bunyavirus* genus, mainly mosquito-transmitted, includes the California group (e.g. California encephalitis, La Crosse). Genus *Phlebovirus* accommodates the important agents of sandfly fever (transmitted by *Phlebotomus*) and Rift Valley fever, both responsible for widespread human disease in Africa. Members of the *Nairovirus* genus, named for the Nairobi sheep disease virus, but also including the agent of Crimean-Congo haemorrhagic fever, are tick-borne. Recently assigned tentatively to the Bunyaviridae family is the Hantaan virus, the cause of the condition which used to be called Korean haemorrhagic fever, but is now referred to as haemorrhagic fever with renal syndrome (HFRS). The agent (review: McCormick and Johnson, 1984) is extremely widely disseminated, causing serious human disease through Northern Asia and Europe, and serological evidence of infection in other continents as well. Rodents, including rats and voles constitute the reservoir; spread possibly occurs by aerosol, not via arthropods.

Retroviruses

Quite large spherical enveloped RNA viruses characterised by a unique morphology, a unique genome, a unique enzyme and a unique life-history (reviews: Bishop, 1978; Weiss *et al.*, 1982). The virion seems to be a helical ribonucleoprotein within an icosahedral capsid within a lipoprotein membrane from which project glycoprotein peplomers. The genome is diploid, consisting of two copies of the same linear molecule of single-stranded positive-sense RNA, base-paired (hydrogen-bonded) at the 5' ends to form an inverted dimer; polyadenylated at the 3' end, capped at the 5' end, with redundant sequences at both ends; a cellular tRNA, which serves as a primer for reverse transcription by the reverse transcriptase (RNA-dependent DNA polymerase) present in the virion. The cDNA so transcribed becomes integrated into the genome of the infected cell and may remain there throughout the lives of that animal and its progeny, being transmitted vertically and inherited in Mendelian fashion as normal cellular genes, and having no detectable effects. These are the 'endogenous' oncoviruses. Some members of the *Oncovirinae* subfamily are oncogenic; 'exogenous' oncoviruses spread horizontally to susceptible vertebrates and may (or may not) induce a malignant tumour—commonly a leukaemia or lymphoma, but sometimes a sarcoma or carcinoma.

Oncoviruses are quite host-specific. Examples are Rous sarcoma virus, mouse mammary tumour virus, Mason-Pfizer monkey virus, and numerous leukaemia and sarcoma viruses of mice and other rodents, chickens and other birds, cattle, cats, monkeys and other primates including man (e.g. T cell leukaemia virus).

The *Spumavirinae* subfamily comprises a number of non-oncogenic 'syncytial' or 'foamy' viruses, while the *Lentivirinae* subfamily embraces some interesting viruses with a triploid genome which cause 'slow infections' of the CNS or lung in sheep (visna, maedi and progressive pneumonia).

Rhabdoviruses

Large bullet-shaped enveloped RNA viruses of helical symmetry (review: Bishop, 1979). RNA, single-stranded, linear, non-segmented, of negative polarity, plus transcriptase. Cytoplasmic multiplication.

The family encompasses viruses from hosts representing all the kingdoms, and includes many that multiply in both plants and insects, or in vertebrates and insects. Arthropod vectors include mosquitoes, sandflies, tabanids, midges, mites, leafhoppers and aphids. Some are transmitted vertically in insects. The plant rhabdoviruses, all of which multiply in aphids or leafhoppers as well, tend to be longer and baciliform (rounded at both ends) rather than bullet-shaped. Well-known examples of mammalian rhabdoviruses include the agents of vesicular stomatitis (horses), bovine ephemeral fever and rabies.

Rabies is native to a number of wild animals including foxes, wolves, jackals, skunks, raccoons, mongooses, and bats; around human settlements in endemic areas it also infects domestic dogs and cats. Spread to man is via saliva, usually by bite from a rabid animal. Virtually 100% lethal unless the infected individual is vaccinated promptly.

Filoviruses

Extraordinarily long pleomorphic, sometimes branched, U-shaped or circular, filamentous enveloped RNA viruses somewhat resembling rhabdoviruses in their internal structure (review: Kiley *et al.*, 1982). Easily visible by light microscopy. Single molecule of ssRNA, probably of negative sense. Cytoplasmic multiplication.

This tentative family contains the exotic viruses, Marburg and Ebola, indigenous to Africa. Their natural hosts are not known, although Marburg virus was first recovered from monkeys from which human contacts had contracted a highly lethal haemorrhagic fever in the course of using their kidneys for the manufacture of poliovaccine.

Reoviruses

Medium-sized icosahedral double-shelled non-enveloped viruses with a unique genome consisting of 10–12 linear molecules of double-stranded RNA, each being a separate gene associated with a transcriptase (reviews: Joklik, 1983; Compans and Bishop, 1983). Cytoplasmic multiplication. Includes members of the cytoplasmic polyhedrosis group which are well-known viruses of insects, whereas the *Phytoreovirus* and *Fijivirus* genera multiply in both plants and insects.

There are three mammalian genera. Members of the *Reovirus* genus occur in birds and mammals, including man; the three human serotypes multiply in the enteric and respiratory tracts but induce no known disease. The *Orbivirus* genus (review: Verwoerd *et al.*, 1979) contains a large number of arboviruses including those causing Colorado tick fever in man (vector: tick), bluetongue in sheep (vector: *Culicoides*), and African horse sickness (vector unknown). The *Rotavirus* genus comprises a large number of agents, all causing diarrhoea. Almost every mammalian species to be carefully searched seems to have its own rotavirus. At least three human serotypes constitute the major cause of gastroenteritis in infants world-wide (review: Holmes, 1979; Estes *et al.*, 1983).

Birnaviruses

Medium-sized icosahedral single-shelled non-enveloped viruses with a genome consisting of two molecules of double-stranded RNA. Cytoplasmic multiplication. Found in birds, fish, molluscs and insects, e.g. infectious bursal disease virus of chickens, infectious pancreatic necrosis virus of fish, *Drosophila* X virus.

Nodaviruses

Small, naked, icosahedral RNA viruses containing two ssRNA molecules of positive polarity. Cytoplasmic multiplication. Though all have been recovered only from insects in nature, one virus, Nodamura, also grows in infant mice and cultured vertebrate cells.

Agents of subacute spongiform encephalopathies

May or may not be viruses; so far not shown to contain nucleic acid. Very small infectious agents, highly resistant to heat, ionising radiation and various nucleases and other chemicals damaging to nucleic acids; non-immunogenic (review: Kimberlin, 1981).

A common feature of the proposed members of this putative family is that they all produce slow infections with incubation periods measured in months or even years leading inexorably to death from a degenerative condition of the brain characterised by a 'spongiform' appearance (vacuolation) (review: Gajdusek, 1977).

THE MULTIPLICATION OF VIRUSES

It is not appropriate to devote a whole chapter of this book to the biochemistry of viral replication, a vast, specialised and rapidly moving subject to which several multivolume treatises have been devoted. Interested readers are referred to *Comprehensive Virology*, vols. 1–18 Fraenkel-Conrat and Wagner, 1974–83), *The Viruses*, several volumes (Fraenkel-Conrat and Wagner, 1982–), *The Replication of Negative-Strand Viruses* (Bishop and Compans, 1981), *The Molecular Biology of Tumor Viruses. DNA Tumor Viruses* (Tooze, 1980), *RNA Tumor Viruses* (Weiss *et al.*, 1982).

Nevertheless, we do consider it relevant to present here a concise synopsis of the salient features of viral multiplication in so far as they contribute to our understanding of viral pathogenesis and immunology at the molecular level. To render the task tractable we have taken some artistic licence—using broad strokes of the brush we paint a composite picture highlighting the key common features of viral replication rather than the minutiae of detail that distinguish each of the 20 families. Certain well studied viruses are taken as models to illustrate the important distinctions between the strategies governing the expression of the distinct types of viral genome.

Fig. 1.2 illustrates in a stylised and greatly simplified diagram the major steps in the multiplication of a 'typical' mammalian virus. Following attachment, the virion is taken up by its host cell and is partially uncoated to expose the viral genome. Certain 'early' viral genes are transcribed into messenger RNA which may then be processed in a number of ways, including splicing. The early gene-products translated from this mRNA are of two main types: proteins that shut down cellular nucleic acid and protein synthesis and regulate the expression of the

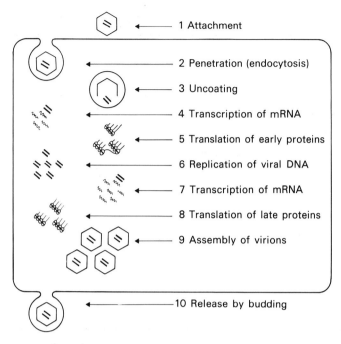

Fig. 1.2. The viral multiplication cycle—a stylised and greatly simplified diagram summarising the key steps in the multiplication of a 'typical' DNA virus. Courtesy of Fenner & White (1976) *Medical Virology*, 2nd edn. Academic Press, New York.

viral genome, and enzymes required for the replication of viral nucleic acid. Following viral nucleic acid (NA) replication, 'late' viral genes become available for transcription. The late proteins are principally structural proteins for incorporation into new virions; some of these are subject to post-translational glycosylation and/or cleavage. Assembly of icosahedral virions occurs in the nucleus or cytoplasm, depending on the particular family. Enveloped viruses, on the other hand, are completed only as they 'bud' through cellular (usually plasma) membrane. Each infected cell yields several thousand new virions over a period of several hours.

Some of the more obvious differences between the families of mammalian viruses in respect of their multiplication are set out in Table 1.3. It will be noted that, with some families, many of the crucial events take place in the cell nucleus, while others multiply exclusively within the cytoplasm (and, in some cases, can multiply successfully in enucleated cells). Some acquire an envelope by budding. The 'eclipse period' or 'latent period' (between infection and production of the first new virion) may be as short as two hours or as long as 24 hours. Some shut down the synthesis of cellular macromolecules very effectively whereas others

Table 1.3. Characteristics of multiplication of selected viruses.

Family	Example	Site of NA replication	Eclipse period (hours)	Budding	Cell shut-down
Papovaviridae	SV40	N	15	–	–
Adenoviridae	Human type 2	N	12	–	+
Herpesviridae	Herpes simplex	N	5	N	+
Poxviridae	Vaccinia	C	5	GP	+
Picornaviridae	Poliovirus	C	$2\frac{1}{2}$	–	+
Togaviridae	Sindbis	C	$2\frac{1}{2}$	P	+
Orthomyxoviridae	Influenza A	N	3	P	+
Paramyxoviridae	NDV	C	4	P	+
Retroviridae	Avian leukosis	N	10	P	–
Rhabdoviridae	VSV	C	$2\frac{1}{2}$	P	+
Reoviridae	Reovirus 3	C	5	–	+

N = nucleus; C = cytoplasm; P = plasma membrane; G = Golgi apparatus.

do not. Indeed, some viruses are 'non-cytocidal', and others actually induce the cell to divide, or even 'transform' it to the malignant state.

Strategy of expression of the viral genome

The story of viral multiplication is the story of the expression of the information contained within the viral genome. While Fig. 1.2 adequately summarises the way in which the genome of a DNA virus is transcribed, translated and replicated, the plot must be modified somewhat to cater for RNA viruses. Moreover, there are very important differences between viruses containing single-stranded rather than double-stranded NA, and between viruses with RNA of positive or negative polarity. Evolution has left us with a quite remarkable diversity of types of viral genome, each with its own unique strategy of replication. With characteristic perspicacity Baltimore (1971) identified the nub of the matter. To make protein one must first have mRNA; hence, either viral RNA must itself be mRNA, or it must be transcribed into mRNA by a transcriptase carried in the virion. Fig. 1.3 illustrates the strategies employed by the six basic classes of viral genome to transcribe mRNA.

There are subtle variations on these basic themes (review: Strauss & Strauss, 1983). The genome of some viruses is in the form of a single polycistronic chromosome, while that of others is segmented into several

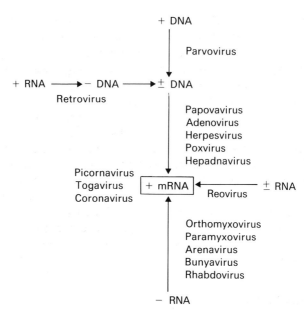

Fig. 1.3. Six basic strategies for transcribing messenger RNA from different types of viral genome. Modified from Baltimore (1971) *Bacteriol. Rev.* **35**, 235.

molecules each of which may (or may not) comprise a separate gene. Messenger RNA transcribed from polycistronic genomes in particular may (or may not) be subsequently cleaved enzymatically, with or without splicing (see p. 26), into gene-length mRNAs for translation into individual proteins. Alternatively, polycistronic mRNA can be directly translated into a 'polyprotein' which is then cleaved by proteases into the individual functional proteins. Furthermore, in the interests of genetic economy, the genome of some viruses may be read in different ways to code for different proteins; there are examples of functional mRNA being transcribed from both strands of dsDNA, from overlapping regions of one strand, or from the same sequence being read in different 'frames'. One can only marvel at the astonishing variety of alternative scenarios Nature has come up with to convert a minimal amount of viral genetic information into the maximum number of (often multifunctional) proteins (Table 1.4).

Each step in the viral multiplication cycle will now be discussed in somewhat more detail.

Attachment (adsorption)

Because virions and cells are both negatively charged at physiological pH, they tend to repel one another, but random collisions do occur and initial (reversible) attachment may be facilitated by cations. Firm binding, however, requires the presence of receptors for the virus on the plasma membrane (reviews: Lonberg-Holm and Philipson, 1981; Poste and Nicolson, 1977). For instance, orthomyxo- and paramyxoviruses bind via an envelope protein known as the haemagglutinin (HA) to glycoproteins or glycolipids with oligosaccharide side-chains terminating in N-acetylneuraminic acid (sialic acid). Numerous other examples are discussed in Chapter 5 in the context of the importance of receptors in determining the host range and/or tissue tropism of viruses. For instance, polioviruses infect primate, not non-primate, cells because only the former carry a receptor for the relevant viral capsid protein. While there is a degree of specificity about the recognition of particular receptors by particular viruses, many quite different viruses may utilise the same receptor (Lonberg-Holm and Philipson, 1981); no doubt viruses have evolved to make opportunistic use of a limited number of membrane glycoproteins which of course would have quite unrelated functions of benefit to the cell.

Uptake (penetration)

Longstanding controversy surrounds the question of how the virion enters the cell (review: Dimmock, 1982). Electron microscopic and other data clearly show that virions can enter by at least three different mechanisms: (1) endocytosis, (2) fusion, and (3) translocation. What is unclear, however, is which of these leads to successful infection. The majority of virions entering a cell fail to initiate infection. The conventional wisdom is that most of the particles taken up by endocytosis are degraded by lysosomal enzymes. Nevertheless, recent evidence suggests that this may be the normal route to successful infection by some viruses at least.

Endocytosis. Virtually all mammalian cells, not only those known as phagocytes, are continuously engaged in phagocytosis, pinocytosis, and receptor-mediated (adsorptive) endocytosis—a specific process for the uptake of essential macromolecules. Helenius *et al*. (1980) clarified how viruses exploit this normal cellular function to initiate infection. Semliki Forest virus (SFV) particles were found to attach particularly, but not exclusively, to receptors on microvilli projecting from the cell. Multi-point attachment of several viral glycoprotein molecules tended to cause the receptors to 'patch', concentrating them in the locality. The virions then moved down into 'coated pits'. These pits, coated with clathrin, are continuously being reformed and shortly thereafter folded inwards to produce 'coated vesicles' that enter the cytoplasm and fuse with a lysosome to form what is sometimes called a 'lysosomal vesicle' (or secondary lysosome; or phagolysosome when the virion has been taken into the cell in a phagocytic vesicle). At the acid pH (5) established in the vesicle the envelope of endocytosed SFV, VSV or influenza virus fuses with the lysosomal membrane, expelling the viral nucleocapsid into the cytoplasm. This explains how a virion can be uncoated yet escape total degradation by the lysosome's hydrolytic enzymes. The whole process seems to resemble closely that whereby many large molecules, such as hormones, are taken up by cells yet avoid degradation in lysosomes.

Recent studies with influenza virus have identified a pH 5-mediated conformational change in the cleaved form of the haemagglutinin (HA) molecule which enables fusion to occur between the viral envelope and the membrane of the secondary lysosome (Skehel *et al.*, 1982; Yoshimura *et al.*, 1982).

Fusion with plasma membrane. The F (fusion) glycoprotein of paramyxoviruses, in its cleaved form, enables the envelope of these viruses to fuse directly with the plasma membrane of cells, even at pH 7. This may allow the nucleocapsid to be released directly into the cytoplasm. Though a number of enveloped viruses display a capacity to fuse mammalian cells or to lyse erythrocytes, it is not clear whether this is the normal way in which they infect cells.

Translocation. Some non-enveloped icosahedral viruses appear to be capable of passing directly through the plasma membrane. Again, we do not know whether this is an atypical event.

Uncoating

In order that at least the early viral genes may become available for transcription it is necessary that the virions be at least partially uncoated. In the case of viruses that enter the cell by fusion of their envelope with either the plasma membrane or the membrane of a lysosomal vesicle, it can be said that uncoating coincides with entry—the nucleocapsid is discharged directly into the cytoplasm. Transcription is initiated off viral RNA still associated with nucleoprotein in at least some types of tubular nucleocapsid. This does not explain how the genome of icosahedral viruses becomes available for transcription. Because virus particles are often visualised within phagosomes it has been surmised for many years that lysosomal enzymes remove the coat of the virion. Indeed, the infectivity of reovirus is greatly enhanced by partial removal of the outer coat with protease *in vitro* to produce 'subviral particles (Silverstein *et al.*, 1974) and mRNA can be transcribed from such subviral particles *in vitro*. One might have imagined that digestion of the coat of a virion by lysosomal proteases and/or lipases would also expose the viral genome to destruction by lysosomal nucleases, or so disturb the orientation of the viral transcriptase with respect to its NA that the particle would be rendered non-infectious.

A quite different possibility is raised by work initiated by Mandel (1967) and pursued by de Sena and Torian (1980) with poliovirus. It was shown that the process of attachment of virion to HeLa cells, or to a particular component extracted from their membranes, leads to a conformational change in the capsid of the virion, resulting successively in the loss of capsid proteins VP4 then VP2, and rendering the particle susceptible to proteases and RNAse. It is tempting to postulate that, for icosahedral viruses, the attachment step itself triggers the process of uncoating.

For certain viruses that replicate in the nucleus there is evidence that the later stages of uncoating occur there, rather than in the cytoplasm. We know almost nothing about how this happens, nor indeed how virions, sub-viral particles or viral macromolecules are transported from cytoplasm to nucleus and back again.

Transcription

In the case of ssRNA viruses of positive polarity (picornaviruses, togaviruses and coronaviruses) the viral RNA itself binds directly to ribosomes and is translated into protein without the need for any prior transcriptional step (Fig. 1.3, Table 1.4). All other classes of viral genome must be transcribed to mRNA. In the case of certain DNA viruses that replicate in the nucleus (adenoviruses, herpesviruses, and papovaviruses, as well as the ssDNA parvoviruses, which utilise a dsDNA intermediate for transcription of mRNA) the cellular DNA-dependent RNA polymerase II is employed for this purpose. All other viruses require unique and specific types of transcriptase which are not only virus-coded but must be carried into the cell as an integral component of the infecting virion in order that transcription can proceed at all (review: Bishop, 1977). Of course, cytoplasmic dsDNA viruses (poxviruses and iridoviruses) carry a DNA-dependent RNA polymerase, whereas dsRNA viruses (reoviruses) have dsRNA-dependent RNA polymerase, while ssRNA viruses of negative polarity, otherwise known as 'negative-stranded' or 'minus-stranded' viruses (orthomyxoviruses, paramyxoviruses, rhabdoviruses, arenaviruses, bunyaviruses) require a ssRNA-dependent RNA polymerase.

In 1978 Fiers and his colleagues presented us with the first complete description of the genome of an animal virus. Analysis of the 5224 nucleotide-pair sequence of the circular dsDNA molecule of the papovavirus SV40 and its transcription programme revealed some remarkable facts. Firstly, the early genes and the late genes are transcribed, by the host-cell's RNA polymerase II, in opposite directions, from different strands of the DNA. Secondly, certain genes overlap, so

Table 1.4. Strategy of expression of viral genome.

Family	Viral nucleic acid					Messenger RNA	
	Type	Strands	Polarity	Segments	Transcriptase in virion	Monocistronic[a]	Spliced
Papovaviridae	DNA	2	±	1	−	+	+
Adenoviridae	DNA	2	±	1	−	+	+
Herpesviridae	DNA	2	±	1	−	+	+
Poxviridae	DNA	2	±	1	+	+	+
Picornaviridae	RNA	1	+	1	−	−	−
Togaviridae	RNA	1	+	1	−	−	−
Orthomyxoviridae	RNA	1	−	8	+	+	±
Paramyxoviridae	RNA	1	−	1	+	+	−
Retroviridae	RNA	1	+	2(diploid)	+	+	+
Rhabdoviridae	RNA	1	−	1	+	+	−
Reoviridae	RNA	2	±	10–12	+	+	−

[a]Monocistronic mRNA is derived from a non-segmented genome by post-transcriptional cleavage, with or without subsequent splicing. In the case of the picornaviruses and togaviruses, polycistronic mRNA is translated into a polyprotein which is then cleaved stepwise into individual functional proteins. With other viruses, post-translational cleavage of certain structural proteins may occur at a late stage in maturation of the virion.

that their products share part of their amino acid sequences in common; this applies to the N-terminal sequence of the early proteins known as 'small-t' and 'large-T', and also to a large common region of the late proteins VP2 and VP3. Thirdly, some regions of the viral DNA are read in two overlapping reading frames, so that two completely different amino acid sequences (VP1, cf VP2 & 3) are obtained. Fourthly, at least 15% of the viral DNA consists of intervening sequences ('introns'), which are transcribed but never translated into protein because they are excised from the primary transcript; indeed, up to three distinct proteins can result from mRNAs derived from a common primary transcript by different splicing protocols (Fiers *et al.*, 1978; Sambrook, 1983).

Sophisticated studies with adenoviruses (reviews: Sambrook, 1983; Sharp, 1984) have elucidated the nature of the mechanisms that regulate the expression of viral genomes. These operate principally, but not exclusively, at the level of transcription. Because of the complications arising from post-transcriptional cleavage of mRNA and post-translational cleavage of precursor proteins in eukaryotic cells, it is no longer adequate to talk of a 'gene' and its 'gene-product'. More appropriate perhaps is to think in terms of the 'transcription unit', i.e. that region of the genome beginning with the transcription initiation site, extending right through to the transcription termination site, and including all introns and exons in between. 'Simple' transcription units may be defined as those encoding only a single protein, whereas 'complex' transcription units code for more than one (review: Darnell, 1982). There are nine adenovirus transcription units, each controlled by a separate promoter. At different stages of the viral multiplication cycle, 'pre-early', 'early', 'intermediate' and 'late', the various transcription units are transcribed in a given temporal sequence. This reflects differences in promoter strengths. For example, after viral DNA replication, there is a 50-fold increase in the rate of transcription from the major late promoter (MLP) relative to the early promoter (EIb). Various virus-coded proteins have been shown to selectively stimulate or suppress initiation of transcription from particular promoters, allowing coordinate regulation of the block of mRNAs within a single transcription unit. A second, less common mechanism of transcriptional control operates at the point of termination rather than initiation of transcription. Transcripts controlled by the P16 promoter terminate at a particular point early in infection but read through this termination site later in infection to produce a range of longer transcripts with different polyadenylation sites.

Transcription from RNA viral genomes is generally not as rigorously regulated as with DNA viruses. In particular, the temporal separation into early genes transcribed before the replication of viral nucleic acid, and late genes transcribed thereafter is not nearly so clear.

Post-transcriptional processing of mRNA. Primary RNA transcripts from eukaryotic DNA are subject to a series of post-transcriptional alterations in the nucleus, known as 'processing', prior to export to the cytoplasm as mature mRNA (review: Darnell, 1982). First, a 'cap', consisting of 7-methyl guanosine (m^7Gppp) is added to the 5' terminus of the primary transcript; the cap is thought to facilitate the formation of a stable initiation complex on the ribosome. Second, a sequence of 50–200 adenylate residues is added to the 3' end; this 'poly(A)' 'tail' appears to stabilise mRNA against degradation in the cytoplasm. Third, a methyl group is added at the 6 position to about 1% of the adenylate residues throughout the mRNA. Fourth, particular non-coding intervening sequences (introns), which begin with GU, end with AG, and contain stop codons, are cleaved (by endonucleases) from the primary transcript and the exposed ends of the remaining exons reunited (by ligases)—a procedure known as 'splicing' (review: Crick, 1979).

The first three of these post-transcriptional events are seen with RNA transcripts from both DNA and RNA mammalian viruses. However, splicing seems to be restricted to those DNA viruses that multiply in the nucleus, plus the retroviruses, which are characterised by the transcription of mRNA from an integrated cDNA template (see Weiss *et al.*, 1982), and the orthomyxoviruses, which have a special involvement with the nucleus (see below). Splicing is another important mechanism for regulating gene expression in nuclear DNA viruses. A given RNA transcript can have two or more splicing sites and be spliced in several different ways to produce a variety of mRNA species coding for distinct proteins; both the preferred poly(A) site and the splicing pattern may change in a systematic fashion as infection proceeds (review: Flint, 1981).

Yet another level of regulation is the rate of degradation of mRNA. Not only do different mRNA species display different half-lives but the half-life of a given mRNA species may change as the viral multiplication cycle progresses.

Mention should be made of a unique requirement for the initiation of synthesis of mRNA from the negative-stranded RNA virus, influenza. A virion-associated endonuclease amputates a short segment from the capped 5'-terminus of eukaryotic (cellular) mRNA; the viral transcriptase then utilises this small fragment as a primer to initiate the transcription of viral mRNA (reviews: Krug, 1981; Lamb and Choppin, 1983).

Translation

Capped and polyadenylated monocistronic viral mRNAs, following splicing when necessary, bind to ribosomes in the cell cytoplasm and are translated into protein in essentially the same fashion as eukaryotic mRNA, presumably utilising cellular tRNAs and initiation factors. The sequence of events has been closely studied for reovirus (review: Kozak, 1981). Each monocistronic mRNA molecule binds via its capped 5'-terminus to the 40S ribosomal subunit, which then moves along the mRNA molecule until stopped at the initiator codon (AUG), presumably by the secondary structure of the mRNA. The 60S ribosomal subunit now binds also, together with methionyl transfer RNA and various initiation factors. Translation then proceeds. Despite the fact that mRNA is transcribed from all the monocistronic dsRNA reovirus genes at the same rate, there are pronounced differences in the amounts of each protein made, indicating the existence of some mechanism of regulation at the level of translation (Joklik, 1981).

In the special case of the plus-stranded picornaviruses and togaviruses, where the polycistronic vRNA is translated directly into a single giant polyprotein, proteases cleave the polypeptide in a defined sequence into smaller proteins. The first cleavage steps are carried out by cellular protease(s) while the polyprotein is still nascent on the polyribosome; a virus-coded protease makes later cuts. Some of the intermediates exist only ephemerally; others have important functions but are subsequently cleaved to produce smaller proteins with other functions.

As mentioned earlier, the proteins translated from the transcripts of early viral genes include enzymes and other proteins, e.g. the papovavirus large-T antigen, required for the replication of viral NA, as well as proteins that shut down host cell RNA and protein synthesis. The function of most early viral proteins, however, is still unknown. Several, no doubt, have important regulatory functions in controlling the transcription of the viral genome.

The late viral proteins are translated from late mRNA, most of which is transcribed only following the replication of the viral NA. Most of the late proteins are structural proteins which are intended for incorporation into new virions (but they are often made in considerable excess). Some of these double as regulatory proteins that shut off the transcription—and perhaps in some instances, the translation—of cellular or early viral genes.

Newly synthesised viral proteins must migrate to the various sites in the cell where they are needed, e.g. back into the nucleus in the case of those viruses that replicate there. Whether this occurs solely by random diffusion or by some sort of active or guided transport, perhaps involving the cytoskeleton, is unknown. In the special case of glycoproteins, the polypeptide backbone is translated on membrane-bound ribosomes, i.e. in rough endoplasmic reticulum; various co- and post-translational modifications, including acylation, proteolytic cleavage, and addition and subtraction of sugars, occur sequentially as the protein moves in vesicles to the Golgi apparatus thence to the plasma membrane (see p. 30).

Replication of viral nucleic acid

DNA replication. The papovavirus genome, with its associated cellular histones, morphologically resembles chromatin. Its replication also closely mimics the replication of eukaryotic chromosomal DNA and utilises host cell enzymes, probably including DNA polymerase α (review: Challberg and Kelly, 1982). An early viral protein, the large-T antigen, binds to three adjacent sites in the 'control' region of the viral genome, initiating replication of the DNA. Thereafter, no other virus-coded protein appears to be required. Replication of this circular dsDNA commences from a unique palindromic origin on the viral chromosome and proceeds simultaneously in both directions at the same rate. At each growing fork, both continuous and discontinuous DNA synthesis occurs (on leading and lagging strands respectively). As in the replication of mammalian DNA, the discontinuous synthesis of the lagging strand involves repeated synthesis of short oligoribonucleotide primers, which in turn initiate short nascent strands of DNA; these 'Okazaki fragments' are then covalently joined to form the growing nascent strand.

The replication of adenovirus DNA is somewhat simpler, but quite different. Adenovirus DNA is linear, the 5' ends of the two strands being mirror images of one another (terminally repeated inverted sequences) and being covalently linked to a protein molecule. Uniquely, the primer for adenoviral DNA synthesis is not another nucleic acid but this virus-coded protein, adenovirus terminal protein (pTP). DNA replication proceeds from both ends, continuously but asynchronously, in a 5' to 3' direction, using cellular DNA polymerases α and γ, and does not require the synthesis of Okazaki fragments.

RNA replication. Replication of RNA is, as far as we know, a phenomenon unique to viruses. Transcription of RNA from an RNA template requires a type of enzyme not found in mammalian cells, namely an RNA-dependent RNA polymerase. Such enzymes must therefore be virus-coded. It is not yet certain whether the polymerase required to transcribe (+)RNA from a (−)RNA template is necessarily different from that needed to make (−)RNA from (+)RNA. Both are essential because the replication of viral RNA (vRNA) first requires the synthesis of complementary RNA (cRNA), which then serves as a template for making more vRNA. Where the vRNA is of negative polarity (orthomyxo-, paramyxo-, rhabdo-, arena-, bunyaviruses) the cRNA will be of positive polarity and the RNA polymerase involved may be the same transcriptase as is responsible for transcription of mRNA. Note however that, whereas the primary transcript from such (−)vRNA is subsequently cleaved (in many cases) to produce mRNA, some must remain uncleaved to serve as a full-length template for vRNA synthesis. In the case of the plus-stranded viruses (picorna-, toga-, coronaviruses) the cRNA is minus-stranded; the polymerase responsible for making vRNA from the cRNA template is sometimes called 'replicase', but this laboratory jargon can cause confusion. Several replicase molecules can operate on a single cRNA template to transcribe a number of molecules of vRNA simultaneously. The resulting structure, known as the 'replicative intermediate' (RI) is therefore partially double-stranded, with single-stranded tails. Initiation of replication of picornavirus RNA, like that of adenovirus DNA, requires a protein, rather than a ribonucleoside triphosphate, as primer (Baron and Baltimore, 1982). This small protein, VPg, is covalently attached to the 5'-terminus of nascent $(+)$ and $(-)$ RNA strands, as well as vRNA, but not mRNA. Little is known about what determines whether a given picornavirus plus-stranded RNA molecule will be directed firstly to a 'replication complex', bound to smooth endoplasmic reticulum, where it serves as a template for transcription by RNA-dependent RNA polymerase into minus-stranded cRNA; or secondly to a polyribosome, free in the cytoplasm or on rough endoplasmic reticulum, where it serves as mRNA for translation into polyprotein; or thirdly to a 'procapsid', with which it associates to form a virion.

Assembly (morphogenesis)

Structural proteins of simple icosahedral viruses can aggregate spontaneously to form capsomers, which in turn may assemble into empty 'procapsids'. Somehow, the viral nucleic acid now enters this structure. Completion of the virion often involves proteolytic cleavage of one or more species of capsid protein.

One of the best studied examples is the picornavirus. The precursor protein NCVP1a aggregates to form pentamers, within which each of the five NCVP1a molecules is then cleaved into VP0, VP1 and VP3. Twelve such pentamers now aggregate into a 'procapsid' which associates with a viral RNA molecule to form a 'provirion'. A final proteolytic event cleaves each of the VP0 molecules into VP2 and VP4, so that the mature virion is a dodecahedron with 60 capsomers, each of which is made up of one molecule each of VP1, 2, 3 and 4 (Rueckert, 1976).

The mechanism of entry of viral nucleic acid into a preconstructed empty viral capsid has been elucidated for adenovirus. One end of the viral DNA molecule is characterised by a nucleotide sequence ('packing sequence') which enables the DNA to enter the procapsid. Then certain proteins are cleaved, surrounding the DNA with a histone-like core.

Glycosylation and budding. All mammalian viruses with tubular nucleocapsids, as well as some with icosahedral nucleocapsids, acquire an envelope by budding through cellular membrane, usually plasma membrane (reviews: Simons and Garoff, 1980; Garoff *et al.*, 1982). Since such envelopes always contain viral glycoproteins (review: Compans and Klenk, 1979) we will begin by discussing the mechanism of glycosylation of these proteins (reviews: Klenk and Rott, 1980; Garoff *et al.*, 1982).

Much of our understanding of the glycosylation of viral proteins comes from studies with the rhabdovirus VSV (Rothman and Lodish, 1977) and the togavirus SFV (Garoff *et al.*, 1982). The fact that essentially comparable results have been obtained with ortho- and paramyxoviruses (Klenk and Rott, 1980) suggests that the essential steps are much the same for all enveloped viruses, hence again a composite picture can be presented here. Once more we shall see that viruses exploit existing cellular pathways—in this case, those normally used for the synthesis and export of secretory and membrane glycoproteins.

The amino-terminal end of viral envelope proteins initially contains a sequence of 15–30 hydrophobic amino acids, known as the 'signal sequence', which characterises the protein as one destined for insertion into membrane and/or export from the cell. The hydrophobicity of the signal sequence facilitates binding of the growing polypeptide chain to a receptor site on the cytoplasmic side of the rough endoplasmic reticulum (RER) and its passage through the lipid bilayer to the luminal side. A signal peptidase then removes the signal sequence. Oligosaccharides are added to the nascent polypeptide in the lumen of the RER (Rothman and Lodish, 1977) by what now seems to be the standard mechanism for attaching sugars to asparagine, namely *en bloc* transfer of a mannose-rich 'core' of preformed oligosaccharides from a lipid-linked intermediate, an oligosaccharide pyrophosphoryldolichol. Glucose residues are then removed by glycosidases, a process known as 'trimming' of the core. At this stage the viral glycoprotein is transported from the RER to the Golgi apparatus, probably inside a coated vesicle (Rothman and Fine, 1980). Here the core carbohydrate is further modified by the removal of several mannose residues, and the addition of further N-acetyl-glucosamine, plus galactose, then the terminal sugars, sialic acid and fucose. The completed oligosaccharide side chains are a mixture of the 'simple' ('high mannose') and the 'complex' types. Also while in the Golgi apparatus the glycoprotein becomes acylated, i.e. fatty acids, such as methyl palmitate, are covalently attached to the hydrophobic membrane-attachment end of the molecule (Schmidt, 1982). Another coated vesicle now transports the glycoprotein to the plasma membrane. At about this time a cellular protease cleaves the protein into two polypeptide chains, which nevertheless remain covalently linked together by internal disulphide bonds. This final cleavage step is analogous to the maturation of many prohormones and blood proproteins. While it is not essential for the release of new virions (indeed, is not effected by certain types of host cell), it is absolutely essential for the production of infectious virions—certainly in the case of the orthomyxoviruses, which require cleavage of the haemagglutinin (Lazarowitz and Choppin, 1975) and the paramyxoviruses, which require cleavage of both the HN and the fusion (F) glycoprotein (see Klenk and Rott, 1980). Following fusion of the coated vesicle with the plasma membrane, the hydrophilic N-terminal end of the amphipathic glycoprotein now finds itself projecting from the external surface of the membrane, while the hydrophobic domain near the C-terminal end remains anchored in the lipid bilayer. Gething and Sambrook (1981) and Sveda et al. (1982) demonstrated that such viral envelope glycoproteins can be converted to secretory glycoproteins by removing the portion of the gene that codes for this 'anchor sequence'.

One fascinating aspect of the transport of glycoproteins around the cell in coated vesicles (Pearse and Bretscher, 1981) is the question of what 'sorting signals' determine the destination of particular glycoproteins. Rodriguez-Boulan and Sabatini (1978) demonstrated that different viruses bud from different domains in the plasma membrane of polarised epithelial cells, e.g. some from the apical and others from the basolateral surface, while yet others bud from intracytoplasmic smooth ER or from nuclear membrane. Presumably some feature of the molecule serves as a 'postal address' ('zip code').

Budding is a form of exocytosis (reviews: Simons and Garoff, 1980; Garoff et al., 1982). The process begins with the insertion of the newly completed viral glycoprotein. Because proteins are free to move laterally in the 'sea of lipid' that constitutes the plasma membrane, cellular proteins are displaced from the patch of membrane into which viral glycoproteins have been inserted. It is not known for certain whether there is any selection of particular lipids for incorporation into the viral envelope, but, to all intents and purposes, the mix of phospholipids, glycolipids and cholesterol is essentially the same as that characterising the membrane of that particular type of host cell. The monomeric, cleaved viral glycoprotein molecules associate into oligomers, to form the typical rod-shaped peplomer or 'spike' with a prominent hydrophilic domain projecting from the external side of the membrane, a hydrophobic domain spanning the membrane near the C-terminal end, and a short hydrophilic sequence right at the C-terminus which projects slightly into the cytoplasm. In the special case of the icosahedral togaviruses, each protein molecule of the viral nucleocapsid binds directly to the C-terminal end of a glycoprotein oligomer. Multivalent attachment of numerous spikes, each to an underlying molecule on the surface of the icosahedron moulds the membrane around the nucleocapsid, forcing it to bulge progressively outwards until finally the nucleocapsid is completely enclosed in a tightly fitting envelope and the new virion buds off into the outside world. The more typical enveloped virus has a tubular nucleocapsid, which does not bind directly to viral glycoprotein but to a 'matrix' (M) protein which has first attached to the cytoplasmic side of the membrane beneath patches of aggregated viral glycoprotein. The putative role of the cytoskeleton in the process of budding is still to be established.

Uniquely, the envelope of the icosahedral DNA herpesviruses is acquired by budding through the inner nuclear membrane; the virus then is thought to pass directly from the space between the two nuclear membranes to the exterior of the cell via cytoplasmic channels. The envelope of the complex DNA poxviruses is not acquired by a typical budding process, but by de novo synthesis of an inner 'membrane' followed by acquisition of a true envelope during passage through the Golgi apparatus to the plasma membrane.

Inhibition of synthesis of cellular macromolecules

Some viruses, but by no means all, shut down the synthesis of cellular protein, and indirectly also that of cellular RNA and DNA (reviews: Burke and Russell, 1975; Tamm, 1975; Shatkin, 1983). The mechanism(s) are not clearly understood. In those cases where the inhibition of cellular protein synthesis develops gradually and only late in the viral multiplication cycle, it is possibly due simply to competition for ribosomes by the large excess of viral mRNA. Even when viral mRNA is not in excess, it may have a selective advantage in binding to ribosomes and initiating translation (Joklik, 1981). A special case is the inactivation during poliovirus infection of a cap-binding protein that is required for the initiation of translation of all cellular messengers (Trachsel et al., 1980); polio RNA is unusual in having no m^7G cap and being translated quite satisfactorily without it. The mRNAs of most other viruses, like eukaryotic mRNAs, are capped, but there is some evidence that late in reovirus infection, uncapped mRNA can be translated (Skup and Millward, 1980). Late shutdown of cellular protein synthesis by adenovirus is at least partially due to inhibition of the transport of cellular mRNA out of the nucleus (Beltz and Flint, 1979), while certain herpesviruses actually bring about selective degradation of cellular mRNA. Furthermore, the gross distortion of the topological arrangement of DNA seen in the nucleus of cells late in the multiplication cycle of many viruses might well explain the decrease in transcription of cellular mRNA demonstrable at that time. Inhibition of cellular DNA synthesis is doubtless also a secondary consequence of inhibition of protein synthesis.

The role of virus-coded proteins in cell shutdown seems to differ from virus to virus. Capsid proteins of some viruses, e.g. adenoviruses, are toxic for cells and may be responsible for the cytocidal effects seen late in infection (or early, following infection at high multiplicity). Yet other viruses seem to code for proteins still to be identified, which selectively inhibit the translation of eukaryotic mRNA. This subject will be discussed further in Chapter 4.

Abortive replication

We have described 'productive' infection of a 'permissive' cell by a typical 'cytocidal' virus. However, some cells are 'non-permissive' for particular viruses. This can be so for any of a number of reasons, e.g. absence of the appropriate receptor, so that infection is not initiated. Viral replication may be blocked because of the absence of a cellular enzyme essential for the full replication of that virus. Such a virus–cell interaction will be 'non-productive', i.e. 'abortive'. The subject is discussed in Chapter 5, under the heading of Host Determinants of Resistance. Depending upon the point in the cycle at which viral multiplication is blocked, certain steps may be successfully accomplished. The extreme case is that of the cell that lacks only the protease to cleave the glycoprotein in the envelope of the virion; here the whole multiplication cycle is completed, and virions are produced, but they are non-infectious.

Abortive replication can also occur in a fully permissive cell, if there is a defect in the viral genome. Cells that support the multiplication of some viruses may not support that of a virus lacking the gene for an essential enzyme. Temperature-sensitive mutants can be classified into 'complementation groups' according to which viral gene contains the *ts* lesion; such mutants have been exploited to determine the function of each viral gene by identifying the particular biochemical step at which the multiplication of each mutant is blocked (Fenner, 1969; Fields and Jaenisch, 1980).

Some viruses are only conditionally defective, in that they can multiply in certain cell types, or in the presence of a 'helper' virus. The best known example is that of the adeno-associated viruses (AAV), comprising the *Dependovirus* genus of the Parvoviridae family. As the name implies, these viruses depend for their replication upon a particular protein coded by a helper virus (adenovirus) multiplying in the same cell (Ward and Tattersall, 1978). In monkey cells, human adenoviruses will multiply only in the presence of a helper virus, SV40; some of the progeny of such mixed infections are recombinants known as 'adenovirus-SV40 hybrids' (Rowe, 1967). Several sarcomagenic retroviruses require a leukaemia virus to code for a particular envelope glycoprotein (Weiss *et al.*, 1982).

Defective interfering (DI) particles. A common byproduct of viral multiplication is a type of defective virion known as a DI particle (reviews: Huang and Baltimore, 1977; Perrault, 1981). DI particles have the following properties: (1) the genome is defective, as it contains at least one deletion; hence the particle is non-infectious; (2) nevertheless, the particle can replicate in the presence of homologous infectious virus, which serves as a helper; (3) the DI particle interferes with the replication of infectious virus.

DI particles, originally called 'incomplete virus', were first described as the principal product of cells infected with influenza virus at high multiplicity; the ratio of incomplete to infectious particles in the yield increased dramatically on serial passage of the progeny. Since then, DI particles have been produced under similar conditions from virtually all families of RNA viruses and some DNA viruses also. In the case of influenza and other viruses with segmented genomes (e.g. reovirus), the defective virions lack one or more of the largest viral genes and contain instead small segments consisting of an incomplete portion of the missing genes. Similarly, in the case of viruses with a non-segmented genome, the DI particles are found to contain RNA which is greatly abbreviated in length—as little as one third of the original sequence in the 'T' (truncated) particles of VSV (a rhabdovirus).

Sequencing studies have revealed an amazing diversity of structural rearrangements, in addition to simple deletions, in the RNA of DI particles from different viral families, and even from cloned stocks of a given parental virus. Most can be explained by the '(promiscuous) leaping polymerase complex' model (Perrault, 1981) which emphasises the facility (promiscuity) with which the viral replicase is able to terminate synthesis, leap to another site and resume synthesis, upstream or downstream, forwards or backwards, on the same or a different RNA strand, so giving rise to internal deletions, repeats, copy-back or snap-back RNAs, and so forth.

DI particles morphologically resemble the homologous parent virus, being somewhat smaller but having a comparable envelope or capsid. This suggests that the physical and chemical constraints on the packaging of nucleic acid into virions are not extremely rigorous. Indeed, by way of contrast with incomplete virus, polyploidy (multiple genomes) is not uncommonly observed as an aberration of replication of enveloped RNA viruses, while co-infection with quite different viruses can give rise to transcapsidation or phenotypic mixing (Fenner *et al.*, 1974). One of the mysteries of virology is how, in the case of viruses with segmented genomes (orthomyxoviruses, arenaviruses, bunyaviruses, reoviruses, birnaviruses, nodaviruses), the newly synthesised virion succeeds in incorporating exactly one molecule of each of its several genes.

The tendency of DI particles to increase preferentially with passage is presumed to be explicable as follows. The shortened RNA molecules that characterise DI particles (1) require less time to be replicated, (2) are less often diverted to serve as templates for transcription of mRNA, and (3) have enhanced affinity for the viral replicase, so giving them a competitive advantage over their full-length counterparts from infectious virus. Hence, it can be seen why DI particles interfere with the replication of the parental virus with progressively greater efficiency on passage.

Clearly, the mechanisms that generate DI particles might also be involved in the generation of viable variants and, in this sense, play an important role in the evolution of viruses. For instance, strand-switching by the viral replicase is presumably responsible for the intramolecular genetic recombination that occurs at low frequency between different but related viruses infecting the same cell (see Fenner *et al.*, 1974; Perrault, 1981). The possible role of DI particles in persistent viral infections (review: Holland *et al.*, 1980) is discussed in Chapter 6.

Transformation by oncogenic viruses

Many herpesviruses and retroviruses cause cancer under natural conditions in animals or birds, while several papovaviruses and adenoviruses are oncogenic when injected into baby rodents. These oncogenic viruses are also capable of transforming cultured cells to the malignant state. Such transformed cells, as well as those in naturally occurring and induced tumours, have been brilliantly investigated using the most sophisticated tools of modern molecular biology to elucidate the role of the viral genome in carcinogenesis. Cancer virology is now a self-sufficient discipline practised by highly skilled and specialised professionals, while papers and books devoted to this super-specialty are appearing at an ever increasing rate. Hence it is quite unnecessary for us to devote space in this book to a subject that is so comprehensively reviewed elsewhere. We simply refer the reader to the following major recent books: Tooze (1980), Weiss *et al.* (1982), Klein (1980; 1982–4), Nahmias *et al.* (1981), Rapp (1980), Epstein and Achong (1979), Essex *et al.* (1980).

Nevertheless, we cannot resist the temptation to mention, albeit briefly, some of the startling new findings that have recently revolutionised tumour virology and, after decades of frustration, have generated a feeling of genuine optimism about the possibility of solving the riddle of cancer at last. We refer, of course, to the new understanding of oncogenes (reviews: Bishop, 1982; 1983; Weinberg, 1982).

Oncogenes have been defined as those genes that confer oncogenicity on certain retroviruses. It is now clear that normal cells in fact contain upwards of 20 'cellular oncogenes' or 'proto-oncogenes' that very closely resemble viral oncogenes, in their nucleotide sequence and in respect of the protein for which they code. The proteins encoded by several known oncogenes are protein kinases which phosphorylate proteins at tyrosine residues. Others have quite different properties, but all are assumed to play a role in the growth or differentiation of normal cells. New evidence suggests that cancer can result from the unrestrained expression of a normal cellular oncogene, or from a mutation in an oncogene.

Because integration of viral cDNA into the host cell's chromosomes constitutes an essential step in the replication of all retroviruses, they are uniquely placed to pick up (transduce) cellular genes. A cellular proto-oncogene is thus incorporated by recombination into the genome of a previously non-oncogenic retrovirus. The oncogene may mutate, thus rendering the virus highly oncogenic. Regardless, if upon subsequent infection of a new host cell, the oncogene is inserted in the wrong spot, it may thereafter be transcribed in unrestrained fashion. Translocation of proto-oncogenes may also be effected by viruses other than retroviruses. Furthermore, integration of the cDNA of even a 'non-oncogenic' retrovirus can activate a normal cellular proto-oncogene in the immediate vicinity.

The only retrovirus to be shown so far to be directly responsible for a human cancer is the human T-cell leukaemia/lymphoma virus (Reitz *et al.*, 1983). Prominent candidates from other families include the herpesvirus, EB virus (Burkitt lymphoma and nasopharyngeal carcinoma—see Epstein and Achong, 1979; Rapp, 1980; Nahmias *et al.*, 1981), the papillomaviruses (see Lancaster and Olson, 1982), and hepatitis B virus (hepatocellular carcinoma—see Szmuness *et al.*, 1982). Some aspects of human infections with these potentially oncogenic viruses will be discussed in Chapter 6.

This attempt to produce a single synthetic picture of viral multiplication has, of necessity, glossed over important differences between individual viruses. Each family boasts its own unique and fascinating replication strategy—as well as its own vast literature! Even the task of selecting the most generally useful recent reviews to which to refer the interested reader is nigh impossible. Nevertheless, we offer the following short list as a starting point.

Papovaviruses:	Sambrook (1981);
Adenoviruses:	Sambrook (1981); Sharp (1984); Ginsberg (1984);
Herpesviruses:	Roizman (1982–84); Nahmias *et al.* (1981);
Poxviruses:	Dales and Pogo (1981);
Hepadnaviruses:	Marion and Robinson (1983); Szmuness *et al.*, (1982);
Parvoviruses:	Berns (1983);
Picornaviruses:	Perez-Bercoff (1979); Rueckert (1976);
Caliciviruses:	Schaffer (1979);
Togaviruses:	Garoff *et al.* (1982); Schlesinger (1980);
Orthomyxoviruses:	Lamb and Choppin (1983); Bishop and Compans (1981);

Paramyxoviruses:	Choppin and Compans (1975); Klenk and Rott (1980);
Coronaviruses:	Siddell *et al.* (1983);
Arenaviruses:	Rawls and Leung (1979);
Bunyaviruses:	Bishop and Shope (1979);
Retroviruses:	Weiss *et al.* (1982);
Rhabdoviruses:	Bishop (1979);
Reoviruses:	Joklik (1983).

SELECTED READING

Alberts, B., Bray, D., Lewis, J., Raff, M., Roberts, K., and Watson, J. D. (1983). *Molecular Biology of the Cell*. Garland, New York.

Andrewes, C., Pereira, H. G., and Wildy, P. (1978). *Viruses of Vertebrates*, 4th edn. Baillière Tindall, London.

Baltimore, D. (1971). Expression of animal virus genomes. *Bacteriol. Rev.* **35**, 235.

Bishop, D. H. L. and Compans, R. W. (eds.) (1981). *The Replication of Negative-Strand Viruses*. Elsevier, Amsterdam.

Bishop, J. M. (1982). Oncogenes. *Sci. Am.* **246**, 68.

Bishop, J. M. (1983). Cellular oncogenes and retroviruses. *Ann. Rev. Biochem.* **52**, 301.

Darnell, J. E. (1982). Variety in the level of gene control in eukaryotic cells. *Nature* **297**, 365.

Essex, M., Todaro, G., and zur Hausen, H. (eds.) (1980). *Viruses in Naturally Occurring Cancers*. Cold Spring Harbor Laboratory, New York.

Fenner, F., McAuslan, B. R., Mims, C. A., Sambrook, J., and White, D. O. (1974). *The Biology of Animal Viruses*, 2nd edn. Academic Press, New York.

Fields, B. and Jaenisch, R. (eds.) (1980). *Animal Virus Genetics*. Academic Press, New York.

Fiers, W., Contreras, R., Haegeman, G., Rogiers, R., van de Voorde, A., van Heuverswyn, H., van Herreweghe, J., Volckaert, G., and Ysebaert, M. (1978). Complete nucleotide sequence of SV40 DNA. *Nature* **273**, 113.

Fraenkel-Conrat, H. and Wagner, R. R. (eds.) (1974–83). *Comprehensive Virology*, vols. 1–18. Plenum Press, New York.

Gluzman, Y. (ed.) (1982). *Eukaryotic Viral Vectors*. Cold Spring Harbor Laboratory, New York.

Joklik, W. K. (1981). Structure and function of the reovirus genome. *Microbiol. Rev.* **45**, 483.

Klenk, H.-D. and Rott, R. (1980). Cotranslational and posttranslational processing of viral glycoproteins. *Curr. Top. Microbiol. Immunol.* **90**, 19.

Lonberg-Holm, K. and Philipson, L. (1981). *Animal Virus Receptors. Series B: Receptors and Recognition*. Chapman and Hall, London.

McGeogh, D. J. (1981). Structural analysis of animal virus genomes. *J. Gen. Virol.* **55**, 1.

Maniatis, T., Fritsch, E. F., and Sambrook, J. (1982). *Molecular Cloning: a Laboratory Manual*. Cold Spring Harbor Laboratory, New York.

Matthews, R. E. F. (1982). Classification and Nomenclature of Viruses. Fourth

Report of the International Committee on Taxonomy of Viruses. *Intervirology* **17**, 1–200.

Palese, P. and Roizman, B. (eds.) (1980). Genetic Variation of Viruses. *Annals. NY Acad. Sci.* **354**.

Shatkin, A. J. (ed.) (1981). *Initiation Signals in Viral Gene Expression*. Springer-Verlag, Berlin.

Simons, K., Garoff, H., and Helenius, A. (1982). How an animal virus gets into and out of its host cell. *Sci. Amer.* **246**, 46.

Strauss, E. G. and Strauss, J. H. (1983). Replication strategies of the single stranded RNA viruses of eukaryotes. *Current Top. Microbiol. Immunol.* **105**, 1.

Tooze, J. (1980). *The Molecular Biology of Tumor Viruses. DNA Tumor Viruses*. Cold Spring Harbor Laboratory, New York.

Weiss, R. A., Teich, N., Varmus, H. E., and Coffin, J. (eds.) (1982). *RNA Tumor Viruses*. Cold Spring Harbor Laboratory, New York.

White, D. O. and Fenner, F. J. (1985). *Medical Virology*, 3rd edn. Academic Press, New York.

Chapter Two
Infection and the Spread of Viruses Through the Body

During a viral infection there are certain obligatory stages that must be completed if the virus is to spread successfully from one individual to another and thus survive in nature. These stages in the infectious process, which are similar for all microorganisms whether protozoa, fungi, bacteria, rickettsiae, chlamydiae or viruses, are as follows:

1 Initial infection of the host. This involves penetration into host tissue or attachment of virus to the first susceptible cells on the body surface.

2 Spread of the infection either locally or through the body, with multiplication.

3 Shedding to the exterior.

These stages are often completed without causing disease in the host, i.e. the infection is 'subclinical' or 'inapparent'. The incubation period is usually defined as the period between initial infection and the production of disease.

Just as a virus infection in the cell cannot be understood without a knowledge of cell structure, physiology, biochemistry and function, so a virus infection in the intact vertebrate host cannot be understood without a knowledge of bodily structure, physiology, biochemistry and function. In this chapter the stages in the infectious process will be described with examples. The immune response and other host resistance factors will be discussed in Chapter 3. The mechanisms of production of tissue damage and disease and the determinants of virulence will be described in Chapters 4 and 5.

ROUTES OF ENTRY

In order to infect the vertebrate host, a virus must first attach to and infect cells somewhere on the body surface. It is also possible for the virus to be carried mechanically through a body surface where there is a breach in its continuity. The host can usefully be represented as a set of body surfaces. At each surface a sheet of epithelial cells separates host tissues from the outside world (Figure 2.1). The outer surface proper is covered by skin which has a relatively impermeable, dry, horny outer layer, and often fur or feathers. This dry protective skin cannot cover all

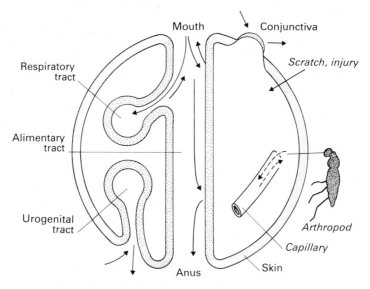

Fig. 2.1. Body surfaces as sites of virus infection and shedding.

body surfaces. In the alimentary canal, where food must be digested and absorbed, the surface lining consists of one or more layers of living cells. In the lungs also, living cells are required where gaseous exchanges take place with the outside world. Another discontinuity in the protective covering of skin is the urogenital tract where urine and sexual products are secreted and released to the exterior. Finally in the eye the skin is replaced by a transparent layer of living cells forming the conjunctiva.

As indicated in Chapter 1, infection of epithelial or other cells generally occurs following interaction between a particular viral surface protein and a receptor on the plasma membrane of the cell (Dimmock, 1982). Molecules acting as receptors presumably serve some useful function and have not been produced for the benefit of viruses. Although there have been many studies with cultured cells, the existence and importance of receptors *in vivo* tends to be assumed rather than formally demonstrated. Examples of specific attachments that are important in pathogenesis are included in Table 2.1.

Skin

This is the largest organ in the body and since its outer layers are composed of dead cells it acts as an important barrier to the entry of viruses. It can be penetrated at sites of damage. Hepatitis B virus in man can be introduced into the body by the contaminated needle of the acupuncturist, tattooist, ear-piercer, dentist or doctor. Biting arthropods, including mosquitoes, mites, ticks and sandflies penetrate the skin during feeding and introduce infection either because their saliva is infected or because their mouthparts are contaminated with the virus. Mechanical transfer by contaminated mouthparts takes place with myxoma virus, fleas or mosquitoes passively carrying the virus from one infected rabbit to another. On the other hand, in yellow fever the virus actually multiplies in the arthropod, hence there is an incubation period in the mosquito before it is ready to transmit the virus via its saliva to a susceptible vertebrate host. These are the characteristics that define the true 'arboviruses'.

Rabies is the classical viral disease introduced into a susceptible animal at the site of skin damage caused by a bite from another animal. Virus is shed in the saliva of infected dogs, wolves, skunks and vampire bats and the bites of these animals, in contrast to those of mosquitoes, are generally noticed. In other infections via the skin, the site of injury may be unnoticed, as is often the case when the human wart virus and other papillomaviruses initiate infection in the skin.

Viruses entering the body through the skin can infect epidermal cells (vaccinia virus), the underlying dermal cells (myxoma virus), deeper tissues such as muscles and nerves (rabies virus), or even gain entry

Table 2.1. Examples of specific attachments of virus to cells.

Virus	Cell	Mechanism
Influenza	Respiratory epithelial cell (mammal)	Viral haemagglutinin binds to neuraminic acid-containing glycoprotein on cell (1)
	Intestinal epithelial cell (birds)	
Parainfluenza 1 (Sendai)	Respiratory epithelial cell	H-N glycoprotein in viral envelope binds to specific glycoside on cell (2)
Coronavirus Rhinovirus	Nasal epithelium	Envelope or capsid protein of virus binds to receptor on cell
Poliovirus	Not known; primate cells only	Minor protein (VP_4) on virus reacts with cell receptor (3)
Coxsackievirus	Respiratory or intestinal tract	Viral capsid protein binds to receptor on cell (4)
Rotavirus	Intestinal epithelial cell	Protein from outer capsid binds to receptor on cell (5)
Reovirus	T lymphocyte, neurone	Haemagglutinin ($\sigma 1$, a minor outer capsid protein of virus) binds to receptor on cell (6)
Adenovirus	Conjunctival, pharyngeal or respiratory epithelial cell	Penton fibre binds to receptor on cell (7)
Rabies	Neuromuscular junction	Envelope protein binds to acetylcholine receptor ? (8)
EB virus	B lymphocyte	Envelope protein binds to receptor closely associated with C_3 receptor (9)

(1) Gottschalk *et al.*, 1972; (2) Markwell *et al.*, 1981; (3) McLaren *et al.*, 1959; (4) Crowell and Philipson, 1971; (5) Bastardo *et al.*, 1981; (6) Fields, 1982; (7) Philipson *et al.*, 1968; (8) Lentz *et al.*, 1982; (9) Wells *et al.*, 1983.

into the blood if a mosquito's proboscis enters a blood vessel and emits a puff of infected saliva (arboviruses, Gordon and Lumsden, 1939).

Respiratory tract

Effective cleansing mechanisms keep the respiratory tract clean by removing inhaled particles (Newhouse et al. 1976; McNabb and Tomasi, 1981), and normally the lungs are almost sterile. Infections take place in spite of the operation of these cleansing mechanisms. A mucociliary blanket lines the nasal cavity and most of the lower respiratory tract. This consists of ciliated cells and mucus, the latter produced from single secretory cells (goblet cells) and from subepithelial glands. Inhaled foreign particles deposited on this surface are entrapped in mucus, carried from the nasal cavity (upper respiratory tract) or from the lungs (lower respiratory tract) to the back of the throat and then swallowed (Fig. 2.2). In the terminal portions of the lower respiratory tract are alveoli, the sites of gaseous exchange, where the mucociliary sheet is absent. The alveoli are lined by epithelial cells and also by highly phago-cytic alveolar macrophages. The fate of inhaled particles depends on their size. Larger visible particles are filtered off by hairs lining the nos-trils. Particles 10 μm or greater in diameter tend to be deposited on the mucosa covering the turbinate bones, which project into the nasal cavity and act as baffle plates. Smaller particles (5 μm or less) are likely to enter the lungs, some of them reaching the alveoli.

If an inhaled virus particle is to initiate infection in the respiratory tract it must first avoid being caught up in mucus, carried to the back of the throat and swallowed. If it reaches the alveoli and encounters an alveolar macrophage it must either resist phagocytosis, or submit to phagocytosis but then survive and multiply rather than be digested and killed. Highly successful myxoviruses such as influenza make a specific and firm attachment via their haemagglutinin to complementary neuraminic acid-containing receptors on the surface of respiratory epithelial cells (Fig. 2.3). Quite possibly one of the functions of the viral neuraminidase is to liberate virions from neuraminic acid-containing inhibitor, analogous to the cell receptor, which is plentiful in mucus. Specific gangliosides have been identified as host cell receptors for Sendai virus (Markwell et al., 1981). Following this initial attachment there is a fusion of viral envelope and cell membrane, the nucleocapsid enters the cell, and viral replication takes place. Probably all viruses that infect the host via the mucociliary lining of the respiratory tract do so by attaching to specific receptors which enable them to enter sus-ceptible cells rather than be carried away in the surface film of mucus.

A few viruses such as pig cytomegalovirus, avoid destruction by alveolar macrophages and infect them. Indeed, alveolar macrophage cultures are used in the standard assay system for this virus, which does

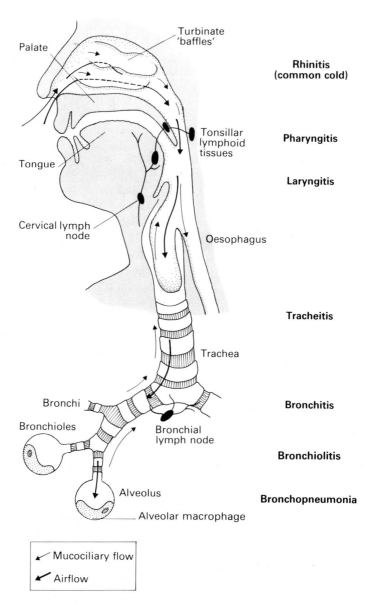

Rhinitis (common cold)

Pharyngitis

Laryngitis

Tracheitis

Bronchitis

Bronchiolitis

Bronchopneumonia

Palate

Turbinate 'baffles'

Tonsillar lymphoid tissues

Tongue

Cervical lymph node

Oesophagus

Trachea

Bronchi

Bronchioles

Bronchial lymph node

Alveolus

Alveolar macrophage

Mucociliary flow

Airflow

Fig. 2.2. Mechanisms of infection in the respiratory tract.

not replicate so well in macrophages from blood, bone marrow or peritoneal cavity (Watt *et al.*, 1973). Influenza virus infects alveolar macrophages of man and mouse but in these cells the replication cycle is abortive (Rodgers and Mims, 1981; 1982). Viral antigens are produced but infectious virus is not released. Mouse alveolar macrophages are

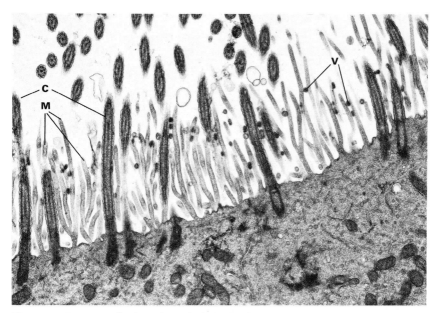

Fig. 2.3. Portion of ciliated epithelial cell from organ culture of guinea pig trachea after incubation with influenza virus for 1 hour at 4°C. Electron micrograph of thin section showing virus particles (V) attached to cilia (C) and to microvilli (M). The fluid between the cilia is watery, the viscous mucoid layer lying above the cilia. Courtesy of R. Dourmashkin.

infected by parainfluenza 1 (Sendai) virus, but there too the infection is abortive.

Oropharynx and intestinal tract

Cleansing mechanisms in the oropharynx are the regular flow of saliva and the action of the tongue and cheeks. The mouth and throat are important sites of entry of viruses into the body. A sore throat is a common symptom in many virus infections, suggesting early growth of virus in epithelial or underlying cells with accompanying inflammation. Surprisingly little is known about the replication and behaviour of viruses in the oropharynx.

In the intestinal tract the general flow of contents acts as a cleansing mechanism, but the walls of the intestine are constantly in motion, and particles move about a good deal while they are being carried downstream. A mucus film lines the mucosa and, as in the respiratory tract, unless virus particles attach firmly to the surface of epithelial cells they are unlikely to have the opportunity to initiate infection. Successful enteric viruses make the most of chance encounters with intestinal epithelial cells by forming firm unions with specific receptors on the susceptible cell surface, allowing time for penetration of virus (examples are included in Table 2.1). Infection of intestinal epithelial cells has not often been studied *in vivo*. Rotaviruses infect intestinal epithelial cells in mice (Little and Shadduck, 1982) and other species, as do many parvoviruses such as feline panleukopenia virus in cats, and coronaviruses such as transmissible gastroenteritis virus in pigs. Worthington and Graney (1973) introduced adenovirus 3 into ileal loops of newborn rats and within five minutes virus particles were seen by electron microscopy in tubules and vesicles of intestinal adsorptive cells. Particles were subsequently seen in cysternae and supranuclear vacuoles but it is not clear whether this led to a productive infection.

As well as infecting epithelial cells, virus particles can be taken up passively from the intestinal lumen. This can be shown by experiments with inert (non-replicating) particles and probably involves specialised areas of the intestine. When rats drink water containing large amounts of bacteriophage T_7 (diameter 30 nm) intact infectious phages are recoverable from thoracic duct lymph within 20 minutes (Mims, 1964). The phenomenon is also seen with infectious viruses such as reovirus type 1 in mice. Large amounts of virus ($>10^8$ pfu) were injected into closed ileal loops of one-week-old mice and the disposition of virus studied at intervals by thin section electron microscopy (Wolfe *et al.*, 1981). Within 30 minutes intact virions were visible on the surface of certain specialised surface cells (M cells) overlying Peyer's patches (collections of lymphoid tissue) in the ileum, and after one hour the virus particles were inside smooth-surfaced cytoplasmic vesicles within these cells. Particles were not seen in ordinary epithelial cells or in goblet (mucus-producing) cells. The M cells appear to hand over virus particles to adjacent mononuclear cells for antigen-processing or replication (see Chapter 3), and some of the particles probably enter local lymphatics.

The likelihood of infection is affected not only by the movement of the intestinal contents but also by the presence of acid, bile, proteolytic enzymes and mucus. Mucus gives mechanical protection to epithelial cells and contains secretory IgA antibodies. Unless a virus is relatively resistant to acid and bile it is unlikely to establish a successful enteric infection and be shed in large amounts in the faeces. Hepatitis A virus and the other enteroviruses (coxsackieviruses, echoviruses and polioviruses) are all acid-resistant, in contrast to other picornaviruses that infect via the oropharynx or respiratory tract (rhinoviruses, foot and mouth disease virus) which are sensitive to acid. Bile salts solubilise lipids and disrupt virus envelopes, which is doubtless why very few enveloped viruses frequent the alimentary tract.

Urogenital tract

The urinary tract is regularly flushed with urine which acts as a physical cleansing mechanism, and invading microorganisms must first and

foremost avoid being washed out during urination. There are few viruses that regularly initiate infection in the urethra. The surfaces of the
genital tract, however, have less effective cleansing mechanisms and are
quite commonly infected by direct mucosal contact during the course of
sexual activity. Examples include herpes simplex type 2 and genital
papillomaviruses (especially HPV6, 11, 16, 18) which are now among the
commonest sexually transmitted infections in man.

Conjunctiva

A continuous flow of secretion (tears), together with the wiping action
of the lids, keep the conjunctiva moist and clean. Viruses alighting on
this surface must make specific attachments to conjunctival cells if they
are to avoid being washed away. This is an uncommon route of infection
for viruses, although it can occur when there is conjunctival injury.
Adenovirus 8, for instance, can be transmitted from eye to eye by the
physician in the course of removing foreign bodies from this site. Other
viruses such as measles and certain adenoviruses sometimes infect the
conjunctiva from the 'inside' after spreading through the body to the
eye, and are then shed to the exterior in tears. Conjunctivitis is not seen
until after an incubation period of a week or more during which time the
virus has been spreading and replicating elsewhere in the body. This is
in contrast to the acute haemorrhagic conjunctivitis due to enterovirus
70 which appears after an incubation period of only 24 hours (Higgins,
1982); in this case the conjunctiva itself can be assumed to be the site of
initial infection.

MECHANISMS OF SPREAD IN THE BODY

Local spread on epithelial surfaces

Many viruses multiply in epithelial cells at the site of entry into the
body, produce a spreading infection in the epithelium, and are then
shed directly to the exterior. These events can occur quite rapidly when
the epithelium is covered with a layer of liquid, as in infections of
respiratory and alimentary tracts by rhinoviruses, coronaviruses,
influenza viruses and rotaviruses. There is little or no invasion of underlying tissues, and the incubation period, in contrast to infections where
the virus spreads through the body and multiplies in distant sites, is not
more than a few days (Table 2.2). Things are different in the skin, however, and here the infection spreads mostly by the sequential infection of
neighbouring cells. Papillomaviruses infect the basal layer of epidermal
cells where the replication cycle is incomplete; virions and viral antigens
develop only as cells move towards the skin surface and become
keratinised (Noyes and Mellors, 1957; Almeida et al., 1962). It is a slow

Table 2.2 Distinction between surface and systemic viral infection.

	SURFACE Infections confined to body surfaces. Incubation period short (usually <1 week)	SYSTEMIC Infections initiated at body surfaces, followed by spread through the body. Long incubation period (usually >1 week)
Respiratory tract	Influenza[a] Parainfluenza Rhinoviruses Coronaviruses[b]	Measles Smallpox Rubella
Oropharynx		Herpes simplex Cytomegalovirus EB virus Mumps
Intestinal tract	Rotaviruses Parvoviruses Enteroviruses[c]	Enteroviruses[c] Adenoviruses[d] Coronaviruses[e]
Skin	Warts Molluscum contagiosum	Arboviruses Rabies
Genital tract	Papillomaviruses	Herpes simplex 2

[a]In mammals.
[b]In man.
[c]Confined to the gut in most individuals, but sometimes invasion of muscle, central nervous system or liver (hepatitis A).
[d]Certain serotypes.
[e]In some animal species.

process and contributes to the longer incubation period of warts. The local spread of ectromelia virus in the skin of mice has been followed after infection by scarification, infected cells being identified by fluorescent antibody staining (Roberts, 1962b). A single focus of infection enlarged slowly over the course of 3–4 days by cell-to-cell spread of infection both in the dermis and epidermis. A similar sequence of events follows the introduction of vaccinia virus into the dermis of man during vaccination against smallpox.

Many respiratory and enteric viruses such as rhinoviruses and rotaviruses are largely confined to epithelial surfaces. They may be carried by lymphatics to local lymph nodes, but do not normally spread through the body or to deeper tissues. The basis for this is not usually known but it may be associated with the following:

1 Temperature sensitivity. Rhinoviruses and human respiratory coronaviruses show optimal growth at 34°C, the temperature of the nasal mucosa, rather than 37°C, the temperature of the body generally.

2 Topography of budding from the epithelial cell. When viruses are liberated only from the external face of epithelial cells (Rodriguez-Boulan and Sabatini, 1978; Boulan and Pendergast, 1980) they are less likely to spread to underlying tissues.

3 Topography of virus production in multilayered epithelium. Papillomaviruses infect the basal layer of epithelial cells in the skin but do not mature until the epithelial cell approaches the body surface. This would restrict spread to underlying tissues.

4 Insusceptibility of cells except at the epithelial surface.

Superficial virus infections generally have incubation periods measured in days rather than weeks and therefore tend to be less affected by more slowly evolving host defences, such as those due to immune responses (see Chapter 3).

Subepithelial invasion and lymphatic spread

After traversing the epithelial layer and its basement membrane and reaching subepithelial tissues (Fig. 2.4), a virus is immediately exposed to:

1 Phagocytic cells.

2 The lymphatic system.

The resident phagocytic cells (histiocytes) are of the macrophage series. If the virus is phagocytosed it will soon be destroyed by acid conditions in the phagosome and by enzymes delivered to the phagosome following lysosomal fusion, unless there is a mechanism by which this fate is avoided. A number of viruses, however, replicate in macrophages, some of them exclusively in macrophages. The subject of viruses and macrophages is dealt with more fully on pp. 53–9.

A complex network of lymphatics lies below the epithelium at body surfaces and free virus particles rapidly enter lymphatic capillaries. They are then carried to local lymph nodes strategically placed to deal with the flow of lymph from these tissues before returning it to the blood. Lymph nodes act as filters, and the local nodes are the sites where immune responses are generated to microbes and their antigens arriving from body surfaces. As they enter the node, viruses are first exposed to macrophages lining the marginal sinus (Fig. 2.4). If the virus is taken up and inactivated, its antigens are subsequently presented to underlying lymphoid cells and the immune response is initiated. The infection progresses no further. If the virus is not inactivated it may infect the macrophages and possibly lymphocytes. This is seen for instance in infections with measles, adenoviruses and various herpesviruses (see Table 6.4). If the virus particles are not taken up in the node they will pass through the node and eventually enter the bloodstream. In either case the lymph node serves then to disseminate rather than confine the infection.

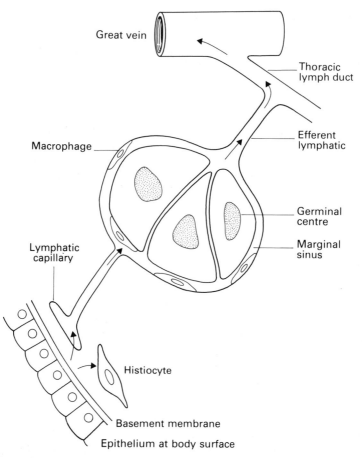

Great vein

Thoracic
lymph duct

Macrophage

Efferent
lymphatic

Germinal
centre

Lymphatic
capillary

Marginal
sinus

Histiocyte

Basement membrane

Epithelium at body surface

Fig. 2.4. Subepithelial invasion and lymphatic spread of viruses.

Macrophages and lymphocytes circulate through the body, those in the skin entering local lymph nodes, and there is also a constant movement of lymphocytes directly from the blood into lymph nodes (see Fig. 3.2). Cells in lymph nodes can travel via the lymph to the bloodstream. If a virus infects these cells without damaging them it can be carried passively round the body in a very short time (see p. 51).

Thus when viruses multiply at the body surface, large numbers enter lymphatics, and the local lymph node becomes an important site at which the infection can be terminated and immune response generated. Sometimes the virus infects and multiplies in lymphatic endothelium (Roberts, 1962b), further increasing the number of virus particles reaching the node. Viruses are not known to enter local blood vessels directly, except perhaps when these are damaged, or pierced by the mouthparts of an infected arthropod. Local blood vessel invasion would theoretically be possible if cells in the walls of capillaries or venules were infected.

The events at the body surface are greatly altered when there is a local inflammatory response. If this occurs early in a viral infection it generally follows tissue damage. But it can also be the sequel to immune events, such as specific interactions between T lymphocytes or antibodies and viral antigens. In the inflammatory response local blood vessels are dilated and their permeability increases. This allows leakage from the blood of immunoglobulins, complement components and other proteins such as fibrinogen, and also the passage of leukocytes into the tissues. The delivery to the infection site of antibodies, complement components, monocytes and lymphocytes can be important for host resistance, especially after the immune response has been generated (see Chapter 3).

Spread by the blood—viraemia

The blood is the most effective and most rapid vehicle for the spread of virus through the body. Once the virus has reached the bloodstream, usually by way of the lymphatic system, it can localise in any part of the body within a minute or two. The first entry of virus into the blood is called primary viraemia. The amount of virus in the blood at any given time may be negligible but it is a common silent event, often known to have taken place only because of the invasion of distant organs. Following further replication in these distant organs the bloodstream is often reinvaded to give a secondary viraemia. This is of larger magnitude, is more easily detected in blood samples, and often leads to infection of a second set of organs. Primary and secondary viraemias are distinct features in the pathogenesis of mousepox, as elucidated in the classic study by Fenner (1948), and also in measles and smallpox (Fig. 2.5), but in other infections they are not distinguishable. To understand viraemia, which is a necessary stage in the pathogenesis of nearly all systemic viral infections, it is necessary to discuss what happens to a virus when it enters the blood (Mims, 1964).

Viruses may be carried free in the plasma, or in the formed elements of the blood, or in more than one of these compartments (Table 2.3). Those carried in leukocytes, generally in monocytes or lymphocytes, are not removed ('cleared') as readily or in the same way as viruses circulating free in the plasma (see next section). Being protected from antibodies and other plasma components they can be carried to distant tissues, especially if the infected cell remains healthy and in the course of its normal migrations moves in and out of the vascular system. For instance, a mononuclear cell infected with measles virus in the subepithelial tissues of the respiratory tract can enter the blood and subsequently localise in the spleen.

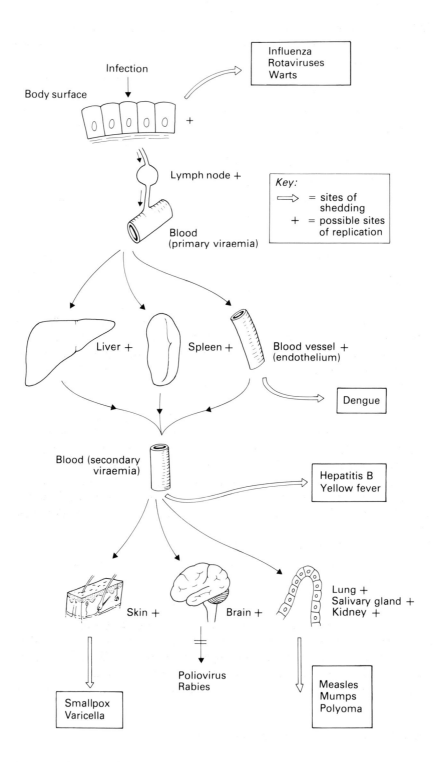

Table 2.3. Carriage of viruses in different compartments of blood[a].

Free in plasma	Cell-associated			
	Monocytes	Lymphocytes	Platelets	Erythrocytes
Poliovirus	LDH	CMV	Murine leukaemia	Colorado tick fever
Togaviruses (e.g. yellow fever)	Ectromelia	EBV	LCM	
	Smallpox	Measles		

[a]Selected examples only; the list is by no means comprehensive.

It is uncommon for viruses to infect erythrocytes. As long as the erythrocyte remains healthy the virus may be protected from antiviral forces, but it has no opportunity to leave the vascular system. Colorado tick fever virus infects erythrocytes in the bone marrow (Oshiro *et al.*, 1978) and in the circulation (Emmons *et al.*, 1972) and this contributes to the viraemia. Many other viruses such as rubella, influenza and parainfluenza attach to the surface of the cells *in vitro* and agglutinate them, but this has not been shown to be important in the infected host. A few viruses such as LCM and certain leukaemia viruses in mice infect megakaryocytes, and therefore the circulating platelets derived from these cells are infected. Platelets are infected more commonly than leukocytes in adult mice inoculated with herpes simplex virus (Forghani and Schmidt, 1983). Infected platelets are not known to be important in the pathogenesis of virus infection.

Viruses carried free in the plasma include picornaviruses and togaviruses such as yellow fever virus. They are exposed to antiviral forces, including antibodies present in plasma. Localisation in organs depends on:
1 Phagocytosis by reticuloendothelial cells, and
2 Ability to adhere to and grow in vascular endothelial cells.

Reticuloendothelial cells: macrophage–virus interactions

The term reticuloendothelial system is old-fashioned but useful. It refers to a 'system' of mononuclear phagocytes (macrophages), widely distributed in the body, and united in their ability to ingest colloidal dyes and inert or infectious particles. Macrophages are professional phagocytes and are present in all major compartments of the body. Those in

Fig. 2.5. The spread of infection through the body.

subepithelial tissues, in the alveoli of the lung and in the sinusoids of the lymphs nodes have been referred to above. Others (reticuloendothelial cells) line the sinusoids of the liver, spleen, bone marrow and adrenals, and remove foreign particles from the blood. The liver macrophages (Kupffer cells) are numerically the most important of these. Larger viruses circulating free in the plasma are generally removed with great efficiency, like inert foreign particles of similar size. Most are removed even during a single passage through the liver. Intravenously injected vaccinia virus for instance is cleared from the blood within a few minutes, whereas smaller sized viruses are cleared less rapidly (Fig. 2.6). Clearance depends on the nature of the virus, and some viruses for unknown reasons are not cleared at all. Serum factors can be important and viruses to which specific antibody and/or complement is attached are more rapidly cleared because macrophages have receptors for the Fc portion of immunoglobulin and for complement. Viruses are also

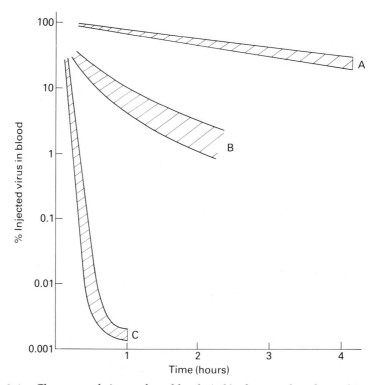

Fig. 2.6. Clearance of viruses from blood. A *No clearance*; but thermal inactivation, e.g. type 1 poliovirus in mice, LCM virus in carrier mice. B *Slow clearance*; with most small viruses—T$_7$ phage (30 nm diam.) in mice or Rift Valley fever virus (30 nm diam.) in mice. C *Rapid clearance*; with larger viruses—vaccinia (250 nm diam.) in mice; or smaller viruses with antibody (and/or complement) attached; or smaller viruses when macrophages are activated.

cleared more rapidly by 'activated' macrophages (see Chapter 3). Following uptake the subsequent course of events depends on the behaviour of the virus in the macrophage. The types of virus-macrophage interaction in the liver for instance, were studied many years ago (Mims, 1964) and found to be important in the pathogenesis of viral infections (Fig. 2.7).

1 No uptake by macrophages. This occurs with certain viruses, and favours persistence of the viraemia.

2 Uptake and destruction by macrophages. This is the fate of most viruses circulating in the plasma. If the viraemia is to be maintained, the virus must enter the blood as fast as it is removed. Such viraemias are prolonged and intensified when uptake ('clearance') by macrophages is diminished. This can be done experimentally by intravenous injection of silica particles or colloidal thorium dioxide (thorotrast), which are taken up by these cells and interfere with their phagocytic activity. The

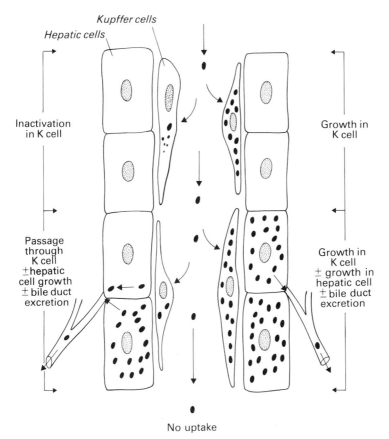

Fig. 2.7. Types of viral behaviour in liver. Endothelial cells have been omitted; in most infections their role is not known.

sustained or increased viraemia produced in this way has been used to demonstrate the dynamics of Semliki Forest virus viraemia (Mims, 1964) and also to promote localisation of circulating yellow fever virus in the mouse brain (Zisman *et al.*, 1971).

3   Uptake and passive transfer from macrophages to hepatic cells. Circulating virus particles are taken up by liver macrophages but fail to establish infection and are passively transferred, perhaps via endothelial cells, to hepatic cells. If the virus cannot grow in hepatic cells things go no further, although the hepatic cells may excrete virus into the bile. This occurs experimentally with poliovirus after intravenous injection into monkeys (Mims, 1964). Viruses that infect hepatic cells, however, may cause hepatitis, in spite of their inability to infect liver macrophages. This is so for certain arthropod-borne viruses such as Rift Valley fever virus (Mims, 1957), which causes enzootic hepatitis in lambs. Virus produced from hepatic cells can be transferred back to the blood (Rift Valley fever virus, hepatitis B in man) and also excreted in bile (hepatitis A in man).

4   Uptake and growth in macrophages and/or endothelial cells. Sometimes macrophages only are infected (LDV in mice) with release of progeny into the blood. The progeny virus particles also have the opportunity to infect hepatic cells. Liver infection in mousepox (see below, and Mims, 1959) and probably in smallpox and yellow fever is caused in this way. There are similar possibilities when infected blood cells localise in liver sinusoids. Kirn and his associates (Gut *et al.*, 1982; Kirn and Keller, 1983) have used Frog virus 3 (FV_3) to study the role of macrophages and endothelial cells lining liver sinusoids. After intravenous injection into rats, FV_3 is taken up by liver macrophages. It fails to multiply at 37°C, but nevertheless destroys macrophages and endothelial cells and causes a fatal hepatitis. The virus does not infect hepatocytes, which are damaged probably as a result of exposure to circulating endotoxin absorbed from the intestine. Rats are 100 times more sensitive to administered endotoxin after destruction of sinusoidal cells by FV_3 and, when they are colectomised to remove the source of endogenous endotoxin, they survive the infection (Gut *et al.*, 1982).

Differences in virus–macrophage interactions may account for differences in the virulence of virus strains, and for differences in host resistance, whether determined by age or by genetic constitution. This is also discussed in Chapter 5. Numerous studies have been made of macrophage susceptibility to viruses, but surprisingly little is known about the cellular basis for resistance or susceptibility. There is a wide spectrum of macrophage responsiveness to be accounted for. At one extreme, the virus (e.g. poliovirus) fails to infect macrophages, and at the other (LDH virus in mice) a subset of macrophages are uniquely susceptible cells in which a highly productive infection is initiated.

Because of their phagocytic prowess and their Fc and C_3 receptors (see Chapter 3), macrophages are likely to ingest virus particles, especially when these are coated with antibody or complement. Specific virus receptors may also be present on the macrophage surface. Daughaday et al. (1981) showed that trypsin-treated human monocytes became insusceptible to dengue virus, except when enhancing antibodies (see Chapter 3) were present. They concluded that virus-specific receptors had been removed by the trypsin, but after combination of virus with enhancing antibody, entry into the cell and infection was mediated by Fc receptors instead. Even if the macrophage is inherently susceptible, the ability of the virus to initiate infection will depend on whether it enters the cell via a virus receptor, via an Fc or C_3 receptor, or by non-specific phagocytosis. There have been few studies of the consequences of fusion of lysosomes and phagosomes, or on the interaction of viruses with lysosomal enzymes and other antimicrobial forces. These matters are known to be important in many bacterial and protozoal infections. In one of the few attempts by virologists to answer these questions, Rager-Zisman et al. (1982) obtained evidence that oxidative metabolism, with generation of oxygen radicals and hydrogen peroxide, was important in the resistance of mouse peritoneal macrophages to vesicular stomatitis virus. Substances such as chloroquine and NH_4Cl rapidly increase lysosomal pH from about 4.7 to 5.5–6.0 (Ohkuma and Poole, 1978), and might be expected to influence the replication of viruses in macrophages. Canning and Fields (1983) found that reovirus shows reduced replication and decreased cytopathic effect in L cells treated with 10 mM NH_4Cl. This could be because of defective uncoating, which for reoviruses is mediated by lysosomal enzymes.

The antiviral actions of macrophages are mostly deduced from in vitro observations. It is difficult to say how important they are in vivo. Also, results may differ according to the age and genetics of the host (see Chapter 5), and the site of origin in the body; indeed, even from a given site there are subpopulations of macrophages that differ in susceptibility (Stueckemann et al., 1982). The state of activation is important. There is an increase in lysosomal enzymes in resident peritoneal macrophages of mice on mere cultivation in serum-containing medium, and activation in vivo by intraperitoneal injection of starch, thioglycollate or casein gives different results from immunological activation by lymphokines. With these reservations in mind, the antiviral actions of macrophages can be categorised as follows:

Macrophages susceptible to infection
1 Completely susceptible—This may lead to destruction of macrophages (ectromelia in mice, see p. 77), or to interference with macrophage function (Sendai virus in mice, LDH virus in mice, see Chapter 5). Antibody can prevent infection after combining with virus (see

Chapter 3) but may enhance infection when smaller amounts of antibody are available. Non-neutralizing antibody can enhance if directed against antigens on the virion surface. Enhancing antibodies have been reported for dengue virus (Halstead, 1979) as discussed in Chapter 4, for arboviruses (Hawkes and Lafferty, 1967; Peiris and Porterfield, 1981), for LDH virus (Cafruny and Plagemann, 1982). Monoclonal antibody studies show that in the case of flaviviruses enhancing antibody reacts with cross-reactive antigenic determinants and can be distinguished from neutralising antibody, but mechanisms are not clear (Peiris et al., 1982; Brandt et al., 1982). Daughaday et al. (1981), studying dengue virus in human peripheral blood monocytes, were able to distinguish infection of cells via (trypsin-sensitive) virus receptors from infection via (trypsin-resistant) Fc receptors.

2   Macrophages susceptible but infection abortive—Little if any infectious progeny is released and hence macrophage infection is a 'dead end' virologically speaking, e.g. Sendai virus in mouse peritoneal macrophages (Mims and Murphy, 1973). Macrophages may be damaged or destroyed, e.g. mouse alveolar macrophages infected with influenza virus (Rodgers and Mims, 1981), and can be thought of as having phagocytosed an invading virus and died in the course of preventing the spread of infection.

3   Macrophages susceptible but become insusceptible following activation mediated immunologically by lymphokines—e.g. vaccinia virus in rabbit macrophages (Buchmeier et al., 1979).

Macrophages insusceptible to infection
Such macrophages are said to display 'intrinsic' antiviral activity. They can also function immunologically or have 'extrinsic' antiviral activity by controlling infection in other cells, as follows:

1   Phagocytosis and degradation of infectious material—important especially in liver.

2   Phagocytosis, 'processing' and 'presentation' of antigens to T cells—Vital immunological role in, e.g. lymph nodes, Peyer's patches, spleen (Chapter 3).

3   Macrophages kill infected cell by interacting with antibodies specifically bound to viral antigens on infected cell surface (Chapter 3), i.e. macrophages act as killer cells (Macfarlan et al., 1977; Smith and Sheppard, 1982).

4   Macrophages secrete arginase and starve replicating virus of arginine (Wildy et al., 1982a), which is essential for the growth of herpesviruses.

5   Macrophages produce interferon locally to protect other cells. Haller (1981) has carried out interesting work using a strain of influenza virus that has been adapted to growth in mouse peritoneal macrophages. Macrophages from different strains of mice show differences in susceptibility depending on the presence of a single gene that determines the

protection against influenza virus induced in macrophages by interferon.

6 Macrophages can prevent the spread of infection in other cells. This is determined experimentally by adding peritoneal macrophages to monolayers of infected cells and testing for a reduction in virus yield or plaque formation. This antiviral effect appears to take place without macrophages destroying the infected cells, or producing interferon. For instance, herpes simplex virus plaque production and virus yield is reduced in the absence of detectable interferon in the culture and in the presence of anti-interferon serum. When the macrophages are removed, plaques develop, showing that it was not a cytotoxic effect (Hayashi *et al.*, 1980; Morse and Morahan, 1981). Macrophages could prevent the spread of infection by promoting the rounding up of infected cells or possibly by affecting protein synthesis in these cells. Although this may occur in monolayer culture, it is not known whether it would be important *in vivo*.

Vascular endothelial cells

If a circulating virus is to invade tissues lacking sinusoids, it must first localise in the endothelium of small blood vessels (capillaries or venules) in that tissue. Here the circulation is slowest and the vessel walls thinnest. The vascular endothelium, together with its basement membrane and adjacent cells, separates the blood from the extravascular tissues and constitutes the blood–tissue junction, often acting as a barrier to the spread of virus into a tissue or organ. The virus can reach tissues from the blood by leaking through, being passively carried through, or by 'growing' through the vessel wall. These alternatives have been studied especially for viruses localising in the central nervous system (see pp. 60–2). They also apply to the localisation of circulating viruses in the salivary glands (mumps), kidney (polyomaviruses), muscle (coxsackie B viruses), respiratory epithelium (measles) or the placenta and foetus (rubella). Vascular endothelial cells are often susceptible to infection *in vivo* (Mims, 1982b) and also *in vitro* (Friedman *et al.*, 1981). The endothelial cells studied *in vitro* are, however, generally from large veins and arteries rather than from the venules and capillaries that would be relevant *in vivo*. The presence of virus receptors on vascular endothelium in a given organ or tissue might determine its susceptibility to infection, but nothing is known of these matters.

Attachment to and uptake of virus by vascular endothelial cells is generally slow compared with reticuloendothelial cells. It is unlikely to occur unless the viraemia is maintained for a long enough period. Neurotropic viruses such as poliovirus or the neurotropic arthropod-borne viruses (Zisman *et al.*, 1971) reach the central nervous system from the blood only when the viraemia is of adequate magnitude and duration. This is also a prerequisite if blood-sucking arthropods are to be infected.

In summary, the sources of virus for the maintenance of viraemia are as follows:

1 Vascular endothelium, as in distemper viral infection of dogs (Coffin and Liu, 1957) or in arthropod-borne viral infections.
2 Reticuloendothelial cells (lactic dehydrogenase virus in mice).
3 Cells adjacent to reticuloendothelial cells (hepatocytes for hepatitis B in man).
4 Blood cells (African swine fever).
5 Tissues from which virus is discharged into the blood via lymph, e.g. striated muscle in coxsackievirus B in man, or experimental Ross River virus infection in mice (Murphy *et al.*, 1973).

Bloodborne invasion of the central nervous system

Circulating viruses invade the central nervous system either after localising in blood vessels in meninges and choroid plexus, neural tissue invasion subsequently taking place from the cerebrospinal fluid (Fig. 2.8), or more directly after localising in blood vessels of the brain and spinal cord (Johnson, 1974). Coxsackie and echovirus infections in man generally cause meningitis rather than encephalitis, and these viruses are recoverable from cerebrospinal fluid. Other viruses (mumps, poliovirus) cause meningitis and also encephalitis and the invasion of the brain via the cerebrospinal fluid has been demonstrated experimentally with mumps virus (Wolinsky *et al.*, 1976) and rat virus (Lipton and Johnson, 1972) in hamsters. Direct and independent invasion of the brain across cerebral blood vessels has been shown, e.g. for poliovirus (Blinzinger *et al.*, 1969) and retroviruses (Swarz *et al.*, 1981).

The mechanism of virus localisation in vessels is unknown. As well as growing in endothelial cells, viruses can leak through, or be passively transferred across the vessel wall by the endothelial cells. Migrating infected leukocytes are able to carry viruses across the vessel wall (Summers *et al.*, 1978) but the importance of this is not known. Passive transfer by endothelial cells or leukocytes is assumed to have occurred when infection of endothelial cells cannot be demonstrated. There are differences in the structure of the vessel wall in different regions. The endothelial cells and basement membrane in cerebral capillaries form a complete barrier between the vessel lumen and extravascular tissues, whereas in the choroid plexus endothelial cells have holes in them (are fenestrated), and the basement membrane is less dense. But these differences, although often referred to in discussions of the 'blood–brain barrier', do not appear by themselves to determine tissue invasion.

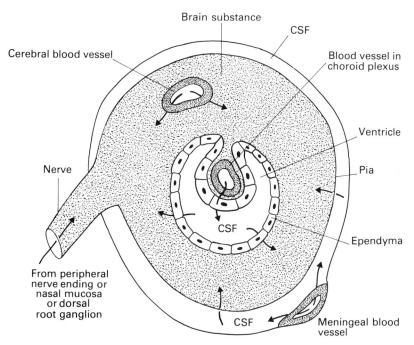

Fig. 2.8. Routes of viral invasion of the central nervous system. CSF-
= Cerebrospinal fluid.

In the central nervous system, as elsewhere, viruses are more likely
to localise in small blood vessels and invade adjacent organs when there
is inflammation. Just as variola virus may localise where the skin is
inflamed by a tight garter to give smallpox lesions at this site, so may a
circulating virus localise in sites of inflammation in the central nervous
system. Yellow fever virus causes lethal disease in adult mice by growing in brain cells after direct intracerebral injection; intraperitoneally
injected virus is harmless, except when intracranial inflammation has
been induced by the intracerebral injection of starch or saline. Fifty years
ago, this was used in a standard mouse protection test for yellow fever
neutralising antibodies in the days before cell culture had been established or infant mice discovered for use in virology (Sawyer and Lloyd,
1931).

Subsequent spread in the CNS can take place via cerebrospinal fluid
(see p. 68), by sequential infection of neural cells, or possibly via the
narrow (10–15 nm) extracellular spaces (Blinzinger and Muller, 1971).
Transit along the extensive axonal and dendritic ramifications of
neurones can be rapid. The different neural cells can now be identified
by immunological and other markers, and the responses of astrocytes,
oligodendrocytes, and of neurones from different sites is being charted
(Johnson, 1980; Kennedy *et al.*, 1983). The subsequent course of the

Infection and the Spread of Viruses Through the Body 61

CNS infection depends on whether the infection kills the cell or more subtly interferes with function, whether or not the virus persists (see Chapter 6), and so on.

Viral invasion of the central nervous system also takes place via peripheral and olfactory nerves (see p. 68).

Bloodborne invasion of placenta and foetus—vertical transmission

Bloodborne invasion of the placenta is particularly important because it can lead to infection of the foetus with results varying from no damage, through typical disease or congenital malformations, to death and abortion (Table 2.4). Localisation of virus in placental (or yolk sac) blood vessels is the necessary preliminary, but the mechanism is not known. As at all blood–tissue junctions, virus can then be carried across, leak across or can grow across the blood vessel wall. The barrier between foetal and maternal blood consists of 1–4 layers of cells, depending on the species of animal and the stage of pregnancy. There is generally a placental focus of infection, as seen with rubella, smallpox and cyto-megalovirus in man, or with primary LCM virus infection in mice (Mims, 1969).

The foetus does not have all the antiviral defences of the postnatal individual and is therefore very susceptible. For many years the chick embryo was the standard laboratory host for a great variety of viruses, and chick and mammalian embryos are still valuable sources of suscep-tible cells in laboratories. Also, because of its accessibility to experimental observation and manipulation the chick embryo has been used in studies of the teratogenic effect of viruses. For instance, neural tube defects are produced when viruses such as NDV are inoculated into 2–3-day-old embryos, at a time when the neural tube has not yet been separated from the overlying ectoderm (Blattner *et al.*, 1973).

But the foetus has considerable ability to repair and compensate for damage, and when the infection is less severe or when the virus is less cytopathogenic, the foetus survives. Often, however, there are congeni-tal defects due to interference with developmental processes. The classic example of viral teratogenesis in man is rubella (Gregg, 1941), but there are many other examples. Most of our understanding of mechanisms has come from comparative studies, especially of togavirus and parvo-virus infections of domestic and experimental animals. Defects are often due to the vulnerability of key organs at certain stages of development as with eyes, ears, brain and heart of the 1–3-month-old human foetus infected with rubella virus (see pp. 79–81).

Parvoviruses show selective growth in mitotically active cells, and provide another example. Kilham's rat virus causes congenital infection in rats, often with foetal death or hepatitis in the newborn, but some of

Table 2.4. Principal viruses infecting the foetus transplacentally[a].

Family	Virus	Host	Effect
Togaviridae	Rubella	Man	Abortion, stillbirth, malformations
	Bovine diarrhoea—mucosal disease	Cow	Cerebellar hypoplasia
	Hog cholera (vaccine strain)	Pig	Malformations
Poxviridae	Variola, vaccinia	Man	Abortion
Herpesviridae	Cytomegalovirus	Man, guinea pig	Malformations
	Equine rhinopneumonitis	Horse	Abortion
Reoviridae	Bluetongue (vaccine strain)	Sheep	Stillbirth, CNS disease
Parvoviridae	HI	Hamster	Foetal death, cerebellar
	RV (rat virus)	Rat	hypoplasia

[a]Various other viruses have been reported to infect the foetus transplacentally. The more common and best studied examples are listed here.

the newborn show cerebellar hypoplasia (Kilham and Margolis, 1966). Experimental infection of newborn hamsters revealed that this was due to selective replication of virus in mitotically active cells of the external germinal layer of the cerebellum. These cells were infected when they were about to migrate deeper into the cerebellum and take up a position below the Purkinje cells. Their destruction by the virus resulted in a grossly hypoplastic cerebellum and gross postural and locomotory defects in the affected hamster (Margolis and Kilham, 1968).

Transplacental transmission is important in human medicine (rubella) and in veterinary medicine (hog cholera, border disease of lambs) because the infected foetus is often aborted or born with reduced viability. This means it is not a significant mechanism for maintaining the infection in the host species. For this the infected foetus must develop more or less normally and survive after birth. There is an occasional exception (e.g. transplacental transmission of malignant catarrhal fever in the wildebeest; Plowright, 1965) but generally the infection is less severe and the opportunities for transmission are greater in the postnatal period. This occurs from maternal milk, saliva, blood or other sources. Infections passing directly from parent to offspring are called 'vertically' transmitted infections (Mims, 1981), in contrast to the 'horizontally' transmitted infections that spread between contemporary individuals.

Vertically transmitted infections include those transmitted directly from parent to offspring via eggs or sperm ('germline transmission'). Certain viruses are uniquely endowed to persist inside cells without seriously disturbing cell functions; fertilisation and embryonic development occurs normally. The infected gamete gives rise to a foetus in which every cell is infected and as long as the immune responses that would eliminate the virus or cause tissue damage are not induced, the infection continues postnatally throughout the life of the individual. Germline transmission is seen in particular with some of the retroviruses, where a reverse transcriptase enables a DNA copy of the viral RNA genome to be synthesised and integrated into the genome of the host. These retroviruses include the leukaemia viruses of mice, cats, cattle, etc. and the leukosis viruses of chickens. They are present in most, perhaps in all vertebrates. In mice retroviral DNA sequences account for 0.04% of the entire host genome (Todaro et al., 1978). The arenavirus, LCM, infects the ovum in mice (Mims, 1966) and can therefore presumably be transmitted via the germline. It infects all cells in the foetus and shows a fluctuating, possibly universal infection of all cells in the adult, but the details and the virological basis for persistence at the cellular level are not known.

Transmission via the germline also occurs in arthropods. Examples include arboviruses transmitted transovarially in their mosquito or tick hosts and sigma (CO_2 sensitivity) virus in drosophila (Mims, 1981).

Many viruses are present in semen (Table 2.5), but in most cases it is not known whether the virus is in secretions from accessory glands or in the sperm cells themselves. Sperm cells are infected with mammary tumour virus in certain strains of mice, but for the most part, viruses in semen are more likely to infect the female during copulation rather than the offspring.

Bloodborne invasion of other organs

Most organs and tissues, from tendons to thymus, from pituitary to prostate, can at times be infected by circulating viruses. A few of the more important ones will be mentioned.

Viral infections of the pancreas have been studied in view of the possible role of viruses in the pathogenesis of juvenile diabetes mellitus.

Table 2.5. Viruses present in semen.

Virus		Host	Comments[a]
Family	Species		
Herpesviridae	Herpes simplex	Human	Virus isolated from prostatic fluid, prostate, vas deferens
	Cytomegalovirus	Human	High titres in fluid rather than sperm; persists for >1 year
	Infectious bovine rhinotracheitis	Cattle	Persists for years in genital tract of bulls
Retroviridae	Mammary tumour virus	Mouse	Transmitted via sperm in some strains of mice
	Bovine leukosis virus	Cattle	Semen is infectious
Reoviridae	Bluetongue	Cattle	Not known whether virus is in fluid or in sperm
Picornaviridae	Foot-and-mouth disease	Cattle	High virus titres in ejaculate of bull
Togaviridae	Border disease	Sheep	Sperm probably infected (also oocytes)
Filoviridae	Marburg	Human	Sexual transmission recorded
	Ebola	Human	Virus present in semen
Hepadnaviridae	Hepatitis B	Human	Virus present in semen

[a]For references see Mims, 1981.

Experimentally in mice, coxsackie B, EMC and other viruses have been shown to infect and damage the islets of Langerhans, sometimes causing a diabetes-like syndrome (Craighead and Steinke, 1971; Notkins, 1977). In man, mumps, congenital rubella (Menser *et al.*, 1978) and coxsackie B (Yoon *et al.*, 1979) virus infection can on occasions lead to diabetes, but it is not known how often these viruses are responsible.

Table 2.6. Viruses and skin lesions.

Virus	Features	Virus in lesion	Shedding to exterior
Measles	Characteristic maculo-papular rash	+	−
Rubella Echoviruses 4, 6, 9, 16 Coxsackieviruses A9, 16, 23	Maculopapular rashes not distinguishable clinically	+	−
Herpes simplex Varicella-zoster Variola Vaccinia Ectromelia[a]	Vesicular rash. Distribution often characteristic	+	+
Vesicular exanthem Foot-and-mouth disease Vesicular stomatitis Coxsackie A16 virus[b]	Vesicles, especially mouth and feet[c]	+	+
Pseudorabies[d]	Self-inflicted skin damage due to pruritis following peripheral nerve invasion	?	−
Chikungunya Ross River Dengue Hepatitis B[e]	Maculopapular rashes, possibly due to immune complexes	?	−
Papilloma[f]	Local benign epidermal tumour	+	+

[a]Other poxviruses cause skin lesions in rabbits (myxomatosis), camels, horses, cows, sheep, goats, elephants and birds.
[b]Hand, foot and mouth disease in man.
[c]Infect pigs (vesicular exanthem); horses, cattle and pigs (vesicular stomatitis); or any cloven-footed animal (foot-and-mouth disease). Mouth and often foot lesions are seen in many other virus infections of animals.
[d]In pigs.
[e]In prodromal stage.
[f]Infect man, cattle, horses. At least 25 distinct viruses cause human skin, laryngeal and genital warts.

Localisation of circulating viruses in salivary glands, mammary glands, kidney tubules and respiratory tract, and subsequent replication in glandular or epithelial cells is the basis for excretion in saliva, milk, urine and respiratory secretions. Cytomegaloviruses were originally called salivary gland viruses and infect salivary glands in mouse, man and other species, generally causing minimal pathological changes. Mumps virus, in contrast, generally causes severe inflammation (parotitis) when it infects parotid salivary glands in man. Viruses that invade kidneys often infect tubular epithelial cells, and are then shed in urine. Examples include polyomaviruses in man and mouse, and cytomegalovirus in man. Pathological changes are minimal, and serious kidney damage in viral infections is usually a result of immune complex deposition (see Chapter 4) rather than local virus replication. Invasion of the respiratory tract from the blood is a feature of many systemic viral infections including smallpox and measles. If the infection fails to reach the air spaces it can cause an interstitial pneumonitis as in K virus infection of mice, in which pulmonary blood vessels show a striking susceptibility to circulating virus (Greenlee, 1979). When the infection spreads to respiratory epithelium, however, bronchitis, pneumonia, etc. can follow, with shedding of virus in respiratory secretions. This is described for measles and other viral infections below.

Localisation in the skin is a feature of many viral infections with rashes, although the localisation of immune complexes rather than infectious virus can be responsible for the rash (Table 2.6). Mechanisms of virus localisation in skin blood vessels and the pathogenesis of rashes are discussed in the descriptions of mousepox and measles (see below). Localisation in feather follicles is necessary for the shedding of Marek's disease virus from infected chickens (Nazarian and Witter, 1970). The distribution of the rash in virus infections is often characteristic. In man, for instance, the smallpox rash is 'centrifugally' distributed, affecting especially the face, arms, hands, legs and feet, whereas in chickenpox it is 'centripetally' distributed, affecting the trunk rather than the extremities. The reason for these differences are unknown. Local dilation of blood vessels can localise a rash such as smallpox but the characteristic distribution in a given infection is unexplained. One possible factor is the presence of virus receptors on vascular endothelial cells in some but not all skin regions, but nothing is known of this. Generalised rashes are a less striking feature of viral infections of animals, and lesions often localise on exposed, hairless areas such as snouts, ears, teats, paws, scrotum and udders.

Myositis is a feature of human infection with many togaviruses, influenza virus and coxsackie B viruses. Viral invasion of striated muscle has been demonstrated in influenza virus infection in man (Ruff and Secrist, 1982), and has long been known to occur in suckling mice. Suckling mice show striking muscle damage in Ross River virus infection (Murphy *et al.*, 1973) and also in infections with coxsackie A virus, reovirus and foot-and-mouth-disease virus. Infection and damage of cardiac muscle is seen in coxsackie B and EMC virus infections of man and laboratory rodents (Woodruff, 1980).

Circulating viruses occasionally invade joints to give arthritis, as seen following natural infection or vaccination with rubella virus (Ogra and Herd, 1971). The epidemic polyarthritis caused by Ross River virus, an arthropod-borne alphavirus (Doherty *et al.*, 1963), is also perhaps due to viral invasion of joints, and the retrovirus responsible for caprine arthritis-encephalitis characteristically invades joints (Crawford *et al.*, 1980).

Spread by cerebrospinal fluid and nerves

Viruses in the blood can reach the central nervous system not only by direct spread across blood vessels but also by traversing the blood–CSF junction in the meninges or choroid plexus (see p. 60, and Fig. 2.8). They can then spread rapidly, passively carried by the flow of fluid, to other parts of the brain and spinal cord.

Rabies and many herpesviruses travel along peripheral nerves. They pass either centripetally from the body surface to the central nervous system (rabies) or sensory ganglia (pseudorabies in pigs, primary herpes simplex infection in man), or centrifugally from the centre to the periphery, as in the reactivation of herpes simplex or varicella-zoster virus in ganglia (Chapter 6). The neural route is not a rapid one. Transection and amputation studies show that both rabies and herpes simplex virus travel in peripheral nerves of mice at up to 10 mm per hour (Baer, 1975; Kristensson *et al.*, 1971). The exact pathway in the nerve varies (Fig. 2.9). Herpes simplex in man travels in either direction in the axon itself, but experimentally in mice it also travels by sequential infection of Schwann cells (Johnson, 1964a). Rabies virus (Murphy, 1977) appears to pass up the axon terminals at the neuromuscular junction (Watson *et al.*, 1981), and there are suggestions that the acetylcholine receptor is also the receptor for rabies virus (Lentz *et al.*, 1982).

Viruses occasionally reach the brain by passing up the olfactory nerve from the olfactory mucosa, and this route appears to be taken by rabies virus when it infects speleologists, the virus derived from the faeces of cave bats forming an infectious aerosol that is inhaled (Constantine, 1971).

Spread by pleural and peritoneal cavities

Rapid spread of virus from one visceral organ to another can take place via the peritoneal or pleural cavity. It is not known whether this is important in naturally occurring infections. Experimentally, viruses

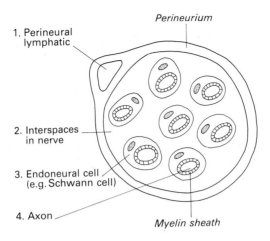

1. Perineural lymphatic

Perineurium

2. Interspaces in nerve

3. Endoneural cell (e.g. Schwann cell)

4. Axon

Myelin sheath

Fig. 2.9. Four possible pathways of viral spread in peripheral nerves.

injected intraperitoneally are delivered to the surface of all organs in the peritoneal cavity (which is lined by macrophages) and also via the draining lymphatics to the blood.

SHEDDING OF VIRUS AND TRANSMISSION

After infecting and multiplying in the host, viruses must then leave the body if fresh individuals are to be infected. Most are shed from body surfaces especially in respiratory secretions and faeces (see Fig. 2.1). Viruses that are transmitted 'biologically' by blood-sucking arthropods, the virus replicating in the arthropod rather than being carried 'mechanically' on mouth parts, have to be present in the blood if they are to infect these arthropods, and can be said to have been shed into the blood. Once shed from the body, transmission to the new host is determined by numerous factors, including the amount of virus shed, its stability, the presence of biting arthropods where these are necessary, and the availability and susceptibility of fresh hosts. It is also influenced by the genetic constitution of both virus and host. The amount of virus shed deserves attention (Table 2.7). The mere fact that virus is present in a secretion or excretion may be of little consequence if the amounts are too small to infect another individual. On the other hand, when infectious material contains 10^7 infectious doses per ml, as with hepatitis B in blood, an invisible quantity of material can initiate infection. Material of low titre may still infect if relatively large volumes are introduced, as with milk transmission of human CMV (Stagno *et al.*, 1980).

Transmission is of major importance in the maintenance of a virus

Table 2.7. Examples of the amount of virus shed from infected hosts.

Virus	Infectious material	Host	Titre/ml or g	Comments	Reference
Rabies	Salivary gland	Fox Dog	$10^{6.9}$ MLD$_{50}$ $10^{5.6}$ MLD$_{50}$	Foxes tend to be more infectious than dogs	Wachendorfer & Frost, 1978
CMV	Saliva	Mouse	10^7 pfu	Important route of transmission	Mims & Gould, 1978
CMV	Milk	Man	10^3 TCID$_{50}$	May be important as large volumes ingested	Stagno et al., 1980
CMV	Semen	Man	$10^{7.7}$ TCID$_{50}$	Venereal transmission	Lang & Kummer, 1972
CMV	Urine	Man	$10^{3.7}$ TCID$_{50}$		Lang & Kummer, 1972
Hepatitis B	Blood	Man	$10^{7.0}$	Volunteer studies	Barker & Murray, 1972
Herpes simplex	Vesicle fluid	Man	$10^{5.3}$ pfu	Infectious virus—antibody complexes	Daniels et al., 1975
Rotavirus	Faeces	Man	10^9–10^{11} particles	Similar viruses infect foals, dogs, pigs, mice, etc.	Flewett & Woode, 1978
Rhinovirus	Nasal secretions	Man	10^6 pfu	Calculation from volunteer studies	Pancic et al., 1980

in nature. The viral properties that give increased transmissibility are not the same as those causing pathogenicity. For instance, certain strains of influenza that are pathogenic for mice are transmitted rather ineffectively, transmission behaving as a separate genetic attribute (Schulman, 1967). Types of transmission are illustrated in Fig. 2.10.

Skin

Many, but not all, viruses that replicate in the skin are shed to the exterior from this site (see Table 2.6, rashes). Virus in skin lesions can infect the mouthparts of a biting arthropod (myxomavirus) or can contaminate the environment (smallpox). Smallpox virus shed from scabs and skin vesicles was a source of infection, but shedding from the respiratory tract was more important during epidemics. Vesicles are also sources of infection in certain herpesvirus infections such as varicella-zoster. Large amounts of virus are spread by direct touch, scratching, etc. from viral papillomas (warts).

Respiratory secretions

For viruses shed from the respiratory tract, transmission often depends on the formation of airborne particles (aerosols) that are infectious. Aerosols are formed especially during coughing or sneezing, to a lesser extent during vocalisations such as barking, talking or singing, and to a minimal extent during breathing. Aerosols are formed more readily when there are excess secretions from infected nasopharynx or lung, and these secretions often induce coughing or sneezing. When a man sneezes up to 20 000 droplets are produced. The droplets evaporate, depending on temperature and relative humidity. The fate of any inhaled particles depends on their size. Many viruses are soon inactivated by drying or exposure to light (e.g. measles, influenza) although some (e.g. smallpox) are more stable. Therefore aerosol transmission usually takes place over short distances, and is especially favoured when susceptible individuals are crowded together or are in enclosed spaces. Respiratory infections spread readily when people are in cities, when chickens are in batteries, or when horses gather at race meetings.

However, respiratory infections are not transmitted only by aerosols. Respiratory secretions often appear in saliva and, in man, secretions from the nose are deposited on hands and handkerchiefs which can then transfer infection to others. In one study with rhinovirus, nasal secretions contained 10^4 $TCID_{50}/ml$, but virus was also transmitted by hand to door knobs, spoons, plastic table tops, etc. (Reed, 1975), where it persisted for at least three hours without much loss of infectivity. Hand-to-hand or doorknob-to-hand transmission is readily demonstrable (Gwaltney and Hendley, 1978), the nose and conjunctiva are

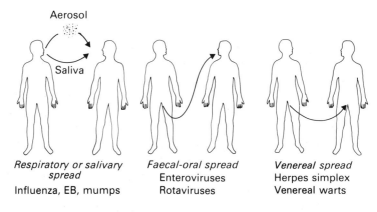

Respiratory or salivary
spread
Influenza, EB, mumps

Faecal-oral spread
Enteroviruses
Rotaviruses

Venereal spread
Herpes simplex
Venereal warts

ZOONOSES
Infection acquired from animals (arthropods, vertebrates).
Human infection controlled by controlling animal infection.

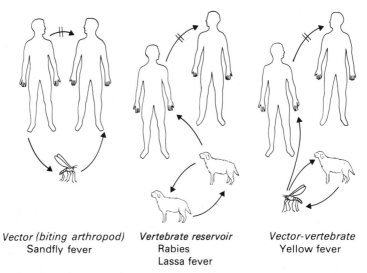

Vector (biting arthropod)
Sandfly fever

Vertebrate reservoir
Rabies
Lassa fever

Vector-vertebrate
Yellow fever

Fig. 2.10. Types of transmission of viral infection in man. Respiratory or salivary spread—not readily controllable. Faecal–oral spread—controllable by public health measures. Venereal spread—control socially difficult. Zoonoses—human infection controlled by controlling vectors, or by controlling animal infection.

regularly visited by the fingers, and it has been suggested that these routes may be as important as aerosols in rhinovirus transmission (Pancic *et al.*, 1980). The route of infection influences the efficiency of transmission. Thus, incredibly, successful infection of volunteers by coxsackievirus A21 was achieved by intranasal administration of less than one $TCID_{50}$, whereas more than 200 $TCID_{50}$ were required on the posterior pharyngeal wall (Buckland *et al.*, 1965).

Saliva

Certain viruses, such as mumps, herpes simplex, EB virus and cyto-megalovirus in man, or rabies in dogs and vampire bats are shed into the oral cavity, often from infected salivary glands (rabies, mumps, CMV). Viruses also reach saliva following infection of the lung or nasal mucosa (see p. 71). In man, the transmission of virus via saliva is influenced by social and sexual habits. Fingers are contaminated by saliva depending on hygiene habits and washing, and can indirectly spread salivary viruses. Direct transmission takes place from mouth to mouth or from mouth to other susceptible sites. EB virus is present in saliva and is transmitted effectively during the first few years of life in developing countries both by indirect and direct methods. At this age the infection causes little or no illness. In developed countries, on the other hand, children often escape infection, which then occurs in adolescence or early adult life during the salivary exchanges that accompany kissing. Infection at this age is more severe and causes glandular fever (see Chapter 6).

Saliva can be transferred directly to other parts of the body during sexual activity, and herpes simplex virus can infect the penis or vaginal introitus in this way. In animals also, salivary spread depends on social activities such as licking, nuzzling, grooming and biting. Rabies (Table 2.7) and foot-and-mouth-disease virus for instance, may be present in large amounts in saliva.

Faeces

Viruses that affect the intestinal tract are shed in faeces and, in most animals and many human communities, there is large-scale recycling of faecal material back into the mouth following faecal contamination of food or water. A more voluminous and more fluid output (diarrhoea) increases the environmental contamination. Viruses transmitted by faeces are generally resistant to acid and bile (see above), but often (e.g. poliovirus) not very resistant to drying. Viruses generally reach the faeces after replicating in intestinal epithelial cells (rotaviruses, corona-viruses, adenoviruses, many enteroviruses) or in throat and sub-epithelial lymphoid tissue (poliovirus). Hepatitis A possibly replicates in intestinal epithelial cells, but in any case replicates in liver cells and presumably enters the intestine after being shed in the bile (Fig. 2.7).

Urine

Urine, like faeces, tends to contaminate food, drink and living space. A number of different viruses are shed in urine after multiplying in tubular epithelial cells in the kidney. These include polyomaviruses in mice and man, cytomegalovirus in man and arenaviruses (e.g. LCM and Lassa virus) in their rodent hosts.

Genital secretions

Viruses shed from the genital tract depend on mucosal contact between susceptible individuals for successful transmission. Herpes simplex type 2 present on the cervix and vagina infects the infant during delivery or the penis during sexual intercourse. An extraordinary variety of interactions between oral, anal and genital mucosae facilitates the transfer of herpes simplex and genital wart viruses in man. Many viruses can be transmitted via semen (Table 2.5). In man, this seems to be a significant route of spread for cytomegalovirus (Lang and Kummer, 1972) and probably hepatitis B.

Milk

Like semen, milk is shed directly into another individual, usually of the same species (Table 2.7). Milk appears to be a route of spread for cytomegalovirus (Stagno *et al.*, 1980), and in some strains of mice mammary tumour virus can be transmitted via the milk. Other viruses shed in milk include mumps, rubella, some of the tick-borne flaviviruses, and caprine arthritis-encephalitis virus, a lentivirus that infects macrophages present in colostrum (Narayan *et al.*, 1983a).

Blood

Shedding into the blood is important for arthropod-borne viral infections, and can also be regarded as a route of transfer to another individual, the foetus, which is parasitic on the host. The foetus is infected when a virus shed into the blood localises in the placenta and enters blood vessels (see Table 2.4).

No shedding

Not all of the virus progeny produced during an infection has an opportunity to be shed to the outside world. Many sites of viral replication are 'non-productive' from this point of view. Some are necessary during the stepwise invasion of the host, for instance, the liver in natural infection of mice with ectromelia virus (Fig. 2.11), or lymphoid tissues in many viral infections (see Chapter 6). Others are true 'dead end' sites, accidental from the virus' point of view because apparently not necessary for successful spread to new hosts. It is often these 'dead end' sites of viral replication that are the cause of major disease in the host, as with polioviruses and arthropod-borne viruses in the brain, coxsackie B vi-

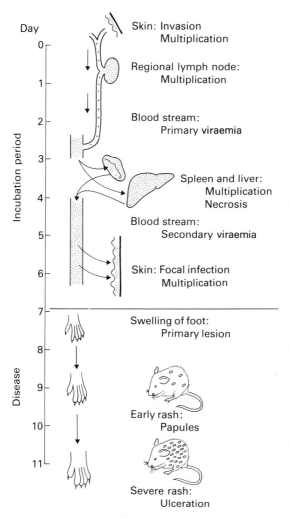

Fig. 2.11. The pathogenesis of infection in mousepox. After Fenner (1948).

ruses in the human heart, or mumps virus in the testicle. Many of the retroviruses and some of the arenaviruses spread from parent to offspring directly by infection of the egg or developing embryo. LCM virus and certain leukaemia viruses behave in this way in mice, infecting the ovum so that all cells in the embryos are infected. This is an important type of vertical transmission, and is often but not always accompanied by shedding of the virus to the outside world, and transmission to other individuals by the horizontal route. The term 'vertical transmission' includes transmission to offspring after birth or hatching (Mims, 1981).

The infectious agent of kuru is not shed to the exterior, and was transmitted only after death of the infected individual, being introduced into the body of a relative during cannibalistic consumption of the carcass (see Chapter 6).

EXAMPLES

To illustrate the principles just described, a more detailed account of the pathogenesis of four viral infections will now be given. Chapter 3 can also be consulted when immunological aspects of these infections are referred to.

Mousepox

This disease is caused by the poxvirus, ectromelia. The basic pathogenesis was elucidated by organ titrations in Fenner's classical work almost four decades ago (Fenner, 1949; see Fig. 2.11). Subsequent studies using immunofluorescence to identify infected cells have confirmed and extended his findings. Following the intradermal injection of a small dose of virus into the feet, there is a regular sequence in the spread, multiplication and shedding of the virus. At the site of infection, the virus multiplies in dermal and epidermal cells, the focus slowly increasing in size by direct spread from cell to cell (Roberts, 1962b). The foot becomes detectably swollen after seven days, partly as a result of local antigen–antibody interactions, marking the end of the incubation period. Meanwhile, the inoculated virus and virus produced by local growth in the skin has entered local lymphatics to reach the local lymph node. It multiplies in lymphatic endothelial cells as well as in macrophages and lymphoid cells in the node. Virus leaving the afferent lymphatics spreads through regional nodes to enter the thoracic duct and thence the large veins to give a primary viraemia.

On first entering the blood, virus is rapidly removed by macrophages lining the liver and spleen sinusoids. These cells are infected, and foci of infection are thus established in liver and spleen about four days after the initial infection. Following further growth the virus is re-seeded into the blood to give the more substantial secondary viraemia. At this stage of the disease, and for reasons that are not clear, the virus localises in the skin and other sites. In the skin, after localising in small blood vessels, the virus infects endothelial and perivascular cells as shown for cowpox virus (Mims, 1968a), then spreads to dermal fibroblasts and histiocytes. Finally, it reaches the epidermis whose layers are sequentially infected. This results in focal necrosis in epidermal cells, and virus-rich blisters or vesicles are formed, from which the virus is shed to the outside world. The skin vesicles soon rupture to form ulcers, which then scab over. The rash is first seen nine days after initial infection when immune responses round the sites of infection lead to the formation of papules. These turn into vesicles, and the rash becomes more severe, with ulceration by eleven days. At the sites of infection in the liver there is focal necrosis, and in very severe infections the liver damage is extensive, mice dying after 8–12 days.

The severity of the infection is determined not only by the dose of virus administered but also by the virus strain and the mouse strain (see Chapter 5). Host defences include macrophages, interferon, antibodies and cell-mediated immunity. They will be dealt with more thoroughly in Chapter 3 but some aspects will be mentioned here.

Macrophages lining the liver sinusoids (Kupffer cells) take up virus from the blood and thus control access of circulating virus to hepatic cells. By restricting or preventing the growth of virus they can protect against liver infection. Roberts (1964b) identified cells by immuno-fluorescence and calculated that when the virulent (Hampstead mouse) strain of ectromelia virus was injected intravenously, more than 50 times as many Kupffer cells were infected than when the same dose of avirulent (Hampstead egg) virus was injected. The average yield of virus per Kupffer cell was also different, being about 15 ID_{50} for the virulent and about 5 ID_{50} for the avirulent strain. Foci of infection were therefore more numerous and liver necrosis more extensive with the virulent strain, although there was no difference in the growth of the two strains of virus once they had reached hepatic cells.

Interferon acts by preventing growth of virus in uninfected cells, and by stimulating NK cells. Antibody to various virus components is detectable in serum after a week, and cell-mediated immune responses appear, mediated by cytotoxic T cells and by delayed hypersensitivity T cells in association with macrophages. Blanden's classic experimental analysis (Blanden, 1970; 1971a; 1971b) showed that cell-mediated responses rather than antibodies are important in resistance and recovery from infection.

The same basic sequence of events has been shown to occur in rabbit-pox in rabbits (Bedson and Duckworth, 1963), myxomatosis in rabbits (Fenner and Woodroofe, 1953) and smallpox in monkeys (Hahon, 1961). A very similar sequence of events occurs in human beings infected with smallpox. Here, after an incubation period of 10–12 days, the illness is ushered in with fever, headache, anorexia, nausea and sometimes a 'prodromal' erythematous rash caused probably by circulating immune complexes. The definitive oropharyngeal and skin lesions appear a few days later. During the incubation period the patient is symptom-free and is not infectious. Smallpox has been one of the major infectious diseases in human history, some strains of virus causing high mortality. Yet almost nothing is known of the causes of illness and death. More extensive virus growth leads to more severe disease but the virus produces no toxins, and organs other than the skin are not very heavily infected. Secondary bacterial infection is sometimes a factor and immunopathological events (see Chapter 4) are thought to be important.

Measles

Measles virus infects susceptible children via the respiratory tract, and is reviewed by Fraser and Martin (1978). Transmission is very effective—probably only a small number of infectious units are needed, and large amounts of virus are shed from infected individuals. At the site of initial infection, multiplication is minimal and indeed has never been detected. The virus enters local lymphatics, either free or associated with mononuclear cells, and reaches local lymph nodes. Here virus multiplication takes place very slowly and there is early spread of infected cells to other lymphoreticular tissues such as the spleen. Infected mononuclear cells give rise to Warthin's multinucleated giant cells, while T lymphocytes, including both suppressor and helper classes, are susceptible to infection when they are mitotically active (Huddlestone *et al.*, 1980).

We are far from having a coherent picture of these early events in lymphoid tissue, but by 5–6 days after initial infection, the virus enters the blood and is now seeded out to all the epithelial surfaces of the body including the oropharynx, conjunctiva, respiratory tract, skin, bladder and alimentary canal (Fig. 2.12). Foci of infection are established in these sites, the virus from local blood vessels spreading towards the epithelial surfaces. At 9–10 days the foci in the respiratory tract and conjunctiva, where there are only one or two layers of epithelial cells, undergo necrosis. There is now an abrupt onset of what appears to be a respiratory illness, and the patient, with running nose and red conjunctivae, sheds large amounts of virus into the environment. Immune responses probably contribute to the respiratory damage, and to the malaise and fever that are seen at this stage and become worse until the appearance of the skin rash. The mucosal sites of virus growth are next to break down, and small ulcers (Koplik's spots) are visible inside the cheek by about day 11, and provide a definite diagnosis. Finally, the characteristic maculopapular rash appears, on average 14 days after initial infection, at which time circulating antibodies become detectable. The fever now falls. This skin rash is largely a result of cell-mediated immune responses to viral antigens, and is not seen in patients with severe T cell deficits. Foci of infection do not spread very far from blood vessels. Vesicles appear microscopically in the epidermis, but the virus does not succeed in growing through the skin and is not shed to the exterior.

The necrotic epithelial areas in nasopharynx and lung give opportunities for secondary bacterial invasion, and bronchopneumonia, otitis media, etc. are frequently striking features of measles. Under certain circumstances adenovirus and herpesvirus pneumonia may come in the

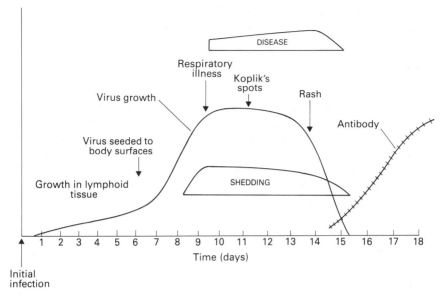

Fig. 2.12. The pathogenesis of measles.

wake of measles (Kaschula *et al.*, 1983). Measles also provides a classic example of the effect of malnutrition on susceptibility to infectious disease (see Chapter 5). Host resistance factors are discussed in Chapter 3.

Rubella

This virus infects the respiratory tract and, like measles, gives no detectable local lesion at the site of initial infection and is not acutely cytopathogenic. It spreads to local lymph nodes and during most of the long and mysterious incubation period there is low-grade multiplication, largely restricted to lymphoreticular tissues including spleen and cervical and occipital lymph nodes. Following this the virus is seeded out to the respiratory tract and skin, where foci of infection are established. About 18 days after initial infection, there are mild respiratory symptoms and malaise. Affected lymph nodes are swollen, and a variable macular rash develops. Virus is shed from the respiratory tract and the patient is infectious but, as in measles, the foci in the skin do not reach the surface. In this infection too, immunological factors contribute to the lesions. In contrast to measles, however, secondary bacterial infection of the foci in the respiratory tract is negligible. Indeed the entire illness is very mild and the infection is often subclinical.

Adults often develop transient arthritis during natural infection with rubella virus or after receiving live virus vaccine (Preblud *et al.*, 1980). At least some of this is due to circulating virus invading joints, and rarely this leads to a more chronic arthritis (Chantler *et al.*, 1981). In pregnant women, however, the virus circulating in the blood can localise in the placenta, leading to infection of the foetus. Until the advent of the vaccine (see Chapter 7), rubella was an important cause of congenital heart disease, deafness, blindness, mental retardation and other malformations. The foetus is especially susceptible during the first three months of pregnancy, but because this virus is not highly cytocidal, the foetus often survives. In contrast to this, the foetus infected with variola or vaccinia virus nearly always dies. Organs are particularly vulnerable to rubella virus when they are first being formed in the embryo. In the 2–3-month-old foetus the heart, brain, eyes and ears are being formed and infection at this critical time leads to defective development in these organs. The foetus may die (abortion) or the infant may be stillborn, but often the defects are not incompatible with life. The affected baby is generally small and the brain also small, with mental retardation. Deafness results from abnormal formation of the organ of Corti. The eyes may be small and cataracts are often present. In the heart the ventricular septum may be imperfectly formed, and the ductus arteriosus may be patent. Other abnormalities are not strictly malformations, including enlarged liver and spleen, purpura, bone changes, immunological changes and late-onset diabetes.

Not all infected foetuses develop abnormally. Data from five prospective studies were used to calculate the mean incidence of congenital defects (Hanshaw and Dudgeon, 1978). This depended on the month of gestation at which maternal rubella occurred and was 15.3% (rubella in first month), 24.6% (second), 17.5% (third), 6.4% (fourth), and 1.7% (fifth month or later). After the fourth month, therefore, infection rarely damages the foetus. The figure for the first month is low, presumably because at this stage of gestation foetal death is a more common sequel to infection.

It is not clear how rubella causes the malformations, but a primary effect on blood vessels seems probable. In human foetal cell cultures infected with rubella virus there is little destruction of cells, but an inhibition of mitotic activity (Rawls and Melnick, 1966). This could account for the small size of affected babies and for the demonstrable decrease in cell numbers (Naeye and Blanc, 1965). The death of a small number of cells or a slowing of their mitotic rate during the critical period of embryonic differentiation might interfere with the formation of key organs.

Infected foetuses produce their own IgM antibodies to the virus, but cell-mediated immune responses are defective and, together with NK responses (Fucillo *et al.*, 1974) remain so postnatally. Further spread in the body is restricted, but there are foci of infection consisting of 'clones' of infected cells (Woods *et al.*, 1966). The infant sheds virus in the urine and stool for several months after birth, in the throat for longer periods, and virus can remain present in affected sites (such as the lens) for years.

Influenza

In man, influenza infection is initiated in the upper or lower respiratory tract when inhaled virus particles attach to epithelial cells. The haemagglutinin molecules projecting from the virus envelope specifically bind to a receptor on the surface of the susceptible cell. The receptor, N-acetylneuraminic acid, is the terminal sugar on the oligosaccharide side-chain of a plasma membrane glycoprotein. After the initial attachment there is fusion of the viral envelope with cell membrane, probably within a phagosome, since it occurs only when the pH falls to 5.0 (Skehel *et al.*, 1982). The nucleocapsid now enters the cytoplasm and virus replication takes place. From these infected cells virus is liberated onto the mucosal surface and spreads rapidly to infect other cells. Carriage of virus in the mucociliary stream tends to spread infection from the lung upwards and from the nasal cavity backwards towards the throat. When secretions increase and become more fluid so that the ciliary beat is less effective, and when cilia are destroyed, the infection can spread in either direction according to gravity. Strong winds blowing across the infected mucosa (coughing or sneezing) will also carry the infection to other areas. Furthermore, in the normal person during sleep there is constant seeding of nasopharyngeal secretions into the lungs, as shown by the behaviour of radiolabelled marker material (Huxley *et al.*, 1978).

Within a few days there are extensive areas of virus growth on the respiratory surfaces. Virus and viral products reaching local lymph nodes (cervical and pulmonary) induce inflammation and this, together with early immune responses, causes swelling. Tonsillar and other lymphoid tissues in the throat become tender as well as swollen. The patient has a sore throat. The infected cells degenerate, become detached, and are carried away in secretions. The infected individual feels unwell (malaise), develops fever, and the excess respiratory secretions cause a running nose, sneezing and often a cough. Damage to ciliated and non-ciliated epithelial cells leaves denuded areas and leads to interruption of mucociliary cleansing mechanisms. The exposed underlying tissues are susceptible to bacterial invasion, especially by the staphylococci, streptococci, etc. that normally live as commensals in the nose. The polymorphs that normally control such bacteria show impaired anti-bacterial functions (Abramson *et al.*, 1982a). Bacterial growth and absorption of bacterial toxins add to the malaise and the fever, and the secretions become more purulent as degenerating polymorphs and other necrotic materials appear in them. Enzymes released from phagocytes make these secretions irritating to the skin around the nose.

The excess secretions are in part an inflammatory response to direct destruction of cells by the virus (see Fig. 4.2). Excess nasal secretions (rhinorrhoea) are also seen in rhinovirus infections, but the constitutional disturbances are generally less marked than with influenza. IgE-mediated immune responses could contribute to the inflammation. Subepithelial mast cells bearing specific antiviral IgE antibodies would release inflammatory mediators when exposed to viral antigens.

Influenza inevitably infects nasal or pulmonary epithelial cells, but little is known about alveolar infection. It is in alveoli that gaseous exchange takes place between air and the blood in alveolar capillaries. If, as a result of infection, this interface is thickened by swollen cells or by an exudation of cells and fluid, the consequences can be serious. As a safeguard the normal lung has an immense capacity to absorb excess fluid. Alveolar infection is seen in the primary influenzal pneumonia that sometimes occurs in the absence of secondary bacterial invasion. Alveoli contain epithelial cells which are known to be infected (Hers and Mulder, 1961), and also surfactant-producing cells and macrophages. Surfactant-producing cells can be infected and this possibly leads to decreased amounts of surfactant which predisposes to local collapse of the lung (Loosli et al., 1975). Both human and mouse alveolar macrophages are very susceptible to influenza virus infection in vitro (Rodgers and Mims, 1981; 1982), although little or no infectious virus is produced. There are conflicting reports about the ability of the infected cells to ingest and kill invading bacteria. In some respiratory virus infections, such as parainfluenza 1 (Sendai) in mice (Heath, 1979), infected alveolar macrophages show impaired antibacterial functions and this seems clearly linked to secondary bacterial infection (Degre, 1970).

Influenza infection is generally restricted to surface epithelial cells. Although the virus spreads locally to lymph nodes, invasion of distant organs does not take place. There are, however, reports of influenza viraemia in man, which is said to be quite common when carefully sought. Also, influenza virus can at times invade the heart and striated muscle. Neuroadapted influenza viruses readily infect these tissues in suckling mice (Wagner, 1955). In man, striated muscle is sometimes involved, especially with influenza B (Ruff and Secrist, 1982).

The pathogenesis of the malaise and fever is not known. Constitutional signs and symptoms might be expected when large amounts of a virus are present in the blood but low level viraemia often occurs during the incubation period in other infections and is generally asymptomatic (see p. 51). It seems unlikely that the products of cell destruction absorbed from the respiratory tract would account for the symptoms. It has been shown that highly purified human α or β interferon, when injected into normal individuals, causes malaise, aches and pains, and fever (Scott et al., 1981). Interferon is produced by infected epithelial cells right from the start and is detectable in respiratory secretions. It presumably enters the blood, and may possibly account for some of the malaise and fever seen in influenza and in other virus infections.

In spite of a great deal of experimental work on influenza virus infections, mostly in laboratory mice, we still have a poor understanding of the factors responsible for pathogenicity in the infected host (Sweet and Smith, 1980; Rott, 1979). This ignorance stands in striking contrast to the sophisticated state of knowledge of the virion and its antigens. Also it is still not clear exactly which factors are responsible for host resistance and recovery from influenza infection. This will be discussed for other viral infections in Chapter 3 but is mentioned here for influenza. Two major problems must be borne in mind when interpreting experiments with influenza virus in mice:

1   When protection is conferred by administering antibody, immune cells, interferon, etc. or when vaccines protect by inducing increased levels of antibody, immune cells, etc., it does not mean that this is the normal mechanism of recovery from acute infections. This proviso also applies to many other virus infections studied experimentally.

2   Influenza in mice differs markedly from influenza in man. In man, influenza generally begins as an upper respiratory infection, whereas mice in most studies are anaesthetised and a volume of inoculum equivalent to half a pint in man is given intranasally. The inoculated material floods directly into the lungs and initiates pneumonic infection.

Antibodies present on the infected respiratory surfaces include secretory IgA and also IgG, especially when inflammatory responses are initiated. Three days after the infection of mice there is a great increase in the number of IgA- and IgM-producing plasma cells in subepithelial tissues and an increase in IgG plasma cells a few days later (Owens *et al.*, 1981). But during primary infection antibodies are not detectable in secretions until eight days, by which time virus replication has already been brought under control. Antibody is formed several days earlier, but is probably complexed to viral antigen in tissues before being detected free in secretions or serum. Interferon is a possible early defence mechanism, being produced by the first infected cells, but it is not easy to assess its importance. Mice treated with anti-interferon serum do not show increased susceptibility to influenza infection (Gresser *et al.*, 1976).

Recent work on mouse influenza has concentrated on specifically reactive T cells. Cytotoxic T (T_c) cells (see Chapter 3), capable of lysing influenza-infected target cells, are generated in the spleen when mice are infected intranasally. They are also present on the infected epithelial surfaces and can be recovered in lung washes (Wyde and Cate, 1978). T_d cells mediating delayed hypersensitivity skin reactions also appear in the spleen. These are capable of mobilising activated macrophages following the liberation of lymphokines. Are T_c cells, T_d cells, or both types of cell important in recovery? Recent work implicates T_c in recovery from infection in man (McMichael *et al.*, 1983), but the picture is confusing (see Chapter 3) and clarification perhaps awaits advances in immunology that will tell us more about T cell classes.

The confusion is of more than academic importance, since it adds to the difficulty of developing effective influenza vaccines (Ada, 1981, and see Chapter 7). Will vaccine-induced protection against infection require the same factors that mediate *recovery* from infection? Which types of immune response (secretory IgA antibodies, cytotoxic T cells, etc.) need to be generated? Other possible factors include NK cells, an early defence mechanism induced by interferon, and macrophages, which have so far not been shown to be determinants of resistance to respiratory infection. In artificial (non-respiratory) experimental infections of mice with an adapted strain of influenza virus, a certain gene confers resistance of interferon-treated macrophages to infection with influenza viruses; resistance on the interferon-treated cells to other viruses is unaffected (Haller, 1981).

The above account refers to influenza in man and in mice. A different picture is seen with influenza infections in birds. Although some strains of virus (e.g. fowl plague) are highly virulent, most cause asymptomatic infections. Infection in ducks primarily involves the intestinal tract (Webster *et al.*, 1978). After replicating in intestinal epithelial cells, the virus is shed in very large amounts in faeces. It is more resistant to thermal inactivation and to acid, being relatively stable at pH 4.0, than are respiratory virus strains from mammals.

SUMMARY

Initiation of infection requires that a virus is carried mechanically through breaks in the body surface (trauma, insect or mammalian bites), or attaches to cells on the body surface. Infection of the oropharynx and conjunctiva, and of respiratory, intestinal and urogenital tracts is discussed in terms of the natural mechanisms protecting these body surfaces, and the attachment of viruses to receptors on susceptible cells. Infections largely confined to body surfaces (such as rhinoviruses, rotaviruses, warts) are contrasted with infections in which invasion of deeper tissues and systemic spread takes place (measles, mumps).

Viraemia follows spread to local lymphatics and lymph nodes. Virus in blood may be cell-associated or free in plasma, and subsequent localisation in tissues depends on interaction of virus with reticuloendothelial macrophages and with vascular endothelium. Virus–macrophage interactions have been extensively studied *in vitro* and in the liver, but less is known about viral infection of vascular endothelium.

The central nervous system is invaded either from the blood across blood vessel walls (poliovirus) or from peripheral nerves (rabies). Subsequent spread takes place via cerebrospinal fluid, by sequential involvement of neural cells, axons, dendrites, or via extracellular spaces.

Infection of the foetus occurs after localisation of circulating virus in the placenta. Foetal tissues are generally very susceptible, and death (abortion, stillbirth) often ensues. Important diseases (congenital rubella, CMV, bluetongue) result from damage which is less severe damage yet interfere with foetal development. Vertical transmission of virus from parent directly to offspring can take place via germline cells as well as via the placenta.

Bloodborne viral invasion of skin causes rashes (rubella, measles) and also enables virus to be shed to the exterior (smallpox, chickenpox). In the same way bloodborne invasion of other organs and tissues causes disease (pancreatitis or diabetes, orchitis, etc.) and can facilitate shedding of virus to the exterior, as when there is invasion of epithelial surfaces in salivary or mammary glands, in conjunctiva, and in respiratory or urogenital tracts.

Transmission to a new host depends on effective shedding of virus into the blood (for arthropod vectors) or from body surfaces. The amount of virus shed, its infectiousness, its stability, and the density and sociosexual habits of the host are important in transmission.

The above principles are illustrated by describing the diseases mousepox, measles, rubella and influenza.

SELECTED READING

Dimmock, N. J. (1982). Initial stages of infection with animal viruses. *J. Gen. Virol.* **59**, 1.

Fraser, K. B. and Martin, S. J. (1978). *Measles Virus and its Biology*. Academic Press, New York.

Heath, R. B. (1979). The pathogenesis of respiratory viral infection. *Postgrad. Med. J.* **55**, 122.

Holmes, I. H. (1979). Viral gastroenteritis. *Progr. Med. Virol.* **25**, 1.

Johnson, R. T. (1982). *Viral Infections of the Nervous System*. Raven Press, New York.

McNabb, P. C. and Tomasi, T. B. (1981). Host defence mechanisms at mucosal surfaces. *Ann. Rev. Microbiol.* **35**, 477.

Mims, C. A. (1964). Aspects of the pathogenesis of virus diseases. *Bact. Rev.* **28**, 30.

Mims, C. A. (1966). The pathogenesis of rashes in virus diseases. *Bact. Rev.* **30**, 739.

Mims, C. A. (1968). Pathogenesis of viral infections of the fetus. *Progr. Med. Virol.* **10**, 194.

Mims, C. A. (1981). Vertical transmission of viruses. *Microbiol. Rev.* **45**, 267.

Mims, C. A. (1982). *The Pathogenesis of Infectious Disease*. Academic Press, New York.

Plotkin, S. A. (1975). Routes of fetal infection and mechanisms of fetal damage. *Am. J. Dis. Child.* **129**, 444.

Sever, J. and White, L. R. (1968). Intrauterine viral infections. *Ann. Rev. Med.* **19**, 471.

Sweet, C. and Smith, H. (1980). Pathogenicity of influenza virus. *Microbiol. Rev.* **44**, 303.

Chapter Three
The Immune Response to Viral Infection

Vertebrates, over the course of hundreds of millions of years, have been continuously exposed to invasion by viruses, bacteria and other parasites. Indeed, it can be argued that the immune system has evolved primarily to deal with these potentially lethal invaders. It comprises a highly efficient early warning system that specifically recognises foreign materials in the body and promptly triggers a range of responses designed to inactivate and restrain the growth of microorganisms, kill parasitised host cells and remove debris. If these responses were completely effective, microbial infections would be few in number and terminated rapidly before much damage had been done. But the defences are not infallible. The rapid rate of evolution of viruses and other parasites ensures that they are always a few steps ahead, exploiting weaknesses in the host's defences. Some viruses are regularly lethal for particular host species; others regularly establish persistent infections, often for life. Moreover, whereas on most occasions the immune response is beneficial to the infected host, aiding recovery and providing resistance to reinfection, it sometimes proves actually harmful, causing inflammation or cell and tissue damage which contributes to the pathological picture. Immunopathology is described more fully in the next chapter. At other times the immune response fails to eliminate the virus. This is what happens in persistent infections, which are the subject of Chapter 6.

This chapter deals with the role of the immune response in recovery from viral infection and resistance to reinfection. We commence with a brief survey of the salient features of modern immunology as relevant to virology. Fuller accounts of the vast and rapidly expanding subject of basic immunology are contained in numerous excellent general texts such as Benacerraf and Unanue (1979), Golub (1981), Lachman and Peters (1982), McConnell *et al*. (1981), Roitt (1980). There are also some useful collections of reviews on particular aspects of viral immunology (Notkins, 1975; Nahmias and O'Reilly, 1982; Fougereau and Dausset, 1980; Möller, 1974; 1981b).

BASIC FEATURES OF THE IMMUNE RESPONSE

The most basic feature of the immune response to a foreign antigen is its specificity for that particular antigen. This exquisite antigen specificity applies both to the antibodies and to the T lymphocytes generated in response to the immunogen. Though the receptors on T and B lymphocytes are not identical, they both display specificity for a particular 'epitope' ('antigenic determinant'). Only the particular clones of T and B cells bearing receptors complementary to a given antigenic determinant will bind and respond to that determinant.

Classically, the immune response was considered to have two arms: (1) the antibody response, referred to as 'humoral immunity', and (2) what we would now recognise as a T lymphocyte-mediated response, known as 'cell-mediated immunity' (CMI). Today, many people use the expression CMI to refer only to T_d and T_c cell-mediated responses and to exclude phenomena mediated by such cells as NK cells, K cells, macrophages, T_h cells or B cells. However, it can be argued that the term 'cell-mediated immunity' is at best confusing and at worst obsolete, following the realisation that cells, including but not exclusively T lymphocytes, are vitally involved in the generation of both the 'humoral' and the 'cell-mediated' response. Indeed, a cardinal feature of the immune response is its dependence on cooperation, usually via soluble mediators, between numerous subsets of cells in an intricate and delicately controlled network. The cells involved in antiviral immune responses are shown diagrammatically in Fig. 3.1.

The first immunologically relevant cell encountered by an invading virus is likely to be a macrophage, strategically situated below an epithelial surface, in a lymph node or in the spleen. Macrophages have numerous functions which will be discussed later, but they play a central role in setting the immune response in motion. The virion is phagocytosed and its coat proteins degraded to smaller peptides which are then, in some unknown way, returned to (or retained on) the plasma membrane and displayed in close association with the Ia (I region-associated, i.e. coded by the Ir (immune response) genes within the MHC complex) antigen molecules on the surface of the macrophage.

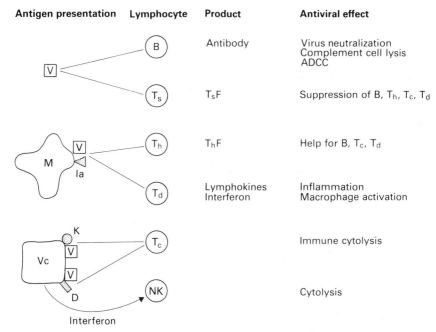

Antigen presentation	Lymphocyte	Product	Antiviral effect
	B	Antibody	Virus neutralization Complement cell lysis ADCC
V	T_s	T_sF	Suppression of B, T_h, T_c, T_d
M V Ia	T_h	T_hF	Help for B, T_c, T_d
	T_d	Lymphokines Interferon	Inflammation Macrophage activation
Vc K V V D	T_c		Immune cytolysis
Interferon	NK		Cytolysis

Fig. 3.1. Cells involved in antiviral immune responses. V = Virus or viral antigen; M = antigen-presenting macrophage; Vc = virus-infected cell.

Only certain Ia^+ subpopulations of macrophages, and probably Langerhans cells and dendritic cells, are able to 'process' and 'present' antigen to T cells.

Lymphocytes are the prime movers in the immune response. There is a constant large-scale recirculation of lymphocytes through the body (Fig. 3.2). About 90% of the recirculation is from blood to lymph nodes via the postcapillary venules and then via lymphatics back to the blood. The rest takes place by cells leaving capillaries in various parts of the body, moving through the tissues, entering lymphatics, passing through local lymph nodes and thus back to the blood. The lymphocytes engaged in this recirculation are mostly T cells. The continuous movement of T cells through tissues and lymph nodes ensures that viruses or viral antigens entering the body sooner or later come into contact with specifically reactive cells.

T lymphocytes ('T cells'), so named because of their dependence on the thymus for their maturation from the pluripotent haemopoietic stem cell, are distinguishable from B lymphocytes (derived from the bursa in birds or its equivalent, the bone marrow, in mammals) not only by their somewhat different antigen-receptors, but also by other surface markers, as well as by completely different functions. Both T and B cells respond to the binding of antigen by differentiating into physiologically

The Immune Response to Viral Infection   89

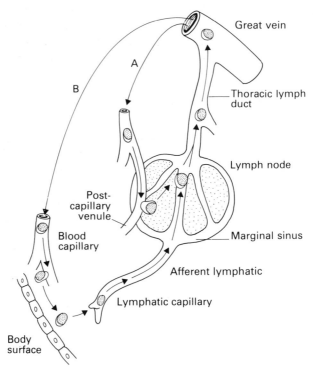

Fig. 3.2. Lymphocyte recirculation. Recirculating lymphocytes in man are mostly T lymphocytes; approximately 90% of recirculation is by route A and 10% by route B.

active lymphoblasts ('blasts') and by dividing to form an enlarged clone of cells ('clonal expansion'), some of which are long-lived and are involved with immunological 'memory'. But there the similarity ends. B blasts (plasma cells) secrete specific antibody, whereas T blasts secrete antigen-specific and non-specific soluble factors known as 'lymphokines' or 'interleukins'. Furthermore, unlike B cells, most T cells cannot bind soluble antigen; they recognise a foreign antigen only when it is presented in association with 'self' MHC (major histocompatibility) antigen on the surface of another cell. Historically, this became known as 'H-2 (or HLA) restriction', in reference to the fact that T lymphocytes cannot recognise foreign (e.g. viral) antigen in association with allogeneic or xenogeneic MHC antigens but are 'restricted' to syngeneic, i.e. histocompatible cells. Of course, such incompatibility never occurs in nature, but the importance of 'restriction' lies in the interpretation that T cells have evidently evolved to recognise, not foreign antigen *per se*, but 'altered self' antigens on the surface of aberrant cells.

Functionally, T lymphocytes are classified as 'helper', 'suppressor', 'cytotoxic' or 'delayed-type hypersensitivity' T cells on the basis of these four distinct physiological activities. Recent evidence suggests that a single cell type can discharge more than one of these functions but that it may recognise viral antigen in association with only a particular class of self MHC antigen (Fig. 3.3). Helper T (T_h or T_H) cells, otherwise known as 'T inducer' cells, recognise foreign (e.g. viral) antigen only in conjunction with self Ia antigen, usually on the surface of a macrophage; various subsets of T_h cells secrete antigen-specific and non-specific 'helper factors' (ThF) that bind to and activate B cells, T_d cells and T_c cells respectively. Cytotoxic T (T_c) cells on the other hand, recognise foreign antigen only in association with self H-2 D, K or L in the mouse (HLA-A, B or C in man); their function is to lyse virus-infected or cancer cells displaying foreign antigen on their surface. 'Delayed-type hypersensitivity' T (Tdth or T_d or T_D) cells, recognise antigen in association with either self Ia antigen (in the mouse; D/DR in man) on the surface of a macrophage or dendritic cell, or in association with self H-2 K, D or L. T_d cells secrete a wide variety of lymphokines which attract and activate macrophages

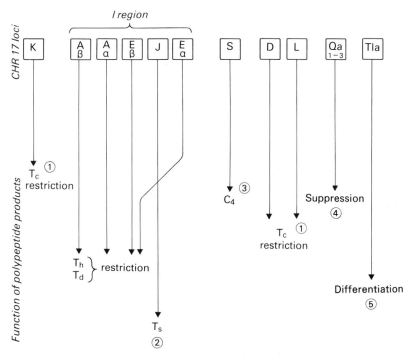

Fig. 3.3. MHC (H2) loci in mouse. DNA cloning methods show that there are more loci than illustrated here. There are three classes of loci, or genes: *class I*—K, D, L, Qa, Tla; *class II*—I region; *class III*—S. KDL antigens displayed on most cells in body. I region (Ia) antigens displayed on antigen-presenting cells. 1 Also may be T_d cell restriction. 2 Suppressor T cells bear I-J. 3 Controls complement activity. 4 T cells with this antigen generate suppressor effects. 5 T cell differentiation antigen.

and other T cells, so greatly augmenting the magnitude of the immune response. Suppressor T (T_s) cells can probably bind viral antigen directly; they secrete antigen-specific and non-specific or idiotype-specific (anti-idiotype) suppressor factors which regulate the immune response by suppressing the activity of B, T_d, T_h or T_c cells in a complex network of interactions yet to be fully elucidated.

Several additional cell types are implicated in the immune response to viral infection. They include NK (natural killer) cells, K (killer) cells and polymorphs. Furthermore, there are important, though immunologically non-specific, molecules other than the lymphokines mentioned so far. The complement system consists of a series of serum components which can be activated, particularly in the presence of antigen–antibody complexes, to 'complement' the immune response. The interferons are a family of proteins with immunomodulatory as well as antiviral effects, the production of which is induced by viral infection of any cell, or antigenic stimulation of lymphocytes. The role of each of these cells and molecules in the immune response to infection by viruses will be described below in more detail.

MOLECULAR BASIS OF VIRAL ANTIGENICITY

Our understanding of the antigenicity and immunogenicity of viral proteins (review: Burns and Allison, 1975) has been revolutionised within the space of the last few years by the concerted application of the techniques of modern molecular biology and immunochemistry to an intensive study of the haemagglutinin (HA) of influenza virus. Laver and Webster opened up the field by characterising the HA molecules from a considerable number of influenza viruses that have arisen sequentially in nature by antigenic drift and shift. First, peptide maps, and subsequently complete cDNA or protein sequences (review: Laver and Air, 1980; Webster *et al.*, 1982; 1984) revealed that the minor antigenic changes characteristic of drift can be attributed to the gradual accumulation of point mutations in the HA gene, expressing themselves as single amino acid substitutions in the primary sequence of the protein. On the other hand, antigenic shift, i.e. the sudden major change that gives rise every 10–20 years to a novel strain of influenza type A resulting in a pandemic, is characterised by the emergence of a completely new human HA subtype, containing dozens of different amino acids and displaying no serological relationship to any recently prevalent human strain. The vital clue to the probable origin of such 'new' subtypes of human influenza virus came with the discovery that their HA molecules closely resemble those found in influenza viruses of birds and animals. This led Webster and Laver (1975) to put forward their hypothesis, now widely accepted, that new subtypes of human influenza type A arise by genetic reassortment resulting in the acquisition by the human virus of the HA (and sometimes the NA) gene from an avian or animal strain (Kilbourne, 1968).

Then Gerhard and his colleagues made a major contribution to immunochemistry with the application of monoclonal antibodies to the antigenic characterisation of viral proteins. Their first approach was to analyse the 'reactivity patterns' (in haemagglutination-inhibition, radio-immunoassay or enzyme immunoassay) of a set of anti-HA monoclonal antibodies, to provide an indication of the diversity of distinguishable antigenic determinants (epitopes) on the HA molecule of different strains of influenza virus (Gerhard and Webster, 1978; Yewdell et al., 1979). Shortly thereafter, the concept of using monoclonal antibodies in a competitive (blocking) radioimmunoassay to enumerate and map the antigenic domains on viral proteins was introduced (Breschkin et al., 1981; Lubeck and Gerhard, 1981). But the most imaginative innovation of all was the exploitation of monoclonal antibodies to select viral mutants in vitro, followed by the sequencing of the HA (or its cDNA) of the mutants to identify the resulting amino acid substitutions (Laver et al., 1981). Such mutants were generally found to contain only a single amino acid substitution, yet this was sufficient to prevent the monoclone in question from binding to the mutant; other monoclones, recognising topographically distinct antigenic sites, could still bind and neutralise the mutant, as could polyclonal antisera against the parent strain.

A milestone in the history of virology was the publication by Wiley et al. (1981) of the first three-dimensional model of a viral protein—again influenza HA (Fig. 3.4). The positions of the particular amino acids known to vary in naturally-occurring or monoclone-selected strains were found to be located predominantly on certain prominent hydrophilic regions on the surface of the exposed 'head' of the molecule. Most of the epitopes occur in a large antigenic area extending from the 'tip' and 'interface' of the molecule to a conspicuous 'loop' a little further down. In so far as all these sites are in the immediate vicinity of the 'cleft' (just left of the 'tip' in Fig. 3.4) which is thought to represent the receptor-binding site, it seems plausible that antibodies binding to any of these epitopes may neutralise the infectivity of the virion (and inhibit haemagglutination) by steric hindrance of adsorption of the virion to cells. The other major antigenic site, the 'hinge', is closer to the site of cleavage of the HA monomer into its two component polypeptides HA_1 and HA_2, which is considered to be vitally involved in the fusion of the infecting virus with (lysosomal?) membrane at pH5 (Skehel et al., 1982; Jackson et al., 1983).

The latest approach to the antigenic characterisation of viruses at the submolecular level is the chemical synthesis of particular segments of the molecule (see Lerner, 1982). Now that the complete nucleotide sequence of genes coding for the HA of several strains of influenza virus is

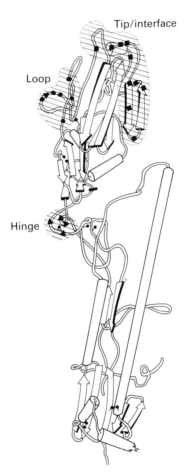

Fig. 3.4. Three-dimensional model of the monomeric HA subunit of the trimeric haemagglutinin molecule of influenza virus. The dots indicate the positions of those amino acids that are substituted in novel strains of influenza virus arising within the H3 subtype either by natural antigenic drift or by *in vitro* selection in the presence of monoclonal antibodies. It will be noted that the epitopes tend to cluster into three or four major antigenic domains on the distal end ('head') of the molecule, designated 'tip', 'loop', 'interface' and 'hinge'. Courtesy of Jackson *et al.* (1983). Modified from Wiley *et al.* (1981) *Nature* **289**, 373–8.

known (see Laver and Air, 1980; Nayak, 1981) it is feasible to synthesise chemically the whole viral protein or any part thereof. The results so far have contained some surprises. Whereas the antigenicity and immuno-genicity of the major presumptive antigenic sites ('loop', 'tip' and 'hinge') is much reduced in such short peptides, presumably as a result of loss of the native tertiary structure of the original conformational determinants (Jackson *et al.*, 1981), some activity is nevertheless demonstrable in peptides representing certain invariate regions of the molecule which are conserved through evolution and are assumed to be non-immunogenic in their native state (N. Green *et al.*, 1982; Müller *et al.*, 1982). The potential significance of these data and their implications for vaccine design are discussed in Chapter 7, together with recent findings with synthetic peptides derived from hepatitis B (Lerner *et al.*, 1981; Dreesman *et al.*, 1982) and foot-and-mouth disease viruses (Bittle *et al.*, 1982).

COMPONENTS OF THE IMMUNE RESPONSE TO VIRUSES

T Lymphocytes

T lymphocytes are most easily distinguished from B lymphocytes and other cells by the presence of certain surface 'markers', namely characteristic antigens recognisable by monoclonal antibodies (Table 3.1). In man these are the so-called OKT antigens, and in mice the Thy-1, Lyt and Qa antigens (review, McKenzie and Potter, 1979). Since far more is known about the immunology of the humble mouse, it will be the subject of most of what follows.

All murine T cells carry Thy-1. Most thymocytes are also Lyt $1^+2^+3^+$ (Ly 123 for short); the short-lived non-recirculating T_1' population retains this phenotype, whereas about 30–35% differentiate into Lyt $1^+2^-3^-$ (Ly 1), and 5–10% into Lyt $1^-2^+3^+$ (Ly 23) cells (see Dutton and Swain, 1982). More properly perhaps these populations should be

Table 3.1. Surface markers of murine lymphocytes.

	Thy 1	Ly 1	Ly 2, 3	I–A	I–J	Ig	FcR[b]	C₃R[c]
T_h	+	+	−	+	−	−	−	−
T_s	+	−	+	+	+	−	−	−
T_c	+	−[a]	+	−	−	−	−	−
T_d	+	+ or −	− or +	+	−	−	−	−
B	−	−	−	+	−	+	+	+
NK	−(±)	−	−	−	−	−	±	−
Mφ	−	−	−	+	−	−	+	+

[a]Some activated T_c claimed to be Ly1$^+$2,3$^+$.
[b]Fc receptor.
[c]C_3 receptor.

designated Ly-1^{high}2, 3^{low} and Ly-1^{low}2, 3^{high}, as these Ly markers are not completely absent from any T cells that are screened by sufficiently sensitive methods. The Ly 1 population includes most of the T_h and T_d cells, called 'inducers' or 'amplifiers' by Cantor and Gershon (1979), while the Ly 23 population contains mainly T_c ('effector' T cells), T_s and some T_d. The Qa antigens, like Lyt, are exclusive to T cells and their expression changes during differentiation (Cantor and Gershon, 1979). Ly 1 'feed-back suppression inducer' cells and Ly 123 'feed-back suppressor' cells are characterised by being Qa-1$^+$. T_s cells generally bear I-J antigen.

Monoclonal antibodies against these surface markers can be used not only to identify particular subpopulations of lymphocytes, e.g. by immunofluorescence, but also to separate them, e.g. by fluorescence-activated cell-sorter (FACS) or by immuno-affinity chromatography, or to remove them, e.g. by antibody/complement lysis. Other surface properties such as adherence or non-adherence to nylon wool, Sephadex or specific-antigen columns can also be exploited, as can characteristics such as radiation-sensitivity or resistance. Nevertheless, physiological variation and technical limitations make it impossible to obtain absolutely pure preparations in the laboratory except by cloning. First, hybridoma technology (fusion of T cells to T lymphoma lines), then transformation of T cells using oncogenic viruses such as radiation leukaemia virus, and now conventional cloning techniques in the presence of interleukin-2 and occasional pulses of antigen (reviews: Möller, 1981a; Feldmann and Schreier, 1982) make it possible today to study uniform populations of lymphocytes originating from a single parent cell. Characterisation of such clones derived from particular subsets of T or B cells specific for particular epitopes on particular antigens from particular viruses constitutes the new methodology of modern immunology. Monoclonal antibodies directed not only against individual viral epitopes but also against various regions of cell surface antigens coded by the MHC complex or against the idiotypes (see pp. 98–9) defining specific antibodies, lymphocyte receptors or lymphokines, provide a second dimension to the technology of the 1980s. Consequently, we can confidently anticipate a quantal leap in our understanding of immunology at the molecular level within the decade.

Already, scrutiny of antigen-specific T cell clones has provided us with major surprises. One of them is that surface markers are not entirely reliable indicators of the specialised function of the cell in question. Such markers change during ontogeny, differentiation, antigen-activation or physiological state. It has also emerged that individual cells may carry out more than one function; for example, cloned T_c cells may effect delayed-hypersensitivity (Lin and Askonas, 1981).

However, there is a solid body of evidence showing that the function of a T cell is closely correlated with the particular type of MHC antigen it expresses on its surface and correspondingly, on the soluble antigen-specific factors it secretes, e.g. I-A and I-E gene-products are expressed on activated helper T cells and their factors, but I-J on suppressor cells and their factors (Fig. 3.3). Moreover, distinct classes of MHC antigen on target cells direct particular classes of T cells to them (Figs. 3.1 and 3.3): H2-K/D/L are recognised (in association with viral antigen) by T_c cells; I-A and I-E by T_h and T_d cells (reviews: Benacerraf and Germain, 1978; Zinkernagel and Doherty, 1979). In this sense the mode of presentation of antigen predetermines the nature of the immune response. Since 'class I' MHC antigens (H-2, K, D, L in the mouse; HLA-A, B, C in man) are present on all cells, viral antigens on the surface of infected cells elicit the T_c response that is required to destroy those target cells. On the other hand, since 'class II' MHC antigens (products of the I region in the mouse, or the D/DR region in man) are present on macrophages and related cells, presentation of viral antigens in this context turns on the T_h cells needed to set in train the antibody synthetic pathway and the T_d cells that augment the immune response by attracting and activating additional cells.

T lymphocytes differentiate into specialised effectors following binding of specific antigen. Clearly, at least two or three steps are involved: antigen-specific recognition, then activation of the cell to differentiate and divide. As a result of cell division the response is amplified, and also memory cells are generated. Little is known about whether separate signals are required to trigger the induction of different physiological functions, or the development of immunological memory. The effector response is generally transient, e.g. T_c and T_d have usually peaked by one week after delivery of antigen, and disappeared by 2–3 weeks. This may be in part attributable to removal, or masking, of the activating agent (antigen) by antibody, but the key to immunoregulation may be the suppressor T cells which are first demonstrable at about the time the other cell types decline in number. Memory T_c, T_d and T_h cells do however, persist for years, and are able to mount a somewhat accelerated response upon subsequent encounter with the same antigen.

T lymphocyte populations seem to contain a larger proportion of cells responding to cross-reactive determinants on the eliciting antigen than do B cells. For example, whereas immunisation with the purified haemagglutinin molecule of a given strain of influenza virus elicits a range of strain-specific antibodies recognising various epitopes, the helper T cells are predominantly, though not exclusively, cross-reactive between strains and even between subtypes (Anders et al., 1981a, b), as are the cytotoxic T cells (Koszinowski et al., 1980) and delayed hypersensitivity T cells (Liew, 1982). As a result, T cell-mediated memory is broader than the spectrum of B cells would suggest. This may provide at least limited protection against reinfection with a different serotype.

T cells act principally via soluble factors ('lymphokines' or 'inter-leukins') which they secrete following antigen-binding (reviews: Tada and Okumura, 1979; Germain and Benacerraf, 1980; Feldmann and Kontiainen, 1981; Feldmann and Schreier, 1982; Möller, 1982). Some of them are antigen-specific factors, others non-specific.

Though dozens of T cell-derived non-specific factors have been described, many of them may be identical and only a few have been really well characterised to date. They might properly be regarded as 'lymphocytotrophic' hormones. Interferons alpha (α) and gamma (γ) are discussed at length in Chapter 4. Interleukin 2 (IL-2), previously known as 'T cell growth factor' (TCGF), is secreted mainly by Lyt 1^+ lymphocytes; it is a mitogen, which promotes the proliferation ('clonal expansion') of antigen-activated T lymphocytes. The 'late-acting T cell-replicating factor' (TRF) is also secreted by Lyt 1^+ lymphocytes but probably acts on B cells, augmenting antibody production. The 'B cell growth factor' (BCGF) amplifies the clone of B cells following their activation. And so on.

The antigen-specific helper and suppressor factors may be T cell receptors or a degraded form thereof, and they constitute the principal mediators of specific T–T cell and T–B cell interactions. Indeed, they can be successfully substituted for T lymphocytes in experimental systems. Each factor is characterised by two distinct components: (1) a variable segment with specificity for antigen, and (2) an I-region gene-product (generally I-A or I-J). The former, designated the 'variable' region by Feldmann and Kontiainen (1981), serves to focus the molecule on to cell-bound, specific antigen; the latter, the 'constant' region, dictates the physiological effector function. Thus, most helper factors carry I-A or I-E, whereas most suppressor factors carry I-J. Some antigen-specific T cell factors are MHC-restricted; others are not.

One of the more fascinating discoveries of modern immunology has been that the unique amino acid sequence that comprises the antigen-combining site in the 'variable' (V) region of an antibody molecule can itself be recognised as a foreign antigen. Hence we mount an 'anti-idiotypic' immune response against the unique 'individual idiotype (IdI)' characterising the antigen-combining site, as well as against the 'cross-reactive idiotypes (IdX)' present on the surrounding framework of the variable region of the H chain (Bona and Hiernaux, 1981). T lymphocytes bearing anti-idiotypic receptors recognise the corresponding idiotype on a particular antibody molecule or on antibody-like (idiotypic) receptors on B cells or other T cells; anti-idiotypic helper factors are secreted and assist the corresponding clone of B cells to make anti-idiotypic antibody, and so on. In theory, the whole process could be extrapolated indefinitely as in a hall of mirrors.

Furthermore, anti-idiotypic antibodies and T cells can either activate or suppress T cells with the corresponding idiotype, depending on other characteristics of the cells and factors involved. The mind boggles at the potential complexity of such a network but it seems to be real, much as predicted by Jerne (1974) many years ago when he perceived the need for such a mechanism to regulate an immune response which would otherwise run out of control, because of the cascade effect of the numerous known amplifying signals. Idiotype/anti-idiotype interactions contribute to an intricate web of positive and negative feed-back controls that regulate all aspects of the immune response (Cantor and Gershon, 1979; Bona and Hiernaux, 1981; Germain and Benacerraf, 1981). This cybernetic nightmare is too involved to discuss in a short monograph on virology but we will later provide just a vignette by outlining the postulated role of idiotypic and anti-idiotypic suppressor T lymphocytes and their soluble factors.

Cytotoxic T cells. Cytotoxic T (T_c) cells kill cells displaying 'foreign' antigen on their surface, including cancer cells and virus-infected cells (review: Blanden, 1974). While it has been long recognised that virus-coded glycoproteins are incorporated into the plasma membrane of cells infected with viruses that subsequently acquire an envelope by budding, it has only recently become clear that viral antigens are also expressed on the surface of cells infected with certain non-budding viruses such as adenoviruses, papovaviruses and reoviruses, rendering these cells also susceptible to T_c-mediated cytolysis (Inada and Uetake, 1978; Fields and Greene, 1982). Because at least some viral protein appears in the membrane before any virions have been produced, lysis of the cell at this stage, or shortly thereafter, brings viral replication to a halt—nipping infection in the bud, as it were. The phenomenon is readily demonstrable in cultured cells, using the release of ^{51}Cr as an assay for cytolysis.

In 1974 Zinkernagel and Doherty reported a most unexpected discovery that has had wide-ranging implications for immunology. They observed that virus-infected cells could be lysed only by T_c derived from an animal histocompatible with the target cell, specifically in the K/D region of the H-2 complex in the mouse (Zinkernagel and Doherty, 1974), since extended to include the L region (Ciavarra and Forman, 1982). The observation has been widely confirmed in other animals, including man, where the 'MHC restriction' is to the HLA-A, B, C antigen complex (reviews: Doherty *et al.*, 1976; Zinkernagel and Doherty, 1979; Möller, 1981b). Sophisticated studies with inbred congenic, recombinant and mutant strains as well as chimaeric and neonatally tolerant mice have since confirmed that the effector cell recognises neither the viral antigen nor MHC antigen alone, but both in association ('associative recognition'). A given clone of T_c cells recognises viral antigen in conjunction with H-2 K or D, but not both. Some viral proteins can associate with K or with D, while others can associate with only one of them. The I region of the MHC complex appears not to be involved at all. The phenomenon can be mimicked by incorporating purified proteins into liposomes (Koszinowski et al., 1980). Mixtures of liposomes containing only viral glycoprotein with others containing only H-2 antigen cannot induce T_c cells; the two antigens must be present in close apposition in the same liposome. Moreover, uninfected histocompatible cells can be rendered susceptible to virus-induced T_c cells by fusion with liposomes containing viral antigen (Koszinowski et al., 1980).

A fundamental question still to be resolved, however, is whether the T cell carries two distinct receptors (one recognising the MHC and the other separately recognising the viral antigen) or only one (recognising both epitopes, situated close together, or alternatively recognising a composite epitope or 'neoantigenic determinant' spanning the putative viral-MHC complex). These are sometimes called the 'dual recognition' and 'altered self' hypotheses (Zinkernagel and Doherty, 1979). The resolution of the dilemma is important because it may shed light on the nature of the T cell receptor. It is evident that the T cell receptor is not the same as that of the B cell. Even suppressor T cells, which have been reported to bind soluble antigen, as well as to share a common idiotype with the corresponding B cell, do not necessarily have the same antigenic repertoire as do B cells. Indeed, it has been proposed that the current diversity of T cell receptors may have evolved by somatic mutation from V genes encoding receptors recognising the body's own MHC antigen (Zinkernagel and Doherty, 1979). Recent data from several laboratories indicate that the structure of the T cell receptor will soon be known (see Williams, 1984).

In most viral infections, specific T_c cell activity is demonstrable after 3–4 days, reaches a peak after about a week, and declines to a very low level by two weeks; thereafter, memory T_c cells persist essentially for life, in the mouse at least (Blanden, 1974; Ashman, 1982). The cytotoxic T cell response is therefore seen to be an early defence mechanism, developing well ahead of the antibody response. Furthermore, since T_c receptors cannot bind free viral antigen their access to infected cells is not blocked.

Delayed-type hypersensitivity T cells. DTH is a T cell-mediated inflammatory reaction characterised by infiltration of mononuclear cells. The T_d cells respond to antigen by proliferating and releasing lymphokines which attract macrophages to the site and induce them to proliferate (review: Liew, 1982). The classical demonstration of DTH, in the form of swelling of the footpad or ear of a mouse 1–2 days after local intradermal inoculation of antigen may seem unsophisticated, yet it is not clear that in vitro assays such as inhibition of migration of macrophages as a result of secretion of MIF by lymphocytes, or proliferation of lymphocytes in response to antigen as monitored by ^{3}H-thymidine incorporation, are measuring the same phenomenon. The classical DTH response, moreover, is proving to be more complex than had been thought (Askenase and van Loveren, 1983). There is evidence for an early phase of the response, in which serotonin released from mast cells (sensitised by an antigen-specific factor from T cells) acts on local blood vessels and promotes the influx of T cells that mediate the classical (second) phase of the response as described.

The classical T_d (Tdth) cell is Lyt $1^+2^-3^-$, and IA (or I-E) restricted. However, it is now clear that there is a distinct T_d population which is Lyt $1^-2^+3^+$, and K/D restricted. Ada *et al.* (1981) refer to cells with the first set of characteristics (which also display T_h activity) as class I, and the second (which also display T_c activity) as class II cells. It had not been appreciated that a T_h or T_c cell could produce a typical DTH response until cloned T_h and T_c cell lines were demonstrated to display both properties (Lin and Askonas, 1981). One must now ask whether there is in fact any such thing as a distinct T_d cell. It may well be that T cells of any class (T_h, T_c or perhaps T_s) can respond to antigen by proliferation and production of lymphokines attracting macrophages, hence cause swelling on inoculation with antigen into the footpad of a mouse.

The DTH response is subject to both help and suppression by particular subsets of T_h and T_s cells, both of which appear to be Lyt $1^+2^-3^-$ (Greene and Weiner, 1980; Leung and Ada, 1981; Liew and Russell, 1980). The T_s(dth) precursors are eliminated by cyclophosphamide, which no doubt accounts for the well-known experimental observation that DTH is augmented by cyclophosphamide pretreatment. The fact that inoculation of mice with ultraviolet-inactivated influenza virus gives a much greater DTH response than does live virus (Ada *et al.*, 1981) suggests that the DTH response is suppressed in normal infection. Liew (1982), pointing to the observation of Ada *et al.* (1981) that adoptive transfer of class I cells to influenza virus-infected mice actually accelerates their demise, asserts that '. . . there is little evidence that DTH is an important arm of the immune response against viral infections'. We would qualify this conclusion somewhat: DTH is probably of vital importance in attracting macrophages and T cells in the critical early phase of the immune response to viruses, but is, and needs to be, suppressed after this task has been accomplished.

Helper T cells. Most viral antigens, like the majority of non-viral antigens, are 'T-dependent' (Burns *et al.*, 1975), i.e. they require 'help' from T lymphocytes to induce a satisfactory antibody response. These helper T (T_h or T_H) cells are Lyt $1^+2^-3^-$ lymphocytes which recognise viral antigen presented only in conjunction with histocompatible I-A (and perhaps sometimes I-E) gene-products on the surface of a macrophage, Langerhans cell or dendritic cell (reviews: Unanue, 1981; Dutton and Swain, 1982). Interleukin 1 (IL-1) secreted by the macrophage is required for optimal antigen-induced activation of the T_h cell, which itself then secretes several distinct lymphokines.

Current opinion is that there are at least two subsets of the T_h cells providing help for B cells. T_{h1} cells are thought to secrete an Ia^+, V_H-bearing, i.e. antigen-specific (Id^+) helper factor, and T_{h2} cells to secrete one or more non-specific helper factors (reviews: Tada and Okumura, 1979; Germain and Benacerraf, 1980; Dutton and Swain, 1982; Feldmann and Schreier, 1982; Möller, 1982). There now appear to be a number of distinct non-specific helper factors, including IL-2, TRF and BCGF (B cell growth factor), which augment the antibody response to any antigen in the manner discussed earlier. Of course, non-specific helper factors induced by any antigenic determinant can help antibody responses to the same or any other determinant. Commonly, T_h cells recognise 'carrier' epitopes on a viral protein, thus secreting non-specific T_hF which helps B cells that recognise the epitope on the 'hapten' moiety of that (or another) viral protein, to make anti-hapten antibody. The antigen-specific T_hF, on the other hand, is presumed to bind only to specific antigen-bearing B lymphocytes and to trigger their division and differentiation into antibody-producing plasma cells.

Little is known about the signals that determine the isotype of the immunoglobulin produced by any given B cell. It is likely that certain helper factors are Ig class-specific, hence are able to bind to and activate only those B cells bearing receptors of the same Ig class or subclass. There is a striking and therapeutically important analogy in a non-antigen-specific, IgE-specific suppressor factor secreted by a T cell hybridoma, which binds only to IgE-bearing B cells and selectively suppresses IgE antibody synthesis (Kishimoto *et al.*, 1982).

Helper T cells, probably of still different subsets, also augment T_c (Ashman and Müllbacher, 1979) and T_d (Leung and Ada, 1981) responses to viral infections.

Suppressor T cells. The most recently recognised T lymphocytes are known as suppressor T (T_s) cells because they suppress the activity of B, T_h, T_d or T_c cells (reviews: Gershon, 1974; Cantor and Gershon, 1979; Germain and Benacerraf, 1981). Suppressors probably play a key role in regulation of the immune response, by turning off the positive 'effector' T cells after they have fulfilled their function and are no longer needed. They are not, however, the only modulators capable of immuno-suppression (or 'tolerance', which is sometimes a manifestation of suppression); antibodies, interferons and prostaglandins are also involved. Interferon-gamma, which is produced by T_s cells following activation by antigen, suppresses antibody production as well as certain other arms of the immune response (see Chapter 5). Prostaglandin E2 seems to be required for expression of T_s function. In general, T_s responses are preferentially turned on in experimental animals by inoculation of virus orally, or of high doses of UV-inactivated virus systemically.

The classical Lyt $1^-2^+3^+$ T_s cell in the mouse is distinguished from all other cells by being I-J$^+$. More recently it has become apparent that this is but one subset of T_s cells involved in an intricate network of T_s cells and their secreted products. Germain and Benacerraf (1981) have put together a working model which, though likely to be proven incomplete or even wrong in certain details, is presented in outline here to give an idea of the complexity of the networks that are now emerging in immunology.

Antigen, perhaps in soluble form, perhaps macrophage-associated, is presented to a Lyt 1^+ or Lyt $1^+2^+3^+$, Ia (I-J)$^+$, cyclophosphamide-sensitive, antigen-specific 'pre T_{s1}' cell, thus activating it to become a mature afferent suppressor cell, 'T_{s1}', which secretes an idiotypic (Id$^+$, anti-antigen), I-J$^+$ factor, T_sF_1. T_sF_1 is assumed to trigger a second subset of cells, 'pre-T_{s2}' (Lyt $1^+2^+3^+$, I-J$^+$) to differentiate into Lyt $1^-2^+3^+$, I-J$^+$, T_{s2} cells whose receptors may be either anti-antigen or anti-idiotype. Hence the I-J$^+$, I-J restricted soluble factor, T_sF_2 they secrete is *either* anti-antigen *or* anti-idiotype. T_sF_2 is presumed to trigger a third cell, 'T_{s3}', which is an antigen-primed, Lyt $1^+2^+3^+$, I-J$^+$, Id$^+$, cyclo-phosphamide-sensitive cell (perhaps in fact a mature T_{s1} cell), to secrete a non-specific effector molecule with suppressor activity. It is not known what determines whether T_{s2} are anti-idiotype or anti-antigen, nor what is the relative importance of the two. Indeed, the natural role of anti-idiotypic cells, soluble factors and antibodies is one of the major unre-solved questions of immunology awaiting clarification during the 1980s.

As if this were not sufficiently complex, Gershon *et al*. (1981) have also described 'contrasuppressor' cells (Green *et al*., 1983). For some years it has been known that oral administration of antigen elicits an IgA antibody response in the gut while simultaneously producing 'systemic tolerance' (suppression of the IgG response) to the same antigen; teleo-logically, this type of microenvironmental immune regulation may have evolved as a means of minimising the development of allergies to foods while still permitting immunological memory to be expressed. The mechanism now appears to be as follows. Helper T cells in Peyer's patches are able to induce a local IgA response because contra-suppressor cells, which are plentiful in that locality, suppress the local IgA-isotype-specific T_s cells. The 'contrasuppressor-inducer' cell is Ly-1^-2^+, I-J$^+$, Qa-1^+; it secretes a soluble factor, Ly-2 TcsiF, which acts on an Ly-1^+2^+, I-J$^+$, Qa-1^+ acceptor cell (D. R. Green *et al*., 1982).

B Lymphocytes

Some of the multipotential haemopoietic 'stem cells' originating from foetal liver and adult bone marrow differentiate via pre-B cells into immature B cells, which are characterised by specific antigen-binding receptors of the IgM isotype, and by receptors for complement (C_3') and for the F_c portion of immunoglobulin, and other cell surface components involved in triggering. On encounter with antigen, the particular clones of B cells bearing receptors (antibody) complementary to any of the several antigenic determinants (epitopes) on that antigen, bind it and, after receiving the appropriate antigen-specific and non-specific signals from helper T cell factors (ThF), respond by division and differentiation into antibody-secreting 'plasma cells'. Each clone of plasma cells secretes antibody of only a single class, specificity and avidity, corresponding to the particular receptors it expresses. Early in the response, when large amounts of antigen are available, there is an opportunity for antigen-reactive B cells to be triggered even if their receptors fit the epitope with relatively poor 'affinity', and hence bind the antigen with low 'avidity'. Later on, when only small amounts of antigen remain, B cells with receptors binding antigen with high affinity are selected, hence the avidity of the antibody secreted increases correspondingly, sometimes 100-fold.

Clonal expansion of B lymphocytes on exposure to antigen also generates a population of memory cells. On re-exposure to the same antigen even years later, these memory cells respond promptly with the production of larger amounts of specific antibody, mainly of the IgG class, after a delay of only a day or two.

Even in the absence of reinfection or of persistent infection, antibodies to a given viral antigen are usually demonstrable in the serum for many years, often for life. For instance, five of six individuals who suffered an attack of yellow fever during an epidemic in Virginia, USA in 1855 were found to have circulating antibodies 75 years later despite the total absence of yellow fever from the area ever since (Sawyer, 1931). Similarly, evidence from isolated Eskimo communities in Alaska showed that antibody to poliovirus persisted for 40 years in the absence of any possible re-exposure. Since the half-life of IgG in man is only about 25 days, these observations indicate that antibody is being synthesised continuously during this long period. The question arises, how do the B cells continue to receive the requisite antigenic stimulus? One possibility is that viral antigens may persist in the body, for instance in follicular dendritic cells, which are known to retain antigen on their surfaces for long periods; such cells may serve as 'antigen turnstiles', repeatedly restimulating sensitised lymphocytes which circulate through lymphoid tissues (Mandel et al., 1980).

Antibody synthesis takes place principally in the spleen and lymph nodes, gut-associated lymphoid tissues (GALT) and bronchus-associated lymphoid tissues (BALT). The spleen and lymph nodes receive foreign antigens via the blood or lymphatics and synthesise antibodies mainly restricted to the IgM (early in the response) and IgG classes. On the other hand, the submucosal ('interstitial') lymphoid concentrations (follicles) of the respiratory and alimentary tracts, such as the tonsils and Peyer's patches, receive antigens directly from the overlying epithelial cells, and make antibodies mainly of the IgA class. Plasma cells are more numerous in the lamina propria of the small intestine than anywhere else in the body and the great majority of these secrete only antibody of the IgA class, directly into the mucus which coats the gut. Indeed, IgA-specific B (and T?) lymphocytes preferentially localise ('home') to submucosal lymphoid tissue such as GALT, BALT and exocrine gland interstitia, for reasons that are not yet entirely clear but may be attributable to complementarity between receptors on these lymphocytes and receptors on submucosal vascular endothelial cells (see Strober et al., 1982). Hence, IgA antibody responses are elicited much more effectively by oral or respiratory delivery than by systemic administration of antigen (see vaccines, Chapter 7). A significant minority of the IgA in mucus secretions can originate in another way, namely by selective transport of the dimeric (and polymeric) forms of circulating IgA, to bile via the liver, to milk via the mammary gland, and to saliva via the salivary glands. Intestinal epithelial cells and the epithelial cells in mammary and salivary glands bear a glycoprotein receptor for the J chain of multimeric IgA and IgM; this receptor, known as the epithelial 'secretory component' (SC), alias 'transport piece', remains associated with the dimeric IgA molecule during its transport through and secretion from these cells.

Antibody

The different classes ('isotypes') of immunoglobulin, with some of their properties, are shown in Table 3.2. The major circulating class of antibody is immunoglobulin G (IgG). It has the basic four-chain immunoglobulin structure in the shape of a Y, as illustrated in Fig. 3.5. There are four subclasses of IgG in man, which differ in the 'constant' region of their heavy chains and consequently in their biological properties such as placental passage, complement fixation and binding to phagocytes. The amounts present in serum are also different. Much antiviral IgG is of the IgG3 subclass (Beck, 1981) and mainly IgG1 and IgG3 responses are seen in varicella-zoster, herpes simplex and CMV infections in man (Sundquist et al., 1983; Linde et al., 1983). The significance of this is not known.

IgM is a polymer built from five of the basic four-chain subunits, and because it is such a large molecule is confined to the vascular system. Its biological importance is firstly that molecule for molecule it has five times the number of antigen-reactive sites as does IgG, and secondly, that it is formed early in the immune response. In the race between replication and spread of virus on the one hand, and generation of an antiviral immune response on the other, such an avid class of antibody that is produced a day or two earlier than other classes may have a

Table 3.2. Properties of immunoglobulin classes in man.

Property	IgG	IgM	IgA[a]	IgE	IgD
Molecular weight	150 000	900 000	385 000 (170 000)	200 000	185 000
Heavy chain	γ	μ	α	ε	δ
Subclasses[d]	γ1,2,3,4	μ1,2	α1,2	—	—
Half life (days)[b]	25	5	(6)[c]	2	3
Percentage of total Ig	80	6	(13)	0.002	0–1
Complement fixation	+	++	±	–	?
Transfer to offspring	via placenta	nil	via milk	nil	nil
Functional significance	Major systemic Ig	Appears early Multivalent	Mucosal antibody	Allergenic responses	Present on B cells

[a]Data for secretory IgA; serum IgA in brackets.
[b]Half life generally shorter for smaller animals, e.g. 2.5 days (IgG) and 0.5 days (IgM) in the mouse.
[c]Strictly speaking, the half life of secretory IgA on mucosal surfaces is measured in minutes rather than days, because it is soon carried away in mucus secretions.
[d]Differ in heavy chains and biological activity.

determining effect on the course of the infection. As the immune response unfolds, IgM antibodies are replaced by IgG. IgM antibodies are also the first to be found during the development of the individual. At 5–6 months' gestation the human foetus, for instance, responds to infection by forming antibodies almost exclusively of the IgM class. Hence the presence of antiviral IgM antibodies in a newborn infant suggests intrauterine infection, because the only maternal antibodies that can pass the placenta to reach the foetus are IgG.

Secretory IgA is the principal immunoglobulin on mucosal surfaces and in milk and colostrum. The common, dimeric form consists of two subunits of the basic four-chain structure with heavy chains of the alpha isotype, plus the linking J (joining) chain and the 'secretory piece' (or secretory component, SC) acquired when the molecule is transferred across the mucosal epithelium. IgA synthesised locally in submucosal tissues following intestinal or respiratory infection lacks this secretory piece. It can enter the blood via lymphatics. In man, most serum IgA is in the monomeric form and of the IgA_1 subclass, whereas most secretory IgA is polymeric and is about equally divided between IgA_1 and IgA_2.

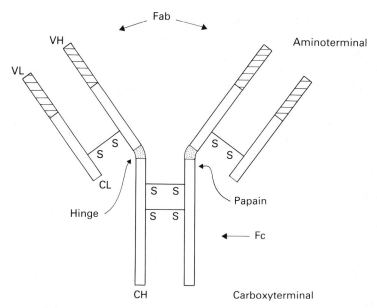

Fig. 3.5. Basic Y-shaped (4 chain) structure of immunoglobulin G molecule. Complex tertiary structure, loops, etc., not shown. VH, VL = region of about 110 amino acids with variable (V) sequence, in heavy (H) and light (L) chains. C = constant regions. Light chains are either κ or λ. Heavy chains are γ for IgG. Hinge region enables arms to swing out to 180° and bridge antigenic sites. Papain digestion of molecule yields two Fab (fragment antigen-binding) portions, and one Fc (fragment crystallisable) portion which confers biological activity on the molecule (placental passage, binding to phagocytes, etc.). Number of disulphide bonds differs in different Ig classes and subclasses. Intrachain disulphide bonds 'pinch' H and L chains into loops or domains.

IgA antibodies are important in resistance to infection of the mucosal surfaces of the body, particularly the respiratory, intestinal and urogenital tracts (Fazekas de St. Groth, 1950; Strober *et al.*, 1982). But the details differ in different species; in sheep for instance, IgG figures as prominently as IgA in secretory immunoglobulins. Secretory Ig transfer in milk and early colostrum is especially important in cows, sheep, horses and other animals in which there is no placental transfer of antibody (Newby *et al.*, 1982).

Specific antibodies can exert antiviral effects via several distinct mechanisms, some involving interaction with the virion itself, others with the virus-infected cell.

Neutralisation of virus. While specific antibody of any class can bind to any accessible epitope on a surface protein of a virion, only those antibodies which bind with reasonably high avidity to particular epitopes on a particular protein in the outer capsid or envelope are capable of neutralising the infectivity of the virion. Antibodies directed against irrelevant or inaccessible epitopes of surface proteins, or against internal proteins of the virion, or virus-coded non-structural proteins (e.g. virus-coded enzymes) can sometimes indirectly exert immunopathological effects but generally play no role in elimination of the infection. In fact, certain non-neutralising antibodies not only form damaging circulating 'immune complexes' (Chapter 5), but may actually impede access of neutralising antibody (Massey and Schochetman, 1981) and enhance the infectivity of the virion for some cells, e.g. macrophages (Chapter 6).

1. Classical neutralisation results when antibody binds to the virion and thereby prevents infection of a susceptible cell (reviews: Mandel, 1979; Della-Porta and Westaway, 1978; Yoshino and Isono, 1978). The mechanism(s) of neutralisation is not fully understood. The particular protein involved is not necessarily the most plentiful on the viral surface; for example, in the case of reovirus, it represents less than 2% of the total mass in the outer capsid (Fields and Weiner, 1977). The key protein is usually the one by which the virion is known to adsorb to receptors on the host cell. But neutralisation is not simply a matter of coating the virion with antibody, nor indeed of blocking attachment to the host cell. Many years ago Fazekas de St. Groth (1962) demonstrated that, except in the presence of such high concentrations of antibody that most or all accessible antigenic sites on the surface of the virion are saturated, neutralised virions attach satisfactorily to susceptible cells. The block occurs at some point following adsorption and entry.

Mandel (1979) first demonstrated how antibody to a surface protein of poliovirus could so distort the conformation of the capsid that enzymes could penetrate and destroy the infectivity of the virion. There emerged the hypothesis that a virion-antibody complex tends to be destroyed by cellular enzymes, presumably in the phagosome, whereas the virion alone is uncoated in a controlled way that generally preserves its infectivity.

Possee *et al*. (1982) have recently taken this one step further by showing that a particular monoclonal antibody to influenza haemagglutinin neutralised the infectivity of the virus without preventing attachment, penetration or uncoating, but inhibited transcription of mRNA by the viral transcriptase. One should not conclude that antibody raised against HA actually binds to the transcriptase; the effect may be indirect, as in Mandel's model. Studies by Webster *et al*. (1982) suggest that monoclonal antibodies binding to different epitopes on the influenza viral HA molecule may neutralise the infectivity of the virion in different ways: those binding near the tip of the molecule, close to the haemagglutinating site (Wiley *et al*., 1981) might indeed block attachment, whereas those binding further down the molecule, near the HA_1/HA_2 cleavage site involved in fusion with host cell membrane (Skehel *et al*., 1982) may block entry/uncoating. Evidently there is more than one mechanism underlying classical neutralisation, perhaps even in a single virus-cell system. Experiments in which the fate of labelled virus particles is followed can be difficult to interpret, because not only infectious but non-infectious particles, always present in excess, are labelled.

Antibody to the haemagglutinin (HN protein) of paramyxoviruses prevents initiation of infection but fails to stop the direct cell-to-cell spread of newly formed virions once infection has been established; the latter is prevented by antibody to the fusion (F) protein (Merz *et al.*, 1980). Similarly, antibody to the neuraminidase (NA) of influenza can inhibit release of progeny from the plasma membrane and significantly slows viral spread (Kilbourne, 1969).

2. *Enhancement of neutralisation by complement* is a well documented phenomenon that itself can occur in a number of different ways which will be discussed below (see Complement).

3. *Enhancement of neutralisation by 'enhancing' antibody* is a more recently described phenomenon (Nemazee and Sato, 1982). Better known perhaps as 'rheumatoid factor' (see Salonen *et al.*, 1980), 'enhancing' antibody is directed against novel epitopes on the immunoglobulin moiety of the virion–antibody complex which are revealed as a consequence of antigen binding. Such antibody, usually of the IgM class, is probably made late in most viral infections, particularly in chronic infections, where antigen–antibody complexes are plentiful. Enhancing antibody presumably strengthens, and consequently perhaps broadens the specificity of antigen–antibody interactions, and also, no doubt, anti-idiotype–antibody complexes. Sometimes complement or anti-rheumatoid factor antibody is needed before enhancement is achieved (Gipson *et al.*, 1974). The term 'enhancing' antibody is also used quite separately to describe enhancement by antibody of viral infection of susceptible cells bearing Fc receptors (see Chapter 6)—the opposite of neutralisation.

4. *Opsonisation and agglutination* of virions by antibody accelerates clearance by phagocytic cells. Agglutination also reduces the number of infectious units.

Immune cytolysis of infected cells. Antibodies may also be involved in the destruction or inhibition of virus-infected host cells by a number of potentially important mechanisms.

1. *Antibody-complement mediated cytotoxicity*, readily demonstrable *in vitro* even at very low concentrations of antibody, is mediated by any antibody that recognises antigen expressed on the surface of an infected cell and that is capable of activating the complement sequence. Such antigens may include not only the envelope proteins of budding viruses but other structural or nonstructural proteins which may be expressed on the plasma membrane (Inada and Uetake, 1977; Fields and Greene, 1982), and even 'neoantigenic determinants' formed by association between viral and MHC proteins (Wylie *et al.*, 1982). Because virus-coded

proteins are expressed on the cell surface before new virions have been produced, 'immune cytolysis' of infected cells could play a major role in elimination of the infection. Sissons and Oldstone (1980), who have studied this system extensively, have concluded that lysis occurs principally via the alternate complement pathway. The phenomenon is discussed in more detail below (see Complement).

2. *Antibody-dependent cell-mediated cytotoxicity (ADCC)* is mediated, in the presence of antibody, by certain types of normal leukocyte. Unlike cytotoxic T lymphocytes, these effector cells are not immunologically specific; they bind only to target cells to which antibody of the IgG class is specifically attached. At least three types of normal leukocyte can effect ADCC in this way because they bear receptors for the Fc end of IgG molecules (FcR). Some are nonB-nonT lymphocytes known as K (killer) cells (Rager-Zisman and Bloom, 1974; Shore *et al.*, 1974), but polymorphs (Rouse *et al.*, 1977) and macrophages (Macfarlan *et al.*, 1977) also mediate the phenomenon very efficiently. Indeed, ADCC was found by Shore *et al.* (1976) to be hundreds of times more efficient per antibody molecule than complement-mediated cytolysis, and hence might be more relevant *in vivo*.

3. *Inhibition of viral multiplication by antibody* to viral antigens expressed on the surface of infected cells can also occur, in the absence of leukocytes or complement, and without involving lysis of the cell (Notkins, 1974). Neither the mechanism nor the *in vivo* significance of the phenomenon is known.

Antibody can also by itself 'modulate' viral antigens expressed on the cell surface, as shown for measles virus by Oldstone and Fujinami (1982). Antibody combines with antigen and the complex is redistributed ('capped') then either shed from the cell as an immune complex or internalised. This does not totally prevent viral multiplication, but interferes with assembly, so that nucleocapsids accumulate in the cytoplasm; when the fusion protein of measles virus is removed from the cell surface in this way, cell-to-cell fusion and spread may be impeded. The phenomenon may be important in virus persistence and is discussed in Chapter 6.

Complement

The classical complement pathway consists of a complicated system of at least 20 distinct proteins and 9 numbered components (C1–C9) present in normal serum (reviews: Cooper, 1979; Hirsch, 1982). It functions by mediating and amplifying immune and inflammatory reactions. The first component (C1) consists of three principal subunits: C1q, C1r and C1s. It is activated after combining with immune complexes (antibody bound to antigen). The immune complex may be free in the tissues or located on the cell surface following the reaction of specific antibody with viral antigen in the plasma membrane. As a result of the combination of the Fab binding site with antigen, Fc sites on the immunoglobulin are slightly altered to expose attachment sites for C1q. Each molecule must bind to at least two Fc sites, which means that there must be several IgG molecules close together in the immune complex. With IgM, several Fc sites are present on a single molecule and IgM therefore activates complement much more efficiently. The activated enzyme C1qrs, a protease, cleaves the next component in the pathway, C4, and so on. The progressive increase in the number of molecules of successive components produces a cascade reaction (Fig. 3.6). A single molecule of activated C1 generates thousands of molecules of the later components and the final response is thus greatly amplified. The later components have various biological activities, including inflammation and cell destruction, so that an immunologically specific reaction at the molecular level can lead to a relatively gross response in the tissues.

When C3b is generated it becomes bound to the antigen–antibody complex, and the whole complex can now attach to C3b receptors present on macrophages and polymorphs. Phospholipase is formed from the last components (C8 and C9), and, if the complex is on the surface of a cell, the phospholipase causes membrane damage and cell lysis.

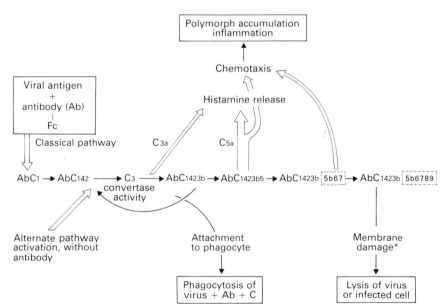

Fig. 3.6. Diagram to show complement activation sequence and antiviral actions. Unfortunately the components were numbered before this sequence of action was elucidated. Histamine release is also termed 'anaphylatoxin activity'.
*Even if the virus is not lysed, its infectivity is reduced when complement components on its surface interfere with adsorption to cells. Complement thus enhances the action of neutralising antibody.

Each activation must be terminated somehow rather than permitted to snowball. The complement sequence is therefore controlled by a number of built-in safety devices in the form of inhibitors and unstable links in the complement chain. The activated components have a short half-life and therefore cannot diffuse through the body and affect distant tissues.

The system just described is the 'classical' complement pathway. A C3 convertase can also be generated independently of antigen–antibody reactions and C142 formation by what are called 'alternate' or 'alternative' complement pathways. The alternative pathway appears to be important in viral infections (reviews: Sissons and Oldstone, 1980; Hirsch, 1982).

Activation of complement by the classical pathway, dependent on specific antigen-antibody interaction, has antiviral effects that can readily be demonstrated *in vitro* (review: Cooper, 1979).

1 Activation of complement following attachment of antibody to virus particles (Radwan and Crawford, 1974) may result in:

(1) Damage to or lysis of the envelope of enveloped virions ('virolysis') resulting in leakage or destruction of viral nucleic acid (Almeida and Waterson, 1969; Schluederberg et al., 1976).

(2) Enhancement of neutralisation of non-enveloped or enveloped viruses by antibody, probably because complement components provide further coverage of viral proteins required for attachment to susceptible cells (Oldstone et al., 1974). In some viral infections the first antibodies that are formed, which are of low avidity as well as low titre, depend on complement for neutralising activity (Yoshino and Isono, 1978; Cooper and Welsh, 1979).

(3) Opsonisation of the virus particle following which it is more readily ingested and disposed of by phagocytes (see Chapters 2 and 5). In the case of macrophages that are susceptible to infection, uptake via C3b receptors perhaps makes infection of the cells less likely.

2 Activation of complement following attachment of antibody to viral antigen on the infected cell surface may result in lysis of that cell. Sometimes this is not sufficient for cell lysis unless the alternative pathway is also activated (Sissons and Oldstone, 1980).

3 Activation following interaction of antibody with viral antigens in tissues leads to inflammation and the accumulation of leukocytes, with possible antiviral effects.

Potentiation of the effect of antibody by complement would be more likely to be important earlier in the course of infection, when antibody is of lower avidity and present in smaller quantities. Some of the above effects, however, can also be mediated following the activation of complement by the alternative pathway, independent of antibody (reviews: Sissons and Oldstone, 1980; Hirsch, 1982). Several viruses, or virus-infected cells, including Sindbis, vesicular stomatitis, measles and RS virus (Smith *et al.*, 1981), directly activate the alternative complement pathway. This is an important phenomenon because it can occur immediately after viral invasion, before immune responses have been generated.

Hence, complement-mediated lysis of infected cells and neutralisation of virus can both occur in the absence of antibody. In the case of RNA tumour viruses, antibody-independent activation of the alternative complement pathway leads to lysis of the virion (Cooper *et al.*, 1976). With Moloney leukaemia virus the C1q component of complement is known to bind the p15E viral protein (Bartholomew *et al.*, 1978). There is also evidence of a more effective activation of the alternative pathway when surface glycoproteins of enveloped viruses lack sialic acid (Hirsch *et al.*, 1981; Hirsch, 1982). The alternative pathway is activated by measles virus-infected cells in the total absence of antibody; lysis of the cells appeared to require the presence of antibody, but not of the complement-binding site, for $F(ab')_2$ was as effective as intact IgG (Sissons and Oldstone, 1980). This is true also for cells infected with mumps, parainfluenza, herpes simplex and other viruses. With measles virus-infected cells, moreover, activation of the classical pathway does not by itself lead to lysis, presumably because there is not enough membrane damage, and lysis only takes place when the alternative pathway also is activated (Cooper and Oldstone, 1983). Perhaps the density of measles virus antigens is too low; with certain other viruses, activation of the classical pathway is enough for lysis. Grewal *et al.* (1980) reported that bovine polymorphs destroy herpes simplex virus-infected bovine cells in the presence of complement, without the need for antibody; presumably, the polymorphs interact with C3b attached to the infected cell surface and kill as a result of activation of the alternative complement pathway.

Macrophages

Cells of the macrophage series play a central role in the immune response to viruses. Their role as scavenger cells, phagocytosing and degrading infectious material, but sometimes susceptible to viral infection, was described in Chapter 2. In Chapter 5 we shall see how the susceptibility of macrophages to productive or abortive infection with certain viruses can influence the susceptibility of the host, and sometimes even determine whether an animal lives or dies. Then in Chapter 6 we shall discuss the role of macrophages in maintaining certain chronic viral infections rather than eliminating them. Here, we will confine our attention to the role of macrophages in the normal immune response. Most of the antiviral activities of macrophages to be described, but not all, could not be expected to operate as effectively against viruses that have evolved the capacity to grow in macrophages and interfere with their function or destroy them.

In considering the so-called 'extrinsic' antiviral activities of macrophages, as well as their 'intrinsic' capacity to digest virions, one must appreciate that the virucidal, cytotoxic, cytostatic and monokine-secreting potential of this diverse class of cells depends very much on the genetics and age of the host, the lineage and state of differentiation of the macrophages, and their state of activation (Morahan, 1980). For instance, macrophages from different sites in the body may display quite distinct antiviral properties (Rodgers and Mims, 1981), as may subpopulations from any given site (Stuekemann *et al.*, 1982). Furthermore, macrophages attracted to the site of infection and 'activated' by lymphokines secreted by T_d lymphocytes acquire a range of new properties (Adams, 1982). These include increased powers of phagocytosis, increased killing of bacteria (Blanden and Mims, 1972), perhaps enhanced efficiency as effector cells, and a tendency towards reduced intrinsic susceptibility to viral multiplication (see Chapters 2 and 5).

Antigen presentation. Once regarded as mere 'accessory cells' of only peripheral interest to immunologists preoccupied with the central problem of immunological specificity, macrophages are now recognised as essential to the determination of that specificity, for only antigen presented in close association with I-A (or sometimes I-E) antigen on the surface of a macrophage is recognised by T_d and T_h cells, hence only in that way does the immune response commence (reviews: Unanue, 1981; Benacerraf and Germain, 1978; Berzofsky, 1980; Dutton and Swain, 1982). It is still not absolutely certain which particular cells of the macrophage/monocyte series are most efficient or most crucial in antigen presentation. Fixed tissue macrophages such as the Kupffer cells of the liver are certainly involved, but evidence is accumulating that Langerhans cells in the skin present antigen to T_h cells and that dendritic cells in lymphoid follicles present antigen to B cells to generate memory. Unlike typical macrophages, these dendritic cells are non-phagocytic and lack Fc receptors; in other respects, including morphology, they resemble macrophages and are Ia$^+$. Indeed, the central requirement is that the presenting cell must express the Ir gene-product; Ia$^-$ macrophages are not involved.

Nor is anything known about the way in which macrophages 'process' antigen before 'presenting' it on their surface. Some degree of proteolytic digestion seems to occur and perhaps some selectivity (by Ia-association?) in the display of particular peptides ('determinant selection', Unanue, 1981; Berzofsky, 1980).

Monokines. Macrophages secrete over 50 soluble products ('monokines'). One of the best known is interleukin-1, which is secreted by both Ia$^+$

and Ia$^-$ macrophages and serves as an essential signal for T cell maturation in response to antigen; this vital hormone now appears to be required for the initiation and amplification of all T cell-dependent immune responses and the inflammatory response (see Möller, 1982; Feldmann and Schreier, 1982). Another monokine is interferon, an immunomodulatory hormone and antiviral agent, discussed at length in Chapter 5.

ADCC. Macrophage-mediated ADCC (Macfarlan *et al.*, 1977; Smith and Sheppard, 1982), mentioned briefly above, is a mechanism whereby these non-specific effectors, once 'armed' with antibody, can specifically kill virus-infected targets. For some viruses the effectiveness of ADCC is enhanced by the fact that macrophages bind directly to viral glycoprotein on the cell surface (Macfarlan and White, 1984).

Direct cytotoxicity. There are indications that adherent, macrophage-like cells can at times preferentially destroy virus-infected cells in the absence of specific antibody. This was shown for vaccinia and herpes simplex virus-infected cells (Chapes and Tompkins, 1979). Similar observations were made with influenza A and Sendai virus-infected target cells by Mak *et al.* (1982), using effector cells more convincingly identified as macrophages. However, the fact that these cells, which acquired maximum cytotoxicity only five days after infection, displayed a degree of immunological specificity (in that they lysed target cells infected with a heterologous serotype of influenza virus considerably less efficiently) suggests that they were armed with antibody and acting via ADCC. In contrast, Letvin *et al.* (1982) showed that macrophages from uninfected mice attach to the haemagglutinin (σ_1 protein) on reovirus type 1 (but not type 3) infected cells, and lyse those cells.

Prevention of viral spread. Macrophages appear to be able to block cell-to-cell spread of herpes simplex virus in monolayers without destroying the cells (Notkins, 1974) and even in the presence of anti-interferon serum (Hayashi *et al.*, 1980; Morse and Morahan, 1981). The mechanism is obscure but may be attributable to reversible inhibition of host metabolism as seems to occur in the 'cytostatic' effect of macrophages on tumour cells. Recently, Wildy *et al.* (1982a) put forward an explanation applicable specifically to herpesviruses, namely that arginase, secreted by macrophages, deprives the cells of arginine essential for the growth of these viruses.

Natural killer cells

Natural killer (NK) cells are immunologically non-specific leukocytes with the capacity to kill tumour cells, virus-infected cells and, to a lesser extent, some normal cells (reviews: Welsh, 1978; Welsh *et al.*, 1979; Haller, 1981; Herberman and Ortaldo, 1981). In 1977 it was discovered that NK cell activity is greatly enhanced within 1–2 days of infection by viruses (Macfarlan *et al.*, 1977; Welsh, 1978; Herberman and Ortaldo, 1981). Virus-induced NK cell activation was subsequently demonstrated to be mediated via interferon (Gidlund *et al.*, 1978; Trinchieri and Santoli, 1978), or directly via viral glycoprotein (Härvast *et al.*, 1980; Casali *et al.*, 1981).

The NK cell has yet to be fully characterised. Indeed there appear to be several types of NK cell; cloned NK cell lines show different surface markers and differ in their ability to kill tumour cells and virus-transformed cells (Hercend *et al.*, 1983). Most 'endogenous' (non-activated) NK cells are small-to-medium lymphocytes which, upon activation, undergo blastogenesis to large, granular lymphocytes, comprising about 5% of the total splenic or peripheral blood leukocytes (Biron and Welsh, 1982). Sensitivity to ^{89}Sr indicates a bone-marrow origin, but the precise lineage is still a mystery. It is not even known whether NK cells differentiate from T lymphocyte or myelomonocytic precursors. They are quite distinct from B lymphocytes, being Ig$^-$, and are certainly not typical T lymphocytes as they are plentiful in athymic mice, though they have been reported to express small amounts of T lymphocyte markers, e.g. Thy 1 in the mouse (Herberman and Ortaldo, 1981), and can differentiate from Ly2$^+$ T cells (Shortman *et al.*, 1983). Nor are they macrophages as they are non-phagocytic and only somewhat adherent to surfaces, but they can (weakly) express Fc receptors for IgG and may at times be capable of acting as K cells via ADCC.

The spontaneous, relatively non-specific cytotoxicity of NK cells is rapidly and dramatically augmented by interferon-inducers, especially viruses. Virus-infected cells and cancer cells are in general, but not exclusively, more susceptible to NK-mediated cytolysis than are normal cells. The basis of this partial selectivity is completely unknown. Recent work suggests that the transferrin receptor, ubiquitous in proliferating metabolically active cells, can be the target for NK-mediated cytolysis (Vodinelich *et al.*, 1983). NK cells do not need to recognise MHC antigens, nor to be armed with antibody, and they certainly demonstrate almost no immunological specificity as we generally understand it. While it is tempting to surmise that they represent the first line of defence against viral infections, persuasive *in vivo* evidence to support such a role is not currently available (see p. 123).

IMMUNOLOGICAL FACTORS IN RECOVERY FROM VIRAL INFECTION

If there is to be recovery from a viral infection it is first necessary that viral multiplication is brought under control. The number of virus particles must be reduced, their spread through the body stopped, or the damage they inflict prevented. The mechanisms leading to recovery from a primary infection are not the same as those responsible for resistance to reinfection. For instance, antibody to measles virus is of prime importance in resistance to reinfection, and susceptible children can be passively protected by injecting antibody; but antibody plays only a small part in recovery from initial infection with measles virus, whereas T cell-mediated immune mechanisms are crucial.

Antibody, CMI, complement, phagocytes and interferon are involved in the response to all viral infections and are together responsible for recovery. These components, illustrated diagrammatically in Fig. 3.7, all normally operate together, and to some extent any attempt to assess their relative importance is an artificial exercise. In only a few instances have the different components been dissected out and separately evaluated. For instance, macrophages play a vital role in both the induction and the expression of CMI. But it has proved remarkably difficult to assign a determinative role *in vivo* for most of the many antiviral immunological mechanisms discussed above. Of course, the fact that a particular cell, substance or phenomenon is unequivocally demonstrated to produce antiviral effects in culture does not shed any light on its importance *in vivo*. The reductionist approach simply allows us to analyse the phenomenon in isolation using relatively defined reagents. Having alerted ourselves in this way to the potential importance of the mechanism in question we must return to the living animal for proof of its biological reality. Yet even this is not sufficient. The fact that one can save the life of an animal by adoptive transfer of primed cytotoxic T

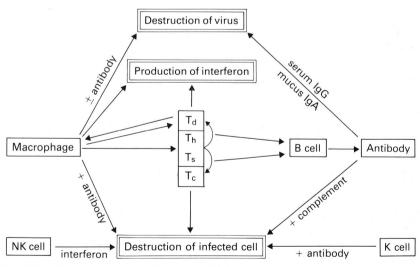

Fig. 3.7. Immune response to virus infection.

cells is dramatic indeed, but does not establish the *relative* importance of this cell in recovery under natural circumstances. For instance, the dosage, timing or state of activation of the artificially transferred cells may be quite out of proportion to the natural counterpart. Or the transferred cell may have a second, more crucial effect or function *in vivo*, or secrete an unknown product. Indeed, the cell may be capable of curing infection yet be of negligible importance in natural infection compared with another mechanism not currently under test.

Various experimental approaches have been used to attack this refractory problem, most of them subject to the reservations expressed above. The first is the least subject to laboratory artefacts, namely simple clinical observation of the occurrence and progress of viral infections in children or animals suffering from congenital immunodeficiencies. There are many such diseases but few of them present as a 'pure' T or B cell deficit. Athymic ('nude') mice, which have almost no T cells, have been widely used to evaluate T cell responses, but T-dependent antibody responses are also affected, and the increased NK activity of these mice must be taken into account. Similarly, attempts have been made to selectively remove one arm of the immune response, but it is often difficult to eliminate one component without affecting the others. For instance, cyclophosphamide and antithymocyte serum have been used to eliminate antibody synthesis and CMI responses respectively, and have provided useful information, but these treatments lack precision, and such experiments often leave ambiguities. An alternative strategy is to ablate completely all immune potential, and then add back one or more of the separate components. Adult mice are thymectomised to eliminate the source of T cells, X-irradiated to eliminate lymphoid cells, and then reconstituted with bone marrow cells to restore haematopoiesis. The separate components of the immune response can now be restored to these animals and the effect on resistance to virus infections studied (Blanden, 1974; Park *et al.*, 1981). But even this heroic type of experimentation has its disadvantages.

Furthermore, it cannot be assumed that all immune responses are useful. They often contribute to pathological changes, and in extreme cases are responsible for severe disease and death, as in the case of adult mice infected with LCM virus. These immunopathological features of viral infection are described in Chapter 4. Also, in many acute viral infections there is a marked although generally temporary depression of antibody or cell-mediated responses to unrelated antigens (Notkins *et al.*, 1970). These are generally viruses that infect lymphocytes or macrophages. It has long been known that when tuberculin-positive individuals develop measles, they temporarily became tuberculin-negative, and that measles exacerbates pre-existing tuberculosis (Christensen *et al.*, 1953). Experimentally, mice infected with LCM (Mims and Wainwright, 1968) or cytomegalovirus (Osborn *et al.*, 1968) for instance, show

reduced capacity to give a primary antibody response to the immu-
nologist's favourite antigen, sheep erythrocytes. Secondary responses
and cell-mediated responses (Howard *et al.*, 1974) can also be affected.

Cell-mediated immunity

The evidence that CMI in general is important in recovery from virus
infections is derived especially from laboratory mice but also from other
species including man. Tissue infiltrates bear the hallmark of CMI: lymphocytes and macrophages. T cell depletion by neonatal thymectomy or
antilymphocyte serum treatment of mice has been shown to increase
susceptibility to ectromelia, herpes simplex, cytomegalovirus, coxsackievirus and other infections (Allison, 1972; Blanden, 1974). Athymic
(nude) mice which are congenitally deficient in T cells are more susceptible to these viral infections. Human beings with severe CMI defects due
to thymic aplasia, lymphoreticular neoplasms (e.g. Hodgkin's disease)
or post-transplant immunosuppression, show increased susceptibility
to vaccinia, varicella-zoster, CMV, HSV, measles and other viral infections. Infants with thymic aplasia suffer from severe CMI deficiency,
although there is a normal antibody response to many antigens. When
they are infected with measles virus there is no rash but an uncontrolled
and progressive growth of virus in the respiratory tract, leading to fatal
giant cell pneumonia (Nahmias *et al.*, 1967). Evidently, in the normal
child, the CMI response controls infection in the lung and also plays a
vital role in the development of the characteristic skin rash. In normal
individuals infected with measles virus, cytotoxic T cells appear (Kreth
et al., 1979), but virus-specific DTH responses have not been studied.
When children are vaccinated against smallpox with vaccinia virus, the
virus grows in epidermal cells at the inoculation site until an immune
inflammatory response at the edges of the lesion after 6–8 days leads to
inhibition of virus growth. The infant with thymic aplasia, however,
does not show this response and the destructive skin lesion continues to
enlarge, occupying an ever-increasing area of the arm and shoulder.
These infants also tend to suffer severe generalised infection with
herpes simplex virus.

There are three or four infections of mice in which the role of CMI
has been well studied. These examples will be discussed to illustrate the
various experimental approaches. Constraints of space compel us to be
highly selective.

Mice show greatly increased susceptibility to ectromelia virus when
T cells are depleted by treatment with antilymphocyte serum (Blanden,
1970). Ectromelia virus normally causes focal liver necrosis (see Chapter
2), but in T cell-depleted mice there is a failure to develop inflammatory
mononuclear cell infiltrations in foci of infection in the liver. The virus
then continues to grow, destroying hepatic cells and causing extensive

liver necrosis and death, in spite of the production of antiviral antibodies and interferon. If immune T cells are transferred to such T-depleted infected animals, there is a prompt cellular infiltration into the foci of infection (Blanden, 1971b) with inhibition of virus growth (Blanden, 1971a). This is partly due to killing of infected hepatic cells by cytotoxic T cells (Blanden and Gardner, 1976), but it was found that the recipient mice were not fully protected if they were irradiated prior to the cell transfer. This appeared to be because (radiation-sensitive) circulating monocytes were necessary for the full expression of the antiviral effect, being recruited into infectious foci presumably following lymphokine production by sensitised T_d cells. In other words, T_d cells and macrophages as well as T_c cells were important.

In the case of LCM virus in mice, where T cell responses can at times be the cause of death (see Chapter 4), it has been shown that immune spleen cells also reduce virus titres when transferred to infected recipients (Blanden and Mims, 1972). The type of T cell responsible for the antiviral effect has not been identified, although it is probably not a cytotoxic T cell (Varho *et al.*, 1981).

The role of CMI has also been extensively studied in herpes simplex virus infection of mice. Early work drew attention to the importance of macrophages (Zisman *et al.*, 1970) and immune spleen cells (Ennis, 1973), but subsequent attempts to dissect out the different components in host resistance have given a complex and at times confusing picture. Cyclophosphamide-treated mice show increased growth of virus in target organs (Rager-Zisman and Allison, 1976). This was prevented by transferring immune spleen cells, the active cells being T cells, as indicated by their sensitivity to antitheta serum plus complement. There was also slight protection when immune serum was given to cyclophosphamide-treated mice, and this was thought to depend on the presence of adherent cells (macrophages). More recently Nash *et al.* (1980) took cells from local lymph nodes after ear infection of mice and transfused them intravenously to mice similarly infected in the ear; titres in the inoculated ear were reduced by up to 1000-fold. But the same group of workers also showed that mice depleted of B cells by injection of antibody to IgM controlled the local infection, but failed to restrict the spread of virus to nerve ganglia as did untreated infected mice (Kapoor *et al.*, 1982a); the treated mice developed no neutralising antibody, but normal DTH responses. Studies on athymic (nude) mice led to similar conclusions about the role of antibody and CMI (Kapoor *et al.*, 1982b). Evidently antibody as well as DTH must be assigned a role in the particular infection, as was also suggested by Worthington *et al.* (1980). Antiviral T_c are said to be not readily demonstrable in herpes simplex-infected mice unless the mice are treated with cyclophosphamide to eliminate suppressors of the T_c response (Pfizenmaier *et al.*, 1977). Nevertheless, Howes *et al.* (1979) studied the H2 restrictions on the transfer of resistance to herpes simplex virus infection by spleen cells. They showed that for early protection (weeks) KD or I region sharing by donor and recipient was necessary, indicating that T_c or T_h or T_d cells were involved. For long-term protection (months), however, I region sharing was necessary, and it was suggested that T_h cells were involved, either by helping antibody production or helping with the generation of other types of T cells. Later evidence (Favila *et al.*, 1982) suggested that the cells operated together with macrophages, or by secreting interferon and activating NK cells. Mice can be made much more susceptible to intraperitoneally injected herpes simplex virus when depleted of macrophages (Zisman *et al.*, 1970) or closely related cells by treatment with ^{89}Sr (Lopez *et al.*, 1980). In their ear infection model, Nash and his colleagues (Nash *et al.*, 1981; Nash and Ashford, 1982) concluded that I and KD sharing was necessary for antiviral defence. The I restriction was explained by suggesting that DTH (rather than helper cells) had a local antiviral action early after infection, the KD restriction accounting for T_c-mediated effects at a later stage. When cloned herpesvirus-specific T_c are adoptively transferred they protect mice from fatal infection (Sethi *et al.*, 1983).

Finally, to make matters even more confusing, Zawatsky *et al.* (1979) reported that T-deficient nude mice of the B6 strain are as resistant to herpes simplex virus infection as their normal litter mates, suggesting that mature T cells are *not* important in antiviral resistance! These workers produced evidence that in this strain of mouse, interferon production was the important factor (Zawatsky *et al.*, 1981), as also indicated by the studies of Lopez (1981). These results, however, were obtained following IP infection of mice and early (non-immune) host defences might be more important following this route of infection than in the ear infection studied by Nash and his colleagues. Further studies will doubtless explain these differences. These conflicting data have been presented partly to illustrate the technical and conceptual difficulties confronting viral immunologists, but equally to emphasise that, in herpes simplex virus infection of mice, host defence mechanisms are complex, depending on the route of infection, age and possibly strain of mouse and strain of virus studied. It is also naive to suppose that the factors responsible for the greater susceptibility of young mice are going to be the same as those responsible for the greater susceptibility of certain strains of mice or that the same factors will determine susceptibility to infection by both the dermal and intraperitoneal route. But T_h, T_c, T_d, antibody, interferon and macrophages have each at some stage or other been invoked. Doubtless they normally operate together, and indeed, antibody and interferon act synergistically in controlling herpes simplex virus replication *in vitro* (Langford *et al.*, 1983), but their relative importance may vary with the circumstances.

CMI defences are undoubtedly important also in resistance to another herpesvirus, cytomegalovirus. In man, when the defences of kidney transplant patients are weakened by immunosuppression, CMV infections are common, with viraemia, fever, and sometimes hepatitis or pneumonitis. This is usually due to reactivation of latent infection; a role for CMI in the control of latent infections will be discussed in Chapter 6. CMI has also been shown to be important in the resistance of mice to primary infection with mouse CMV (Starr and Allison, 1977). Cytotoxic T cells can be demonstrated (Quinnan et al., 1978), DTH is generated (Chong and Mims, 1982) and NK cells are activated (Shellam et al., 1980). We still have little information as to which of these are the most important.

The other virus that has been extensively investigated is influenza (see also Chapter 2). There are substantial differences between the human infection (Couch and Kasel, 1983) and the model infection in mice. Yap et al. (1978) showed that mice could be protected against intranasal challenge by intravenous transfer of immune K/D-restricted T cells, and it was concluded that T_c cells were responsible. Protection conferred in this way is not attributable to NK activity (Wells et al., 1983). However, while it is generally true that T_c are K/D-restricted, and T_h and T_d only I-restricted (Ertl, 1981), it has recently become clear that some T_d cells are K/D, not I, restricted (Zinkernagel, 1976; Ada et al., 1981). Indeed, Leung and Ada (1981) have shown that 'class II' T cells, which are K/D-restricted, Lyt $1^-2^+3^+$ and include cells with T_d and T_c activity, protect mice against influenza, whereas 'class I' T cells, which are I-restricted, Lyt $1^+2^-3^-$, and include cells with T_d and T_h activity, accelerate the death of infected mice. The complexity of the situation is underlined by the finding of Lin and Askonas (1980) that a cloned influenza HA-specific T_c cell line which conferred protection upon adoptive transfer in vivo, as well as lysing influenza-infected target cells in vitro, was subsequently found also to confer DTH skin reactivity to influenza virus (Lin and Askonas, 1981) and to produce interferon after exposure to influenza virus-infected cells in vitro (Morris et al., 1982), so leaving open the question of whether in vivo protection is attributable to T_c, T_d or interferon. This multipotentiality of cloned T cells is a surprise, and needs to be confirmed. Only the systematic examination of the whole range of biological properties of many such clones in vivo and in vitro will reveal whether surface markers as determined with mono-clonal antibodies, or the type of MHC restriction, can reliably identify the physiological phenotype of a T cell, whether T_c and other T cell classes also carry T_d potential, and whether DTH plays an essential role in recovery from infections with viruses. These considerations apply also to the reported transfer of resistance to herpes simplex in mice by means of cloned herpes simplex-specific cytotoxic T cells (Sethi et al., 1983).

Although there is suggestive evidence that natural killer cells are important in defence against viral infection, particularly during the first couple of days, before T_c and antibody emerge, their role is still uncertain. Beige mice, for instance, show little or no NK activity and are about twice as susceptible to mouse CMV in spite of producing higher interferon responses than non-beige mice (Shellam *et al.*, 1980). Also Quinnan *et al.* (1982) showed that hydrocortisone-treated mice, with depressed NK but normal antibody, CMI and interferon responses, were more susceptible to MCMV. On the other hand, B10.BR mice, which generate low NK activity, are nevertheless resistant to MCMV (Bancroft *et al.*, 1981), and nude (T cell deficient) mice with high NK activity are very susceptible to MCMV. But interferon, although it induces increased NK cell activity, has an independent antiviral effect on the susceptible cell (Chong *et al.*, 1983). It is not easy to interpret such experiments because resistance mechanisms are probably multiple, and differ according to the strain of mouse. For instance, although nude CBA mice are 16 times more susceptible to CMV than normal CBA mice, they are still no more susceptible than normal Balb/c mice (Grundy and Melief, 1982). A general antiviral role for NK cells seems doubtful when it is seen that by no means all cells acquire increased susceptibility to NK lysis following infection with viruses (Welsh and Hallenbeck, 1980). On the other hand, some of the evidence for NK cells is persuasive (Bukowski *et al.*, 1983), and in any case there seems no reason why NK cells should be equally important in all viral infections. Indeed, mice depleted of NK cells by treatment with NK-specific antiserum show greatly increased replication of some viruses (mouse CMV, mouse hepatitis virus, vaccinia) but not others (LCM virus). These experiments provide very strong evidence for the importance of NK cells in certain viral infections.

Although it is to be expected that the separate contributions of T_c, T_d and NK cells to antiviral defence will soon be elucidated, the picture could at the same time become more complex, as for example, if T_c are capable of mediating DTH and liberating interferon.

Antibody, complement and interferon

Viruses producing systemic disease characterised by a 'plasma' viraemia, appear to be controlled principally by circulating antibody. This is so in yellow fever or poliomyelitis virus infections. Children with severe hypogammaglobulinaemia recover normally from measles or varicella, or from smallpox vaccination, but are about 10 000 times more likely than normal individuals to develop paralytic disease after vaccination with live poliovirus vaccine (Wyatt, 1973). They have normal CMI and interferon responses, normal phagocytic cells and complement, but cannot produce antibody, which is essential if viral spread to the central nervous system via the bloodstream is to be prevented. The poliovirus infection is of a chronic type in these children because there is also impaired clearance of virus from the brain, in spite of inflammatory responses in affected areas.

Mice become susceptible to intraperitoneally inoculated yellow fever virus when immunosuppressed by cyclophosphamide. Circulating virus then localises in the brain, multiples and causes death. Such cyclophosphamide-treated mice are protected if specific antibody is administered (Zisman *et al.*, 1971). In mice infected intravenously with yellow fever virus, viral invasion of the brain and death were enhanced when macrophages were damaged by treatment with silica. Passively administered antibody, however, still protected by controlling viraemia and preventing infection of the target organ, the brain (Zisman *et al.*, 1971). In a careful study with another togavirus, Sindbis, adult thymectomised, irradiated mice were infected intracerebrally and the protective effect of different factors tested by selective reconstitution of the mice (Park *et al.*, 1981). It was concluded that antibodies as well as macrophages and T cells helped to clear virus from the brain. Even without reconstitution, however, there was a considerable antiviral effect in these mice, indicating that other factors, such as endogenous interferon, were important.

Interesting recent work shows that interferon can act synergistically with specific antibody in controlling infection (Langford *et al.*, 1983). The yield from cells infected with coxsackie A24 and certain other viruses was reduced by either antibody or interferon, but when both were present the antiviral effect was up to a thousand times greater than the sum of their separate effects. Furthermore the protective effect of antiviral antibody was greatly reduced in the presence of antibody to interferon, suggesting that interferon produced by the infected cells enhances the action of antibody. The mechanisms are not known.

In general, antibodies are thought to play a major role in recovery from togavirus, picornavirus and papovavirus infections. But their protective action often depends on the presence of macrophages (Woodruff, 1979), as Rager-Zisman and Allison (1976) had previously found with the herpes simplex virus. Kohl and Loo (1982) have interpreted somewhat analogous data to demonstrate a role for ADCC *in vivo*. They showed that infant mice could be protected against lethal HSV infection after transfer of subneutralising amounts of antibody only if accompanied by normal *human* leukocytes, which, unlike leukocytes from *newborn* mice, can mediate ADCC. On the other hand, Schmaljohn *et al.* (1982) have presented very interesting data which they interpret to support an *in vivo* role for antibody-complement mediated cytolysis. Monoclonal antibody to the E1 glycoprotein of Sindbis virus, which induces complement-mediated lysis of infected cells *in vitro* just as efficiently as does neutralizing antibody directed against the E2 glycoprotein, fails to neutralise virus *in vitro* but protects *in vivo*. Monoclonal antibody studies with Semliki Forest (Boere *et al.*, 1983) and herpes simplex (Balachandran *et al.*, 1982) viruses also suggest a protective role for non-neutralising antibody.

Viral infections that are limited to epithelial surfaces and do not undergo a time-consuming spread of infection through the body have incubation periods of no more than a few days. There is little opportunity for the slowly evolving immune responses to play an important role in recovery, and viral replication is often stopped before there has been a detectable IgA response. On the other hand, it must be remembered that antibodies (IgG or IgA) can be produced locally within a few days after experimental respiratory tract infections, and they would not be detected routinely if bound to viral antigens at this stage. A discussion of antibody and other responses in recovery from infection with influenza virus was given at the end of Chapter 2. Secretory IgA antibodies may aid recovery if the infection lingers on, but it seems probable that interferon, which is produced locally from the outset may be the more important element in recovery. The possible role of T cells has been discussed above.

How important is the complement system *in vivo*? When mice were C3-depleted by treatment with cobra venom factor they showed increased severity of Sindbis and influenza virus infections. In Sindbis virus infection there was prolonged viraemia and increased virus titres in the brain, but the mortality was not affected. Sindbis was also studied in a C5-deficient mouse strain (Hirsch *et al.*, 1980) but these mice showed increased organ titres without any effect on the level of viraemia. C5-deficient mice, or mice treated with cobra venom factor (C3-depleted), showed increased virus titres in the lung and increased mortality following infection with influenza virus (Hicks *et al.*, 1978). While these results suggest a key role for complement in recovery from viral infections *in vivo*, the matter is still unresolved.

Unfortunately there are no studies in man that demonstrate the importance of complement in antiviral resistance. It is often difficult to distinguish between changes in the consumption, activation, synthesis or catabolism of complement components, and the picture is complicated by the extravasation of complement components (Hirsch, 1982). In general, patients with complement deficiency do not show increased susceptibility to viral infections.

IMMUNITY TO REINFECTION

Whereas a plethora of interacting phenomena may contribute to recovery from viral infection, the mechanism of acquired immunity to reinfection with the same agent is probably much simpler. The first line of defence is antibody. If this succeeds in neutralising the challenge, that is the end of the matter. Only if the antibody defences are breached does infection become established; under these circumstances the several mechanisms that contribute to recovery are called into play again, the principal differences on this second occasion being that (1) the dose of infecting virus has been reduced by antibody, and (2) preprimed memory T and B lymphocytes generate a more rapid ('anamnestic') response.

There is abundant evidence of the efficacy of antibody in preventing infection. Passive immunisation with antibody parenterally protects man very satisfactorily against challenge with measles, polio, rabies or hepatitis A virus (see Chapter 7). Furthermore, passive immunity is routinely transmitted from mother to child via maternal antibodies which cross the placenta and protect the newborn infant against most of the infections that the mother experienced. There is also transfer of secretory IgA antibodies via the milk; transfer in colostrum (early milk) is a particularly important route in cows, sheep, horses and other animals in which there is no placental transfer. This maternal 'umbrella' of antibodies lasts for about six months in man, hence the infant encounters many viral infections while still partially protected. Under these circumstances the virus multiplies, but only to a limited extent, stimulating an immune response without causing significant disease. The infant thus acquires active immunity while partially protected by maternal immunity.

Passive immunity acquired from the mother lasts only a few months because of the limited life of immunoglobulin *in vivo*. In contrast, the antibody acquired by active infection with systemic viruses such as measles or polio continues to be synthesised for the life of the individual, and protects against reinfection for many years. This lasting immunity is attributable to serum IgG, which must be encountered during the viraemic stage of reinfection with these viruses.

As a general rule the secretory IgA antibody response is short-lived compared to the serum IgG response. One factor is that secretory IgA antibodies are exported to the outside world, whereas IgG accumulates in the blood as it is produced. Accordingly, resistance to reinfection with respiratory viruses tends to be short-lived. Repeated attacks of common colds or influenza reflect infection with antigenically distinct strains of virus, but even with particular serotypes of parainfluenza virus or with respiratory syncytial virus, reinfections are common.

The immune response to the first infection with a virus can have a dominating influence on subsequent immune responses to antigenically related viruses. The second virus often induces a response that is directed mainly against the antigens of the original virus strain. Thus, the immune response of a human to sequential infections with different strains of influenza type A is dominated by antibody to the antigens characterising the particular strain of influenza type A he first experienced. This phenomenon is called 'original antigenic sin' (Francis, 1955) and is seen not only in influenza but also in enterovirus, paramyxovirus and togavirus infections. The immunological basis or original antigenic sin remains unexplained. It has important implications for interpretation of seroepidemiological studies, for immunopathology (Chapter 4), and particularly for vaccination strategy against diseases such as influenza, under which heading the subject is discussed further in Chapter 7.

SUMMARY

Viruses are powerful immunogens. A single encounter, even sub-clinical, with a virus producing generalised infection, e.g. measles, leads to lifelong production of specific IgG antibody which confers lasting immunity to reinfection with that agent. In contrast, acquired immunity following superficial infections of epithelial surfaces is attributable to specific antibody of the IgA class secreted into the mucus, and is con-siderably less durable. Moreover, respiratory viruses tend to undergo antigenic 'drift' and 'shift', generating a plethora of different strains that display little or no cross-protection.

Sophisticated studies of the amino acid sequence and tertiary structure of the HA molecule of influenza virus mutants arising spontaneously in the field or selected in the laboratory by monoclonal antibodies have provided new insights into the nature of viral antigenic determinants (epitopes). Monoclonal antibodies recognising certain antigenic sites may neutralise the infectivity of the virion by steric hin-drance of its adsorption to the host cell. More commonly, however, neutralising antibodies act upon a later step, e.g. 'fusion' of the viral envelope with the plasma membrane, or with lysosomes at pH 5. Neutralisation of viruses can be augmented by complement or by 'enhancing' antibody binding to novel epitopes on the virion–antibody complex.

In contrast with acquired immunity to reinfection, recovery from first infection is usually not attributable to antibody. Recovery is generally a much more complicated process involving 'cell-mediated immunity' (T cells, macrophages, NK cells), complement, interferons and other lymphokines, as well as antibody.

Cytotoxic T (T_c) cells are Lyt $1^-2^+3^+$ lymphocytes which recognise viral antigen only in association with the glycoprotein coded by the K, D or L gene of the mouse H-2 complex (HLA-A, B or C in man). The molecular mechanism of this 'associative recognition' (or 'MHC restric-tion') is still uncertain. The T cell may carry two distinct receptors (one recognising the MHC and the other separately recognising the viral antigen), or only one (recognising both epitopes, situated close together, or alternatively recognising a composite epitope, or 'neoantigenic determinant' spanning the putative viral-MHC complex). The appropri-ate clones of T_c lymphocytes expand rapidly following encounter with virus-infected cells, reaching a peak of activity after about a week. Because newly synthesised virus-coded proteins are present in the plasma membrane of infected cells before any virions have been produced, destruction of such vulnerable targets by T_c lymphocytes, or indeed by other mechanisms of immune cytolysis (see below), greatly reduces the yield of infectious virus. Adoptive transfer of virus-specific T_c cells to syngeneic infected animals under appropriate experimental conditions can save their lives. This strongly suggests that cytotoxic T cells play a major role in recovery from viral infection.

Another type of T lymphocyte, the T_d cell, has an important role to play in the phenomenon known classically as delayed-type hypersensitivity (DTH). The principal partner in DTH is the macrophage which phagocytoses the incoming virus or virus–antibody complex. After 'processing', viral antigens, presumably in the form of shorter peptides, are 'presented' on the surface of macrophages, dendritic cells or Langerhans cells, in association with Ia antigen in the mouse (D/DR in man). The Ia–viral antigen complex is recognised by Lyt $1^+2^-3^-$ T_d lymphocytes, which respond by proliferating and releasing lymphokines that in turn attract macrophages to the site and induce them to proliferate. Recent studies with T cell clones have revealed that Lyt $1^-2^+3^+$ T_c cells can also mediate DTH. It is generally assumed that DTH is 'a good thing', in that it effectively launches, focusses and augments the immune response via secretion of numerous lymphokines (including interferons) which not only attract macrophages to the danger area but also activate other lymphocytes. However, the resulting infiltration of cells can cause problems and may even be lethal in organs such as lung or brain. Perhaps this is why the DTH response is eventually turned off by suppressor T cells.

Helper T (T_h) cells, also Ly 1^+, also recognise viral antigen presented in conjunction with the I-A (or I-E) gene-product on cells of the macrophage series. Following activation by interleukin 1 (IL-1) they secrete several lymphokines known as 'helper factors' (T_hF). Helper factors fall into two broad classes: antigen-specific and non-specific, e.g. IL-2. Antigen-specific T_hF contain a 'variable' region with specificity for antigen, and a 'constant' region, which is the I-A or I-E gene-product. These T_hF trigger the appropriate clones of B lymphocytes, following binding of viral antigen, to divide and differentiate into antibody-secreting plasma cells.

Suppressor T (T_s) cells regulate the immune response by turning off the effector T cells (T_h, T_c, T_d) after they have fulfilled their function and are no longer needed. The classical $T_{s(2)}$ cell was defined by the surface markers, Lyt $1^-2^+3^+$, I-J$^+$. However, it now appears that this is but one important subset of T_s lymphocytes in a complex pathway. Furthermore, whereas some clones of T_s cells and the factors (T_sF) they secrete are Id$^+$, i.e. bind antigen, others are anti-idiotypic, i.e. bind the antigen-binding site (idiotype) of specific antiviral antibody or of the specific receptor on lymphocytes. Such Id/anti-Id interactions contribute to an intricate web of positive and negative feed-back controls that regulate all aspects of the immune response.

Several more types of cells are involved in the immune response to viral infection even though, unlike T and B lymphocytes, they lack immunological specificity. The seminal role of cells of the macrophage series in Ia-linked presentation of antigen to lymphocytes has been described, as has their phagocytic function and their secretion of monokines. Macrophages can also inhibit cell-to-cell spread of certain viruses, or destroy cells infected with certain viruses *in vitro*. Moreover, when 'armed' with virus-specific antibody, they can lyse virus-infected cells. This phenomenon, known as 'antibody-dependent cell-mediated cytotoxicity' (ADCC), can also be mediated by other cells bearing Fc receptors, notably polymorphs and K cells.

NK (natural killer) cells are immunologically non-specific leukocytes with the capacity to kill tumour cells, virus-infected cells and to a lesser extent, some normal cells. NK cell activity is greatly enhanced within 1–2 days of viral infection. We still know relatively little about their lineage, the basis of their partial selectivity, or their importance in resistance to or recovery from viral disease.

Antibody may contribute to recovery from an established viral infection by pathways other than neutralisation of the infectivity of the virion. Like cytotoxic T cells, antibody can mediate lysis of virus-infected cells (immune cytolysis). ADCC is one such mechanism. The other involves complement rather than non-specific effector cells; binding of antibody to the cell surface triggers the classical complement cascade. The alternative complement pathway may be even more important. Indeed, with certain viruses, complement-mediated lysis of infected cells, neutralisation of virus, and lysis of enveloped virions ('virolysis') can all occur in the absence of antibody.

Though almost all the mechanisms described above have been demonstrated to exert antiviral effects *in vivo* as well as in cultured cells, the relative importance of the contribution each of them makes to the final result is extremely difficult to ascertain, and almost certainly differs from virus to virus, perhaps even from host to host. Furthermore, since immune responses generally depend upon cooperative interplay between different cell types, often via soluble mediators, it is perhaps naive to imagine that we will ever be able to assign a determinative role to T_c cells, T_d cells, NK cells, macrophages, antibody or interferon alone in the case of any viral infection. Nevertheless, useful experimental approaches have included: (1) observation of the occurrence and progress of viral infections in children or animals suffering from congenital immunodeficiencies; (2) ablation of all immune potential by lethal whole-body irradiation and thymectomy, followed by selective reconstitution by adoptive transfer of bone marrow cells and any antigen-primed or unprimed purified cell population one wishes to test; (3) *in vitro* and *in vivo* analysis of the immunological repertoire and physiological potential of cloned populations of T or B cells and monoclonal antibodies. While these and other techniques have clearly established the validity of a number of important phenomena, they have not yet enabled us to be dogmatic about the predominance of any given cell, or indeed any given mechanism, in recovery from viral infection. Such progress as has been made is illustrated by brief descriptions of the cardinal findings with certain viruses that have become popular models for immunological investigations in mice, notably ectromelia, LCM, herpes simplex, cytomegalovirus, Sindbis and influenza.

SELECTED READING

Ada, G. L., Leung, K. N., and Ertl, H. (1981). An analysis of effector T cell generation and function in mice exposed to influenza A or Sendai viruses. *Immunol. Rev.* **58**, 5.

Benacerraf, B. and Germain, R. (1978). The immune response genes of the major histocompatibility complex. *Immunol. Rev.* **38**, 70.

Blanden, R. V. (1974). T cell response to viral and bacterial infection. *Transplant. Rev.* **19**, 56.

Burns, W. H. and Allison, A. C. (1975). Virus infections and the immune responses they elicit. In *The Antigens* (ed. M. Sela), vol. 3, 480–574. Academic Press, New York.

Cantor, H. and Gershon, G. K. (1979). Immunological circuits: cellular composition. *Fed. Proc.* **38**, 2058.

Cooper, N. R. (1979). Humoral immunity to viruses. In *Comprehensive Virology* (eds. H. Fraenkel-Conrat and R. R. Wagner), vol. 15, p. 123. Plenum Press, New York.

Doherty, P. C., Blanden, R. V., and Zinkernagel, R. M. (1976). Specificity of virus-immune effector T cells for H-2K or H-2D compatible interactions: implications for H-antigen diversity. *Transplant. Rev.* **29**, 89.

Dutton, R. W. and Swain, S. L. (1982). Regulation of the immune response: T-cell interactions. *Crit. Rev. Immunol.* **3**, 209.

Fougereau, M. and Dausset, J. (eds.) (1980). *Immunology 80.* Academic Press, New York.

Mandel, B. (1979). Interaction of viruses with neutralizing antibodies. In *Comprehensive Virology* (eds. H. Fraenkel-Conrat and R. R. Wagner), vol. 15, p. 37. Plenum Press, New York.

Möller, G. (ed.) (1974). The Immune Response to Infectious Diseases. *Transplant. Rev.* **19**.

Möller, G. (ed.) (1981a). T Cell Clones. *Immunol. Rev.* **54**.

Möller, G. (ed.) (1981b). MHC Restriction of Anti-Viral Immunity. *Immunol. Rev.* **58**.

Möller, G. (ed.) (1982). Interleukins and Lymphocyte Activation. *Immunol. Rev.* **63**.

Nahmias, A. J. and O'Reilly. R. J. (1982). Immunology of Human Infection, Part 2. Viruses. In *Comprehensive Immunology*, vol. 9. Plenum Press, New York.

Notkins, A. L. (ed.) (1975). *Viral Immunology and Immunopathology*. Academic Press, New York.

Oldstone, M. B. A., Fujinami, R. S., and Lampert, P. W. (1980). Membrane and cytoplasmic changes in virus-infected cells induced by interactions of antiviral antibody with surface viral antigens. *Progr. Med. Virol.* **26**, 45.

Roitt, I. M. (1980). *Essential Immunology*, 4th edition. Blackwell Scientific Publications, Oxford.

Sissons, J. G. and Oldstone, M. B. A. (1980). Antibody-mediated destruction of virus infected cells. *Adv. Immunol.* **29**, 209.

Unanue, E. R. (1981). The regulatory role of macrophages in antigenic stimulation. *Adv. Immunol.* **31**, 1.

Webster, R. G., Laver, W. G., Air, G. M., and Schild, G. C. (1982). Molecular mechanisms of variation in influenza viruses. *Nature* **296**, 115.

Welsh, R. M. (1978). Mouse natural killer cells: induction, specificity and function. *J. Immunol.* **121**, 1631.

Wiley, D. C., Wilson, I. A., and Skehel, J. J. (1981). Structural identification of the antibody binding sites of Hong Kong influenza haemagglutinin and their involvement in antigenic variation. *Nature* **289**, 373.

Zinkernagel, R. M. and Doherty, P. C. (1979). MHC-restricted cytotoxic T cells: studies on the biological role of polymorphic major transplantation antigens determining T-cell restriction—specificity, function and responsiveness. *Adv. Immunol.* **27**, 51.

Chapter Four
Mechanisms of Disease Production

A good deal of cell and tissue damage can take place without the host suffering an overt illness or being aware of the infection. For instance, destruction of a limited number of intestinal epithelial cells or liver cells may not be noticed. These tissues have considerable functional reserves. Even when the damage causes signs or symptoms of illness, the impact on the host depends very much on the tissue involved. Damage to muscle in the leg or stomach for instance, may not be serious. But in the heart, where the very existence of the host depends on a strong muscle contraction continuing to occur every second, the effect of minor damage or functional changes may be catastrophic. The central nervous system is likewise particularly vulnerable to damage. The passage of nerve impulses requires normal function in the neuronal cell membrane, and viruses have important effects on the cell membrane. Also, a degree of cellular or tissue oedema that is tolerable in most tissues may have serious consequences if it occurs in the brain, enclosed in that more or less rigid box, the skull. Therefore encephalitis and meningitis can be associated with more severe illness than might be expected from the histological changes in the tissues. Oedema is a serious matter also in the lung. Oedema fluid or inflammatory cell exudate appears first in the space between the alveolar capillary and the alveolar wall, decreasing the efficiency of gaseous exchange. Respiratory function can also be drastically impaired when fluid or cells accumulate in the alveolar spaces. Pathological changes in blood vessels are important. Cellular damage has profound effects if it involves the endothelial cells of small blood vessels. The resulting circulatory changes can lead to anoxia or necrosis in the tissues supplied by these vessels. *In vitro* experiments give little information about this type of tissue damage.

Despite recent penetrating insights at the molecular level, mechanisms of tissue damage and disease production in the whole animal are still shrouded in mystery. For instance, we do not even know why patients died from smallpox, a disease in which the virus grew almost exclusively in the skin. The same is true for rabbits dying with myxomatosis. A valiant attempt to elucidate the pathophysiological factors in rabbits dying after infection with rabbitpox has been made by Boulter *et al*. (1961). Gumboro disease, caused by infectious bursal disease virus, poses similar problems, and shows tantalising but baffling immunological features. The virus causes a lethal disease in chickens, but its replication is more or less confined to B lymphocytes in the bursa of Fabricius (Becht, 1980). Bursal follicles undergo necrosis and chickens die within 3–4 days, but if the bursa is removed surgically before infection the disease is prevented (Kaufer and Weiss, 1980). The pathogenesis of very minor abnormalities can be equally mysterious, such as the deformed whiskers seen in mice infected with certain leukaemia viruses (Rowe, 1983).

DIRECT DAMAGE AT THE CELLULAR LEVEL

General features of the biochemical changes in cells following virus infection have been referred to in Chapter 1. Mechanisms of cell damage differ for different viruses, and much remains to be learnt (Shatkin, 1983). Many viruses, including picornaviruses, poxviruses and herpesviruses cause a shutdown in cellular macromolecular synthesis and thus directly damage the infected cell (Tamm, 1975). Viral capsid proteins accumulating in the cell during replication possibly have a toxic effect and contribute to cell damage, as suggested by work on adenoviruses (Valentine and Pereira, 1965). There have been reports of inflammatory factors liberated from infected cells (Brier *et al.*, 1970) but their importance is uncertain. Kirn and Keller (1983) have evidence for a toxin from a frog virus (FV$_3$) that kills cells within an hour and may play a role in the pathogenesis of this virus infection in the mouse liver. But toxins are not a feature of virus infections. The so-called 'toxic' effects caused by certain viruses such as influenza under experimental conditions may be due to a single abortive cycle of growth in non-permissive cells (Mims, 1960a; 1960b). However, in the case of the liver necrosis caused in mice by massive intravenous injections of influenza virus there have been reports that non-infectious viral subunits also have this effect (Kato and Okada, 1961). The hepatic lesions and mild cerebral oedema seen in mice infected intravenously with influenza B have been suggested as a model for Reye's syndrome in man (Davis *et al.*, 1983).

The lesions in cells infected with viruses are generally not specific. The most common and potentially reversible change, the oedema seen as 'cloudy swelling' by routine histology, is associated with membrane permeability changes. Changes in the endoplasmic reticulum, mitochondria and polyribosomes are seen by electron microscopy at this stage. These changes probably provide the basis for the 'rounding up' or early CPE seen in cell culture. Further cytopathic effects may be autolytic consequences of leakage of lysosomal enzymes into the cell (Allison, 1967). Later the nuclear chromatin moves to the edge of the nucleus ('margination') and becomes condensed (pyknosis) but the cell has already died by this time.

There are two characteristic types of morphological change produced by certain viruses, and these were recognised by histologists more than 50 years ago. The first are inclusion bodies; these are areas of the cell

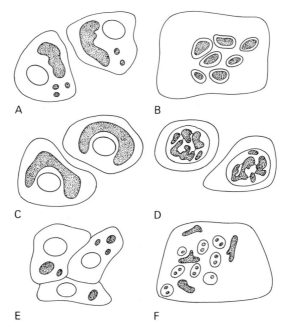

A   B

C   D

E   F

Fig. 4.1. Inclusion bodies in virus-infected cells. A Vaccinia virus—intracytoplasmic acidophilic inclusions. B Herpes simplex virus—intranuclear acidophilic inclusion (Cowdry type A); cell fusion produces syncytium. C Reovirus—perinuclear intracytoplasmic acidophilic inclusion. D Adenovirus—intranuclear basophilic inclusion. E Rabies virus—intracytoplasmic acidophilic inclusions (Negri bodies). F Measles virus—intranuclear and intracytoplasmic acidophilic inclusions; cell fusion produces syncytium. Courtesy of Fenner *et al.* (1974) *The Biology of Animal Viruses*. Academic Press, New York.

with altered staining behaviour that develop during infection (Fig. 4.1). They can represent crystalline arrays of virus particles as in the intranuclear inclusions in papovavirus and adenovirus infections. They may represent virus 'factories' in which viral components are being synthesised and assembled, as elegantly demonstrated for vaccinia virus by Cairns (1960). The intracytoplasmic inclusions (Negri bodies) of rabies virus have a similar origin. Sometimes, however, they are mere collections of surplus viral antigen, as with some of the inclusions seen in poxvirus-infected cells (Ichihashi *et al.*, 1971). The classic Cowdry type A intranuclear inclusions seen after staining of herpesvirus-infected cells are to some extent artefacts (shrinkage of altered chromatin) caused by fixation prior to staining.

The second characteristic morphological change caused by viruses is the formation of multinucleate giant cells. This is generally a result of cell fusion, hence the giant cell is called a 'syncytium'. Syncytia are characteristic of the paramyxoviruses and herpesviruses. Indeed, parainfluenza virus 1 (Sendai) was for many years routinely used by cell biologists to fuse cells together to form 'heterokaryons'—the 'hybridoma' technology that gave us monoclonal antibodies (Kohler and Milstein, 1975) and revolutionised immunology is testimony to this. The paramyxoviruses contain a 'fusion' (F) glycoprotein that is responsible for syncytium production and is required for direct cell to cell spread of these viruses (Merz *et al.*, 1980).

Finally, many viruses cause chromosomal alterations or damage in cultured cells (Nichols, 1970), most of which are assumed to represent late changes resulting from the release of lysosomal enzymes inside the dying cell. However, the specific chromosomal translocations that characterise certain tumours may indicate the site of insertion of cellular ('proto-') oncogenes, e.g. the c-*myc* oncogene in Burkitt lymphoma and in mouse plasmacytomas (Klein, 1983).

Not all viruses kill the cell in which they grow. Many retroviruses and arenaviruses, for example are 'non-cytopathogenic'. Even though they multiply productively, they cause no obvious damage to the host cell, which may continue to divide indefinitely despite the production of thousands of progeny virions. At the extreme, oncogenic viruses, far from destroying the cell, turn it into a malignant cell. On the other hand, some viruses cause subtle changes in cell function in the absence of cell damage (see p. 138).

DIRECT DAMAGE IN THE INFECTED HOST

We have just seen that there is a spectrum of viral pathogenicity at the cellular level, ranging from early death of infected cells to little or no effect on the life or function of the cell. Similar distinctions can be observed *in vivo*.

Poliovirus in the central nervous system provides an example of direct and rapid viral damage at the level of the infected host. When this virus grows in cells it causes an early shutdown of RNA, protein, and DNA synthesis in the cell (see Chapter 1). Within a few hours there is an inevitable cytopathic effect and the cell dies. In the affected host, if enough motor neurones in the spinal cord are infected, damaged and destroyed, the corresponding muscles cannot function and the patient develops paralytic poliomyelitis. Another example of direct viral damage is seen in the common cold when caused by the rhinovirus group of picornaviruses. These viruses infect nasal epithelial cells, and at an early stage the cells round up, fall off the mucosal surface and are carried away, often with their cilia still beating, in a stream of fluid induced by the infection. This leaves areas of raw mucosa, with the exposed underlying tissues inflamed, oedematous and susceptible to infection by the normally harmless resident bacteria (Fig. 4.2).

It must be emphasised, however, that the severity of disease *in vivo* is not necessarily correlated with the cytotoxicity of the virus for cells *in vitro* or *in vivo*. Many viruses that are highly lethal for cultured cells are harmless *in vivo* (e.g. most echoviruses) whereas others that are non-cytocidal *in vitro* cause a lethal disease *in vivo* (e.g. rabies). On the one hand, destruction of cells *in vivo* may cause no symptomatology if their numbers are small or their function is not vital, while on the other hand

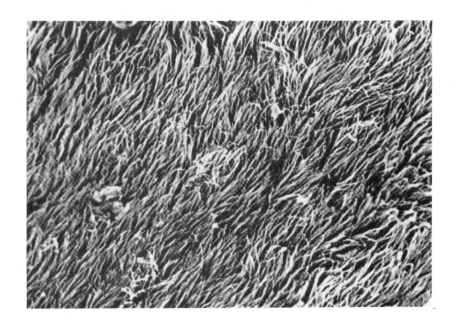

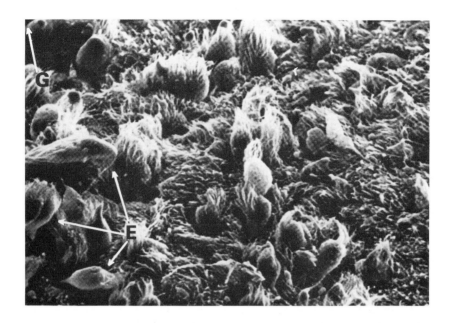

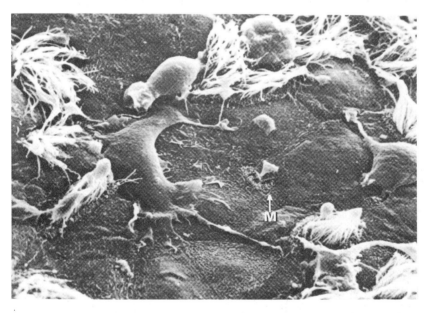

Fig. 4.2. Direct cytopathic effect of rhinovirus on bovine tracheal epithelium *in vitro*, as shown by scanning electron microscopy of organ cultures.
1 Normal appearance: continuous sheet of ciliated cells. Field width 100 μm.
2 Six days after infection: cells rounded up or detached. Field width 180 μm.
3 Six days after infection: macrophages and polymorphs (arrows) scavenging on landscape of rounded ciliated cells and exposed underlying tissues. Field width 100 μm. Courtesy of Reed & Boyle (1972).

cells with a vital function may suffer subtle alterations without morphological damage and give rise to a disease.

Many viruses appear to replicate in cells in the infected host without causing any obvious damage. Examples include lactic dehydrogenase (LDH) virus in macrophages, murine leukaemia viruses and rubella virus in developing embryonic cells, and LCM virus in neural and other cells of the mouse. But there may be important functional changes in infected cells, even if grossly observable properties such as cell morphology and cell division are unaffected. This can be detected especially when 'luxury functions' (Oldstone and Fujinami, 1982) of specialised cells are examined. For instance, LDH virus was so named because it impairs the clearance from the blood of certain endogenous enzymes including lactic dehydrogenase, by mouse macrophages *in vivo*. The infected cells also show impaired antigen presentation (Isakov *et al.*, 1980), but otherwise appear to be quite normal. Rubella virus infects human embryo cells without causing obvious damage, but the growth rate of infected cells is reduced (Rawls, 1968), and this may contribute to impaired growth and morphogenesis of the infected embryo. LCM virus infection of specialised cells such as neuroblastoma cells causes changes in their ability to make or degrade acetylcholine, without affecting growth rate or cloning efficiency (Oldstone *et al.*, 1977). In the brains of LCM carrier mice nearly all neurones are infected and contain LCM virus antigen (Mims, 1966, and see Fig. 6.3), but impaired luxury function might account for the behavioural abnormalities that have been reported in carrier mice (Hotchin and Seegal, 1977). Likewise, LCM virus infection of hybridoma cells is also harmless, but less antibody is produced than in uninfected cells (Oldstone and Fujinami, 1982). LCM virus also provides a fascinating example of impaired luxury functions in infected cells giving rise to major effects in the host. In mice carrying this virus there is infection of growth hormone-producing cells in the anterior pituitary. Although no cytopathic effects are detectable, the output of growth hormone is reduced and as a result of this, mice are runted (Oldstone *et al.*, 1982; Rodriguez *et al.*, 1983c). Rabies virus impairs acetylcholine and other membrane receptor functions in neural cells both *in vitro* and *in vivo* without causing a cytopathic effect (Koschel and Halbach, 1979; Tsiang, 1982).

Before leaving the subject of direct damage by viruses, one supreme example will be given. Here the direct damage is of such a magnitude that a susceptible host dies a mere six hours after infection. Rift Valley fever virus, an arthropod-borne virus of cattle, sheep and man in Africa was injected in extremely large doses intravenously into mice (Mims, 1957). The injected virus passed straight through the Kupffer cells and endothelial cells lining liver sinusoids (see Chapter 2) and infected nearly all hepatic cells. Hepatic cells showed nuclear inclusions within an hour and necrosis by four hours. As the single cycle of growth in hepatic cells was completed, massive liver necrosis took place and mice died only six hours after initial infection. The host defences in the form of local lymph nodes, local tissue phagocytes, etc. are completely overcome by the intravenous route of infection, and by the inability of Kupffer cells to prevent infection of hepatic cells. Direct damage by the replicating virus destroys hepatic cells long before immune or interferon responses have an opportunity to control the infection. This is the summit of virulence, an infectious disease whose incubation period between infection and death is a mere six hours. The experimental situation is artificial but it illustrates direct and lethal damage to host tissues after all host defence mechanisms have been overwhelmed.

INDIRECT DAMAGE VIA THE IMMUNE RESPONSE (IMMUNOPATHOLOGY)

The expression of the immune response necessarily involves a certain amount of inflammation, cell infiltration, lymph node swelling, even tissue destruction, as described in Chapter 2. Such changes caused by the immune response are classed as immunopathological. Sometimes they are very severe, leading to severe disease or death, as in adult mice after primary intracerebral infection with LCM virus, but at other times they play a minimal part in the pathogenesis of disease. There will nearly always be some contribution of the immune response to pathological changes. The mere enlargement of lymphoid organs during infectious diseases is a morphological change that can often be regarded as pathological. The lymph node swelling seen in glandular fever for instance is an immunopathological feature of the disease.

Inflammation causes redness, swelling, pain and sometimes loss of function of the affected part, and can be a major cause of the signs and symptoms of a virus disease. It is often, but not always, generated by immune responses. For instance, inflammatory materials are liberated when cells die, and the inflammatory response can be a result of direct viral damage to small blood vessels.

Four types of hypersensitivity response are traditionally distinguished according to the original classification by Coombs and Gell (Lachmann and Peters, 1982). The distinction between Type II and Type III reactions has become less clear, and we now recognise a wider variety of immune responses (see Chapter 3), many of which may be involved in viral immunopathology. It is nevertheless convenient to describe the phenomena under the original headings (Table 4.1).

Hypersensitivity reactions—type 1

These are anaphylactic reactions, and depend on the reactions of antigens with reaginic (IgE) antibodies attached to mast cells, resulting in

Table 4.1. Immunopathology in viral diseases.

Hypersensivity	Mechanism	Result	Virological example
Type 1 Anaphylactic	Antigen + reaginic (IgE) antibody on mast cells → histamine, etc. release	Anaphylactic shock Bronchospasm Local inflammation	Contribution to certain rashes or wheezing (RSV)
Type 2 Cytotoxic	Antibody + antigen on cell surface → complement activation or ADCC	Lysis of cells bearing viral antigens	Liver cell necrosis in hepatitis B?
Type 3 Immune complex	Antibody + extracellular antigen → complex → complement activation, inflammatory mediators, endogenous pyrogen	*Extravascular complex:* Inflammation ± tissue damage	Edge of smallpox vaccination site?
		Intravascular complex: Complex deposited in glomeruli, joints, small skin vessels, etc. → glomerulonephritis, vasculitis, etc.	Glomerulonephritis in mice carrying LCM virus Prodromal rashes. Fever
Type 4 Cell-mediated (delayed)	Sensitised T lymphocyte reacts with antigen; lymphokines liberated	*Extracellular antigen:* Inflammation, mononuclear accumulation, macrophage activation Tissue damage	Acute LCM viral disease in adult mice? Certain viral rashes
		Antigen on infected cell: T lymphocyte lyses cell	Acute LCM viral disease in adult mice?

the release of histamine and heparin from mast cell granules, and the activation of serotonin and plasma kinins. If the antigen–antibody interaction takes place on a large enough scale in the tissues, the histamine that is released can give rise to anaphylactic shock, the exact features depending on the sensitivity and particular reaction of the species of animal to histamine. This type of immunopathology, although accounting for anaphylactic reactions to horse serum or penicillin, is not known to be important in virus infection. When the antigen-IgE antibody interaction takes place at body surfaces, however, there are local inflammatory events, giving rise to urticaria in the skin and hay fever or asthma in the respiratory tract. This local type of anaphylaxis has not been adequately studied in virus infections but it possibly plays a part in the pathogenesis of the common cold, in respiratory syncytial virus bronchiolitis of infants (McIntosh and Fishaut, 1980; Welliver *et al.*, 1981), or in the pathogenesis of skin rashes in certain viral diseases.

Hypersensitivity reactions—type 2

These are cytolytic or cytotoxic reactions mediated by antibody. Reactions of this type occur when antibody combines with viral antigen on the surface of a tissue cell, activates the complement sequence and causes destruction of the cell (Chapter 3). Antibodies can also sensitise cells for destruction by K (killer) cells, polymorphs or macrophages (ADCC). Clearly the antibody-mediated destruction of infected cells means tissue damage, and could account for some of the liver necrosis in hepatitis B for instance, or in yellow fever. But the importance of these reactions *in vivo* is not known.

There is evidence from transfer experiments that specific antibody can cause early death in mice infected intracerebrally with rabies virus (Prabhakar and Nathanson, 1981). Antibody-treated infected mice do not show the paralysis and focal necrosis usually seen with rabies, but suffer from convulsions and 'toxic' spasms. It is not clear how the antibodies act, nor what type of antibody is involved, but effects on infected neuronal cell membranes might be expected. Rabies-infected cells are susceptible to K cell-mediated antibody-dependent cytotoxicity (ADCC) *in vitro* (Harfast *et al.*, 1977).

Hypersensitivity reactions—type 3

These are immune complex reactions. Combination of antibody with antigen is an important event, initiating inflammatory phenomena that are inevitably involved in the expression of the immune response. These inflammatory phenomena, although most of the time of antimicrobial value (see Chapter 3), are nevertheless immunopathological features of the infection. Immune complex reactions sometimes do a great deal of damage in the infected host. The mechanisms by which antigen–antibody reactions caused inflammation and cell damage are outlined in Fig. 4.3.

When the antigen–antibody reaction takes place in extravascular tissues, there is inflammation and oedema with infiltration of polymorphs. If soluble antigen is injected intradermally into an individual with large amounts of IgG antibody, the antigen–antibody reaction takes place in the walls of skin blood vessels, and causes an inflammatory response. The infiltrating polymorphs degenerate and their lysosomal enzymes cause extensive vascular damage. This is the classical Arthus response. Antigen–antibody reactions in tissues are not usually as serious as this, and milder inflammatory sequelae are more common, as in the case of the red zone seen round the corners of a smallpox vaccination site after 7 or 8 days. In this example circulating antibodies pass through the vessel walls, meet vaccinia viral antigens in the dermal tissues, and an inflammatory response is generated. A similar milder response with less inflammation would result in local leakage of plasma proteins from blood vessels which could be detected visibly if circulating plasma proteins were first coloured by the intravenous injection of Evans blue. This type of reaction would theoretically provide the basis for much of the inflammation and oedema seen after antibodies have been generated.

When the antigen–antibody reaction takes place in the blood to give circulating immune complexes, the sequelae depend to a large extent on the relative proportions of antigen and antibody, and also on antibody affinity. If there is a large excess of antibody, each antigen molecule is covered with antibody and is rapidly removed by reticuloendothelial cells, which have receptors for the Fc portion of the antibody molecule (see Chapter 3). When equal amounts of antigen and antibody combine, lattice structures are formed, and these develop into large aggregates whose size ensures that they are also rapidly removed by reticulo-

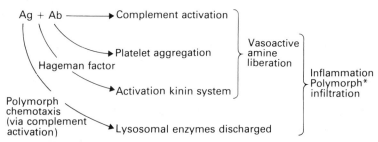

Fig. 4.3. Mechanisms of inflammation and tissue damage induced by antigen-antibody reactions.
*If the reaction continues beyond the acute stage, polymorphs are replaced by mononuclear cells.

endothelial cells. If, however, complexes are formed in antigen excess, and especially if the antibody is of low affinity, the poorly coated antigen molecules are not removed by reticuloendothelial cells. They continue to circulate in the blood and have the opportunity to localise in small blood vessels elsewhere in the body. The mechanisms by which complexes localise is not clear, but they are filtered off in the glomerular capillaries of the kidney. The smallest sized complexes seem to enter the urine, but others are retained in local phagocytic cells (mesangial cells). This is probably the normal mechanism of disposal of such complexes from the body.

Circulating immune complexes are probably formed in most acute virus infections. Viral antigens are often present in the blood and when the immune response has been generated and the first trickle of specific antibody enters the blood, immune complexes are formed in antigen excess. This is generally a transitional stage, soon giving way to antibody excess, as more and more antibody enters the blood and the infection is terminated. Under certain circumstances complexes continue to be formed in the blood and deposited in blood vessels for long periods. This happens in persistent virus infections in which virus particles or antigens are continuously released into the blood but antibody responses are only minimal or of poor quality (low affinity or directed at 'non-critical' sites on the virion). Complexes are deposited in glomeruli over the course of weeks, months or even years. The normal mechanisms for removal are inadequate, and the deposits accumulate just outside the blood vessels together with complement components. Mesangial cells enlarge and multiply, the structure of the basement membrane between glomerular capillary and urinary compartment alters, and as a result of these and other changes, the filtering function of the glomerulus becomes progressively impaired. Proteins leak through into the urine. Eventually many glomeruli cease to produce urine and the individual has chronic glomerulonephritis.

Circulating immune complexes are also deposited in the walls of small blood vessels in the skin and the joints where they may induce inflammatory changes, and also in the choroid plexus. Prodromal rashes seen in exanthematous virus infections and in hepatitis B are probably caused in this way. If the vascular changes are more marked they give rise to the condition called erythema nodosum, with tender red nodules in the skin and deposits of antigen, antibody and complement in vessel walls. When small arteries are severely affected, as in some patients with hepatitis B, this gives rise to periarteritis nodosa.

Immune-complex glomerulonephritis occurs in certain virus infections of animals. The antibodies formed in viral infections generally neutralise any free virus particles and so help to terminate the infection, but sometimes the infection persists (see Chapter 6), antigen continues to be released into the blood and immune complexes are formed over long periods. Persistent viral infections with these characteristics are included in Table 4.2. In each instance complexes are deposited in kidney glomeruli and sometimes in other blood vessels as described above. A classic example is persistent infection of mice with LCM virus following intrauterine or neonatal infection (Buchmeier *et al.*, 1980). The viral antigens are present in the blood and small amounts of antibody of poor affinity are formed (Oldstone and Dixon, 1967), giving rise to circulating immune complexes that are progressively deposited in glomeruli (Oldstone and Dixon, 1969). The outcome depends on the strain of mouse, and there are numerous possible mechanisms for genetic control of susceptibility. For instance, recent work shows that the formation of C1q binding immune complexes in infected mice is under multigenic control (Oldstone *et al.*, 1983). In severe cases this otherwise harmless infection ends with glomerulonephritis, uraemia and death. On the other hand, there are few, if any, pathological changes in mice persistently infected with LDH or leukaemia viruses; this is perhaps because there is a slower rate of immune-complex deposition. Oldstone and Dixon (1971) found that 63.7 µg of IgG could be eluted from each kidney of SWR/J mice carrying LCM virus, whereas only 4.1 µg of IgG per kidney was eluted from the same strain of mice persistently infected with lactic dehydrogenase virus, with a correspondingly low incidence of glomerulonephritis.

In mink persistently infected with Aleutian disease virus, very large amounts of antibody of low neutralising capacity are formed. Immune complexes are present in the blood over long periods, and are deposited in glomeruli and in blood vessels, causing damage that is manifested by glomerulonephritis and sometimes haemorrhage from affected arteries (Porter *et al.*, 1980). During the acute stage of hepatitis B in man, when antibodies against excess circulating viral 'surface' antigen (HB_s Ag) are first synthesised, immune complexes are formed and deposited in glomeruli. But the deposition is short-lived and there is generally no glomerulonephritis, although it may occur (Kohler *et al.*, 1974), and periarteritis nodosa is sometimes seen. Persistent carriers of the antigen do not develop immune-complex phenomena because their antibody is directed against the 'core' antigen (HB_c Ag) which is present in relatively small amounts, rather than against the more plentiful circulating HB_s Ag. Certain arthropod-borne viruses, including Chikungunya and O'nyong-nyong cause illnesses characterised by fever, arthralgia and itchy rashes; these sound as if they could be immune complex in origin, although certain other togaviruses, including Ross River virus and rubella virus, can invade the joint and cause arthralgia or arthritis by more direct mechanisms (Tesh, 1982).

In addition to their local effects, antigen–antibody complexes generate systemic reactions. For instance, the fever that appears at the end of the incubation period in many viral infections is perhaps attributable to

Table 4.2. The deposition of circulating immune complexes in persistent viral infections.

Virus	Host	Kidney deposits	Glomerulonephritis	Vascular deposits
Mouse leukaemia	Mouse	+	±	−
Cat leukaemia	Cat	+	±	−
Lactic dehydrogenase (LDV)	Mouse	+	±	−
Lymphocytic chorio-meningitis (LCM)	Mouse	++	+	±
Aleutian disease (ADV)	Mink	++	+	++
Equine infectious anaemia	Horse	+	+	+
Hepatitis B	Man	+	−	+
Rubella[a]	Man	?	−	?

[a]Circulating immune complexes associated with persistent congenital rubella infection (Coyle et al., 1981) and with progressive rubella panencephalitis (Coyle and Wolinsky, 1981), but pathogenic role unknown.

a large-scale interaction of antibodies with viral antigen, although extensive CMI reactions also cause fever. The febrile response is mediated by endogenous pyrogens liberated from polymorphs and macrophages. Perhaps the characteristic subjective sensations of illness ('malaise') and some of the 'toxic' features of viral diseases are also caused by immune reactions.

Systemic immune complex reactions taking place during certain viral infections may occasionally give rise to a serious condition known as disseminated intravascular coagulation. This is sometimes seen in yellow fever and other arboviral haemorrhagic fevers, and in smallpox. Immune reactions activate the enzymes of the coagulation cascade, leading to histamine release and increased vascular permeability. Fibrin is formed and deposited in kidney, lung, adrenals and pituitary. This causes multiple thromboses with infarcts and there are also scattered haemorrhages because of the depletion of platelets, prothrombin, fibrinogen, etc. Systemic immune-complex reactions were once thought to form the basis for dengue haemorrhagic fever but alternative explanations now seem more likely (see pp. 152–3). Kittens infected with feline infectious peritonitis virus, a coronavirus, have circulating immune complexes (Jacobse-Geels et al., 1982) and develop disseminated intravascular coagulation (Weiss et al., 1980).

Hypersensitivity reactions—type 4

These are T cell-mediated immune (CMI) reactions. The expression of a CMI response involves inflammation, lymphocytic infiltration, macrophage accumulation and macrophage activation resulting from the secretion of lymphokines by T_d cells, as described in Chapter 3. This alone is sufficient to cause pathological changes; for instance, there is evidence that T_d cells contribute to pathology in influenzal pneumonia of mice (Leung and Ada, 1980). Cytotoxic T (T_c) lymphocytes also cause pathological changes by destroying host cells bearing viral antigen on their surface, and are demonstrable in most viral infections. But in spite of the fact that the *in vitro* test system so clearly displays the immunopathological potential of cytotoxic T cells this is not easy to evaluate in the infected host. It may contribute to the tissue damage seen, for instance, in the liver in hepatitis B infection and also in many herpesvirus and poxvirus infections.

But in LCM viral infections of adult mice—the most thoroughly investigated and classic experimental example of cell-mediated immunopathology—the sequence of events is still debatable. When virus is injected intracerebrally into adult mice it grows in the meninges and ependyma and choroid plexus epithelium, but the infected cells do not show the slightest sign of damage or dysfunction. After 7–10 days, however, the mouse develops severe meningitis with cerebral oedema (Doherty and Zinkernagel, 1974) and dies, often during the course of a convulsion. The illness can be completely prevented by adequate immunosuppression with X-irradiation, antilymphocyte serum, cytotoxic drugs or neonatal thymectomy (Lehmann-Grube, 1971; Buchmeier *et al.*, 1980). The lesions are attributable to the mouse's own vigorous CMI reaction to infected cells in meninges, ependyma and choroid plexus epithelium. Lymphocytes, after entering the cerebrospinal fluid and encountering the infected cells, could destroy these cells and generate the inflammatory response and interference with normal neural function that causes the disease. T_c cells that kill LCM-infected target cells *in vitro* are present in the cerebrospinal fluid of infected mice (Zinkernagel and Doherty, 1973). But tissue destruction is not a feature of the neurological disease, and no signs of cell damage were seen in careful electron microscopic studies of infected mouse brains (Walker *et al.*, 1975). Perhaps in this disease the role of T_d cells needs further consideration, as suggested by Thomsen *et al.* (1983). It may be noted that the brain is uniquely vulnerable to inflammation and oedema, as pointed out earlier in this chapter. The infected mouse shows the same type of lesions in scattered foci of infection in the liver and elsewhere, associated with a reduction in recirculating (T) lymphocytes (Wallnerova and Mims, 1971) but the extraneural lesions are not a cause of sickness or death. LCM infection of mice is a classical example of immunopathology in which death itself is entirely due to the cell-mediated immune response of the infected individual. This response, although apparently irrelevant and harmful, nevertheless has useful antiviral effects. It has been shown that immune T cells effectively inhibit viral growth in infected organs (Mims and Blanden, 1972). However, a response that, in most extraneural sites would be useful and appropriate, turns out to be self-destructive when it takes place in the central nervous system. It should be noted that this disease, caused by intracerebral injection of LCM virus into adult mice, is a highly artificial one. Under natural circumstances mice are infected as infants, in whom immunopathological responses are less marked, and by extraneural routes. Even in adult mice, extraneural infection gives rise to immunopathology that has less serious consequences.

When pathological changes are made less severe by immunosuppressive agents, it is generally assumed that immunopathology makes an important contribution to the disease. There has been much experimental work of this nature, such as that just discussed in acute LCM virus infections of the nervous system of mice. Immune responses, however, generally have antiviral actions, and treatment with immunosuppressive agents therefore permits more extensive viral growth and spread. In human diseases such as herpes simplex encephalitis, steroid therapy reduces inflammation and thus leads to clinical improvement, but at the same time the viral infection may become more extensive because immune restraints on viral growth have been weakened. This clinical dilemma will be resolved when a powerful antiviral drug can be administered together with an anti-inflammatory agent.

Another organ especially vulnerable to inflammation, cell infiltration and oedema is the lung. There is considerable evidence that specific T cell responses to influenza virus infection not only contribute to antiviral defence (see Chapter 3) but also cause immunopathology and enhance the severity of the infection in the lung (Ada et al., 1981). Ada et al. presented evidence that 'class II' T cells (Ly 2, displaying cytotoxic, as well as DTH, activity) protected mice against intranasal challenge, whereas 'class I' T cells (Ly 1, displaying helper and DTH activity) actually accelerated the demise of the mouse. Recent work shows that antigen-specific suppression of this delayed hypersensitivity response reduces the severity of the infection (Liew and Russell, 1983). Transfusion of influenza-specific T_d cells enhances the severity of infection, but when they are pre-incubated with T_s cells with specificity for influenzal DTH, the mortality is greatly reduced. Liew and Russell suggest that, in this infection, antigen-specific suppression is beneficial to the host.

One human viral infection in which a strong CMI contribution to pathology seems probable is measles (Burnet, 1968). Children with thymic aplasia show a general failure to develop T lymphocytes and cell-mediated immunity, and suffer a fatal disease if they are infected with measles virus. Instead of the very limited viral growth seen in the respiratory tract of normal children, there is inexorable multiplication of virus in the lung, in spite of some antibody formation, giving rise to a giant-cell pneumonia. This indicates that the CMI response is essential for the control of viral growth. In addition, there is a total absence of the typical measles rash, and this further indicates that the CMI response is essential for the production of the skin lesions in normal children. Children with the B cell deficiency, agammaglobulinaemia, but with intact CMI responses, develop a typical measles rash. There is evidence that cell-mediated immune responses also make a contribution to the rash in poxvirus infections (Pincus and Flick, 1963).

Immune responses to inappropriate antigens

Immunopathology can result from the induction of inappropriate immune responses. The paramyxovirus F glycoprotein acquires its fusion activity following cleavage by a host protease in the membrane of the infected cell. The F protein is responsible for penetration of virions into cells, spread from cell to cell and formation of syncytia. Formaldehyde-inactivated vaccines fail to elicit anti-F antibodies (Norrby et al., 1975). If vaccinees are subsequently infected, they fail to control the spread of virus. This allows large amounts of viral antigen to be produced which react with non-neutralising (anti-HN) antibodies and give immunopathological changes (Choppin and Scheid, 1980). There is thus a failure to protect against infection and a potential for immunopathological events. This is probably the explanation of the more severe atypical disease seen when individuals given killed measles or respiratory syncytial virus vaccines were subsequently infected (McIntosh and Fischaut, 1980). This salutory tale provides something of a warning against the possible dangers of inactivated vaccines, especially against respiratory viruses.

Many chronic viral infections persist in spite of titres of antibody so high that virus–antibody complexes are deposited in the kidneys and arterioles (Table 4.2). The reasons this antibody fails to eliminate the virus may be that it is directed against the wrong antigenic sites on the virion and is therefore non-neutralising (see Chapter 6).

Autoimmunity

If virus-induced immune responses are directed not only against viral antigens and infected cells but also against normal host components, then the stage is set for further immunopathological events, which are classed as 'autoimmune'. In an acute infection this would merely lead to increased tissue damage, but if the infection became chronic or if the autoimmune phenomena continued over a longer period, more extensive tissue damage would be possible. The autoimmune responses could theoretically be induced in the following ways:

1 If the envelope of budding virions bore host-determined as well as viral antigens, anti-host responses might be induced together with anti-viral responses. Generally, in the virus envelope there is a complete replacement of host cell proteins by viral proteins, although Lodish and Potter (1980) reported finding a small amount of cellular protein in highly purified vesicular stomatitis virions. Nevertheless, since the immune system is 'tolerant' of all 'self' antigens, an individual would not be expected to mount a response to 'self' antigens on viruses or on virus infected cells unless epitopes normally hidden were now exposed. It is quite possible that association of viral proteins with cellular proteins in the plasma membrane may result in the presentation of 'forbidden' antigenic determinants on those cellular proteins which are normally not exposed or not optimally presented. The viral antigen could act as a helper (carrier) determinant for a response to the host cell antigen. This could apply as much to cells infected with non-budding as with budding viruses, providing that they express viral antigens on the plasma membrane (Inada and Uetake, 1977).

Some support for this possibility comes from experiments by Bromberg et al. (1982), who found that antibody responses to antigens on mouse thymus cells were increased 30-fold when these cells were infected with herpes simplex, vaccinia or Newcastle disease virus. Many years earlier, Lindenmann and colleagues had shown that the immune response to tumour antigens on cancer cells could be augmented by immunisation with virus-infected cancer cells or their plasma membranes (Lindenmann and Klein, 1967).

2 Following cell destruction by any type of virus, immune responses could be induced against intracellular or other host proteins not normally exposed to the immune system. However, it must be added, undamaged cells would not be expected to be targets for antibodies or lymphocytes directed against such internal cellular proteins.

3 There might be clones of lymphocytes that recognise determinants that happen to be present on both viral and host antigens, so that cross-reactive immune responses are generated. Such a mechanism helps explain the degeneration of neurones and cardiac muscle cells seen in Chagas' disease caused by Trypanosoma cruzi; Wood et al. (1982) obtained a monoclonal antibody that reacted with normal neurones and cardiac muscle cells, as well as with Trypanosoma cruzi. This mechanism probably also explains the observations of Fujinami et al. (1983), who described monoclonal antibodies directed against defined herpes simplex or measles virus proteins that cross-react with an intermediate filament protein (probably vimentin) present in normal uninfected cells.

4 If autoimmune responses are normally kept in check by specific suppressor mechanisms a viral infection might destroy or otherwise affect

these suppressor T cells so as to upset the immunoregulatory balance and allow autoimmunity to become manifest (Paterson et al., 1981).

5   The infected host can form antibody to the idiotype on antiviral antibodies. Anti-idiotype antibody may normally have immuno-regulatory functions, but if directed against antibody to viral surface components it could also react with virus-specific receptors on normal cells. This provides a possible basis for autoimmunity. Nepom et al. (1982) and Noseworthy et al. (1983) showed that antibody to the idiotype on antibody to reovirus 3 haemagglutinin also reacts with normal lymphoid and neural cells.

6   Certain viruses cause polyclonal activation of B cells and some of the antibodies they secrete may react with host tissues and could theoretically cause damage. EB virus infects B cells and 5–6 days after the initial infection IgG secretion is induced in 5–7% of infected cells (Sugden, 1982), which is the probable source of heterophil antibodies and other autoantibodies in this infection.

Possibilities 2–4 have been particularly attractive in theories about the pathogenesis of chronic demyelinating diseases such as multiple sclerosis, and other chronic diseases such as rheumatoid arthritis. In multiple sclerosis for instance, immune responses to oligodendrocytes and myelin are perhaps triggered by virus infections. This does not necessarily require the presence of virus in the lesions (see possibilities 2–6). A convincing example of virus-triggered autoimmunity is seen in young mice infected with reovirus type 1 (Onodera et al., 1981). These mice show transient diabetes and runting; cells in the islets of Langerhans and in the anterior pituitary are infected, and auto-antibodies to insulin and growth hormone are present. Spleen cells from infected mice yield monoclonal antibodies reacting with these host components (Haspel et al., 1983). In experiments with vaccinia virus Dales et al. (1983) found that hybridomas from virus-treated mice produced autoantibody to cytoskeletal components, and one of these antibodies cross-reacted with viral antigens. Reports such as those of Steck et al. (1981), who found that mice infected intracerebrally with a neurotropic strain of vaccinia virus developed antibody to various myelin and oligo-dendrocyte components need confirmation.

Recent work by Watanabe et al. (1983) provides promising evidence for virus-triggered autoimmune disease. Rats were infected with the JHM strain of mouse hepatitis virus, as a result of which they became ill with a demyelinating encephalomyelitis. Their spleen cells were then stimulated in vitro with myelin basic protein and transferred to normal uninfected rats, who developed neural lesions and mild disease. Experimental models of virus-induced demyelinating diseases are surveyed by dal Canto and Rabinowitz (1982).

In most of these types of autoimmunity there will be strong host genetic determinants, operating via immune response (Ir) genes. Auto-immune responses occur in viral infections, but would not necessarily be harmful. It is known that damage to the heart or central nervous system caused by non-infectious agents can give rise to autoantibodies to heart muscle or myelin. Immune responses to peripheral nerve components are seen in Marek's disease in chickens (Pepose *et al.*, 1981) which is often used as a model for acute demyelinating peripheral neuritis in man (Guillain-Barré syndrome). The Guillain-Barré syndrome can follow infection by any of a number of different viruses (EBV, CMV, influenza, BK, mumps, vaccinia, etc.) and it seems highly unlikely that all share antigenic determinants with peripheral nerves, but certain of the other hypotheses may be applicable.

The various possibilities remain as theoretically attractive explanations of certain important diseases of unknown aetiology, and it seems likely that current work by virologists and immunologists in which monoclonal antibodies can be used, will soon provide more definite answers.

OTHER INDIRECT MECHANISMS OF DAMAGE

Hormonal effects

Sometimes in viral infections there are prominent pathological changes which are not attributable to the direct action of the virus nor to inflammation nor to immunopathology. The 'stress' changes mediated by adrenocortical hormones come into this category. Stress is a general term used to describe various noxious influences including cold, heat, starvation, injury, psychological stress and infection. An infectious disease is an important stress and increased corticosteroid secretion by adrenal glands takes place in all severe infections. This is vital for resistance to disease, and resistance is greatly reduced if there is a failure in corticosteroid secretion. Patients with Addison's disease, in whom adrenal glands are destroyed, have to be given corticosteroids in increased doses during infections. On the other hand, administration of excess corticosteroid to normal individuals during infection can increase disease severity. These matters are discussed in Mims (1982a, pp. 251–2). Corticosteroids tend to inhibit the development of inflammatory and immune responses, and have pronounced effects on lymphoid tissues, causing thymic involution and lymphocyte destruction. Thymic involution seen in mice infected intravenously with vaccinia virus is also produced by injections of hydrocortisone, and is prevented by bilateral adrenalectomy (Wallnerova and Mims, 1970).

Other hormonal effects are seen when an endocrine gland is damaged or destroyed. Mice that develop diabetes after infection with EMC or coxsackieviruses show some of the secondary complications of diabetes, an indirect result of the action of the virus on the islets of Langerhan (Notkins, 1977). As mentioned in Chapter 6, growth hormone-producing cells in the pituitary gland are infected in mice carrying LCM virus. The infected cells are not damaged, but the output of growth hormone is reduced, leading to pituitary dwarfism (Oldstone *et al.*, 1983). The obesity syndrome caused by canine distemper virus in mice (Lyons *et al.*, 1982) is in the same category, if we class obesity as a pathological change. Mice develop maximal obesity 16–20 weeks after infection, when they weigh twice as much as uninfected controls, and there is a great increase in the number of adipocytes. The virus, which multiplies in the brain, could theoretically damage or interfere with the function of appetite-controlling centres in the hypothalamus, but so far there is no evidence for this.

Haemorrhage

Pathological changes are sometimes caused in an indirect way as follows. Yellow fever in its severest form is characterised by devastating liver lesions. There is massive mid-zonal liver necrosis following the extensive growth of virus in liver cells, resulting in the jaundice that gives the disease its name. Destruction of the liver also leads to a decrease in the rate of formation of the blood coagulation factor, prothrombin, and infected human beings or monkeys show prolonged coagulation and bleeding times. Haemorrhagic phenomena are therefore characteristic of severe yellow fever, including haemorrhage into the stomach and intestines. In the stomach the appearance of blood is altered by acid, and the vomiting of altered blood gave yellow fever another of its names, 'black vomit disease'.

Haemorrhagic phenomena in virus diseases can also be due to direct damage to blood vessels, as in the reovirus infection responsible for epizootic haemorrhagic disease of deer (Tsai and Karstad, 1973).

Haemorrhage can also be caused by immunologically mediated damage to blood vessels. The haemorrhage and shock of dengue haemorrhagic fever were once thought to be due to systemic immune-complex reactions. Dengue haemorrhagic fever is seen in parts of the world where dengue is endemic, mainly (Halstead, 1979) but not exclusively (Rosen, 1982) in individuals immune to one type of dengue who then become infected with a different serotype of the virus. They have no neutralising antibody against the second virus, but do have non-neutralising antibody directed against other antigens shared by the two serotypes. The cross-reactive non-neutralising antibodies actually (see p. 58) enhance infection of susceptible mononuclear cells by the second virus (Halstead, 1979), so larger amounts of virus and viral antigen are produced. It was thought this unusually large quantity of viral antigen in the blood reacted massively with antibody to cause the haemorrhages, shock, vascular collapse, and often death. Immune-complex reactions activate the enzymes of the coagulation cascade leading to histamine release and increased vascular permeability. Fibrin is formed and is deposited in blood vessels in the kidneys and elsewhere. This causes multiple thromboses with infarcts, and there are also scattered haemorrhages because of the depletion of platelets, prothrombin, fibrinogen, etc. The general increase in capillary permeability leads to shock. However, it has proved difficult to demonstrate this pathophysiological sequence (Petchclai and Saelim, 1978; Halstead, 1981a; 1981b), and the mechanisms are still unclear (Pang and Lam, 1983; Porterfield, 1982). Quite probably the disease is produced by mediators released from sensitised T cells (Pang, 1983) or from macrophages.

Increased clotting times in association with low prothrombin levels and low platelet counts have been reported in Lassa fever virus infections of man (Buckley and Casals, 1978) and in simian haemorrhagic fever (Abildgaard et al., 1975), but here too, the pathophysiological sequence is not known. The pathogenesis of Lassa fever is poorly understood and in man it is not strictly a haemorrhagic disease. The virus replicates especially in liver, lung and adrenal glands, but the pathological changes in these organs do not account for death. In fatal cases 1% or fewer of the liver cells may be necrotic, with minor intestitial changes in the lungs and 90% of adrenal cells morphologically normal (Walker et al., 1982). In this particular disease we know little of inflammatory mediators and complement activation. Perhaps in dengue and in some of the other viral haemorrhagic fevers, virus multiplication in capillary endothelial cells is an important factor in disease production.

Finally, there are a few viral diseases in which platelets are depleted, sometimes as a result of their combination with immune complexes plus complement, giving thrombocytopaenia and a tendency to haemorrhage. Thrombocytopaenic purpura is occasionally seen in congenital rubella and in certain other severe generalised viral infections.

Diarrhoea

The viral diarrhoeas are very important illnesses, especially in developing countries, where diarrhoea is a major cause of death in childhood. The pathogenesis is still not clear but there is an interesting indirect mechanism which appears to be involved. Rotaviruses are known to invade epithelial cells in the small intestine and they cause diarrhoea in man, foals, dogs, pigs, mice, etc. (Flewett and Woode, 1978). Extensive multiplication takes place, and very large amounts of virus are shed in faeces. Intestinal epithelial cells normally produce lactose-digesting enzymes (disaccharidases), and as more and more of these cells are destroyed or functionally impaired, ingested lactose accumulates in the gut. The lactose itself causes an osmotic flux of fluid into the intestines, and it is also fermented by intestinal bacteria to give additional products with osmotic activity. The increased water and salt in the intestinal lumen cause diarrhoea. Lactose intolerance may be important in rotavirus diarrhoea in the unweaned child or very young calf, because the diarrhoea usually stops when milk is withheld and an electrolyte solution substituted. Similar pathogenetic mechanisms would be involved if damage to intestinal epithelial cells led to defective absorption of glucose. Indeed, a general increase in permeability of plasma membranes of infected cells could lead to the passage of water and salts into the intestinal lumen. Other viruses such as the caliciviruses, adenoviruses, and coronaviruses also replicate in the intestinal epithelial cells and cause diarrhoea (Blacklow and Cukor, 1981), possibly by similar pathogenetic mechanisms.

There is another possible mechanism for the pathogenesis of gastrointestinal disease which does not involve local viral replication in the gastrointestinal tract. Haemagglutinating encephalomyelitis virus is a coronavirus infecting pigs, causing 'vomiting and wasting' disease. The vomiting appears to be of neurological origin. Vomiting is induced as a result of viral infection either of ganglia and nerve plexuses in the gastrointestinal wall, or of neurones in the brain stem and spinal cord (Andries and Pensaert, 1980).

Interferon

There is evidence that interferon is able to cause illness in human beings and in animals. Highly purified human alpha interferon has been shown to cause malaise, headaches, myalgia and fever when injected into volunteers (Scott et al., 1981), and large daily doses of beta interferon may give rise to psychiatric symptoms (Rohatiner et al., 1983). Even cloned subtypes of the various interferons obtained by recombinant DNA technology regularly produce these symptoms at high dosage ($>10^7$ units per day). Peripheral neuropathy, myelosuppression (granulocytopaenia, thrombocytopaenia and lymphopaenia) and hepatotoxicity, all generally reversible, are also not infrequent (Gutterman et al., 1982). There have been suggestions that some of the symptoms of influenza and other viral infections could be due to endogenous interferon produced in the infected individual.

A pathogenetic role for interferon is suggested from work on LCM virus infections in mice. In adult mice fatal disease follows viral replication in the brain, but extraneural tissues are also infected. Jacobson et al. (1981) found that pathogenic strains of LCM virus, unlike less virulent strains, induce large amounts of circulating interferon 3–4 days after infection. The less virulent strains became lethal when interferon inducers such as Newcastle disease virus or poly I.poly C were given. However, there is one possible mechanism which would absolve interferon from any directly pathogenic role (Pfau *et al.*, 1982). If circulating interferon reduces viral replication at extraneural sites, the influx of T cells into the infected brain would be greater than had T cells been distributed in addition to numerous extraneural growth sites. This would lead to more severe T cell-mediated immunopathology in the brain, as an indirect result of interferon. But in infant mice LCM-specific T_c are not produced (Doyle *et al.*, 1980) yet here too there are indications that interferon is involved in pathogenicity. The lethality of LCM virus in infant mice is increased by giving interferon (Rivière *et al.*, 1980) and significantly reduced by treatment with anti-interferon serum (Rivière *et al.*, 1977).

An unusual class of acid-labile α-interferons has been found in patients with the 'gay lymphadenopathy syndrome' and the acquired immune deficiency syndrome (AIDS) (de Stefano *et al.*, 1982) or certain auto-immune syndromes, notably lupus erythematosus (Preble *et al.*, 1982), but the significance of these associations is unknown.

It used to be assumed that interferons were non-immunogenic. Recently however, anti-IFN antibodies have been detected in a small number of patients following the administration of interferon (Gutterman *et al.*, 1982). Now it is apparent that this is not an uncommon development in patients receiving HuIFN (α or β), and furthermore, that some patients, especially those suffering from autoimmune disease or cancer, can, less commonly, develop low levels of antibody to their own endogenous interferon (Panem *et al.*, 1982). The short or long-term clinical significance of such antibodies has yet to be evaluated.

SUMMARY

Most viral infections produce no disease at all—they are inapparent (subclinical). This is despite extensive viral replication which leads to a lasting immunity. On the other hand, some organs such as the brain, are especially vulnerable, relatively minor changes often causing major illness in the host. One obvious mechanism of tissue damage is destruction of infected cells, such as ciliated respiratory epithelium (rhinoviruses) or anterior horn cells (polioviruses). But there is no absolute correlation between the severity of the cytopathic effects induced by a given virus in cultured cells and the severity of the disease it induces *in vivo* (e.g. rabies, congenital rubella). More subtle effects on the physiological functions of cells may also be important.

Host immune responses sometimes make a contribution to tissue damage. Type 1 hypersensitivity reactions (IgE-mediated) may be important in certain respiratory viral infections. Type 2(cytotoxic) reactions mediated by antibody and complement are readily demonstrable with virus-infected cells *in vitro*, but are of uncertain importance *in vivo*.

Type 3 (immune-complex) reactions contribute to acute inflammatory phenomena, via activation of complement. Circulating immune-complexes are important, especially in certain persistent viral infections in which antibody fails to control the infection and complexes are deposited in glomeruli (also small blood vessels, joints, etc.) giving rise to chronic glomerulonephritis (LCM in mice, Aleutian disease in mink). Host genetic factors have a decisive influence on the severity of such infections. Type 4 (cell-mediated) reactions, in which sensitised T cells trigger delayed hypersensitivity reactions, lead to inflammation, cell infiltration and tissue damage. Cytotoxic T lymphocytes kill cells infected with viruses and can be demonstrated in many viral infections, yet their immunopathological role *in vivo* is not clearly established. Immune responses that cause pathological changes, and even those that are lethal for the host (primary infection with LCM virus in mice) often have an antiviral action at the same time.

Viral infections sometimes trigger autoimmune responses that may be associated with disease, including perhaps some important conditions of currently unknown aetiology. Possible mechanisms by which viral infections may generate autoimmune disease are discussed.

The role of hormones such as cortisone and interferons in disease production is discussed. In general however, the mechanisms behind pathological phenomena, such as haemorrhage and diarrhoea, are still poorly understood.

SELECTED READING

Bablanian, R. (1975). Structural and functional alterations in cultured cells infected with cytocidal viruses. *Progr. Med. Virol.* **19**, 40.

Halstead, S. B. (1981). The pathogenesis of dengue. Molecular epidemiology in infectious disease. *Am. J. Epidemiol.* **114**, 632.

Hirsch, M. S. and Proffitt, M. R. (1975). Auto-immunity in viral infections. In *Viral Immunology and Immunopathology*, (A. L. Notkins, ed.), pp. 419–34. Academic Press, New York.

Lehmann-Grube, F. (1982). Lymphocytic choriomeningitis virus. In *The Mouse in Biomedical Research*, vol. II (eds. H. L. Foster, J. D. Small and J. G. Fox). Academic Press, New York.

Merz, D. C., Scheid, A. and Choppin, P. W. (1980). Importance of antibodies to the fusion glycoprotein of paramyxoviruses in the prevention of spread of infection, *J. Exp. Med.* **151**, 275.

Mims, C. A. (1982). *The Pathogenesis of Infectious Disease*, 2nd edition. Academic Press, New York.

Oldstone, M. B. A. (1975). Virus neutralization and virus-induced immune complex disease. *Progr. Med. Virol.* **19**, 84.

Rott, R. (1979). Molecular basis of infectivity and pathogenicity of myxovirus. *Arch. Virol.* **59**, 285.

Shatkin, A. J. (1983). Molecular mechanisms of virus-mediated cytopathology. *Phil. Trans. R. Soc. Lond. B* **303**, 167.

Chapter Five
Determinants of Viral Virulence and Host Resistance

The word 'virulence' is used here as a measure of the pathogenicity of a virus, i.e. its ability to cause disease in the infected host. The word is at times used incorrectly to refer to infectiousness (transmissibility) of a virus, but this is a different property which was dealt with in Chapter 2. Highly virulent viruses are not always readily transmissible from individual to individual (e.g. rabies), and readily transmissible viruses may not be very virulent (e.g. rhinoviruses). A measure of virulence is given by the dose of virus required to cause disease or death (Table 5.1). This figure differs for different hosts because a wide range of factors, genetic and non-genetic, immunological and non-immunological, influence resistance of a host to a given virus. Indeed, the virulence of a virus and the susceptibility/resistance of the host cannot be considered in isolation—it is their interaction that is relevant. Avirulent viruses may be capable of causing serious disease or death if administered experimentally via an atypical route, or in very large dosage, as is the case of avirulent ectromelia virus given by the footpad route to susceptible Bagg mice. Even a virulent strain may need to be given in large doses to cause disease in resistant animals, as in the case of virulent ectromelia virus given by the footpad route to resistant C57 B1 mice (Schell, 1960).

There is a wide range of pathogenicity. At one extreme the infection is harmless, asymptomatic, with very low pathogenicity. This is so for many common virus infections such as LDH virus in the mouse or CMV in man. Even when a virus has a recognised clinical disease associated with it, as in the case of poliomyelitis or mumps, there is a great range of host responses, and many infections are asymptomatic, an antibody response being the only evidence of infection. At the other extreme

Table 5.1. Examples of the dose of virus required to produce infection, disease or death.

Virus	Host	Route of infection	Minimal infectious (ID) disease-producing(DD) or lethal dose (LD)		Comments	Reference
Rhinovirus	Man	Nasal	$0.03\ TCID_{50}$	(ID)	Sensitivity of nasal epithelium greater than pharynx	Couch et al., 1966;
Coxsackievirus A21	Man	Nasal	$<1\ TCID_{50}$	(ID)		Buckland et al., 1965
		Conjunctiva	$<16\ TCID_{50}$	(ID)		
		Pharynx	$>200\ TCID_{50}$	(ID)		
Ectromelia (virulent strain)	Mouse (C57 B1 or WEHI)	Footpad	1–2 virions	(ID)	Host resistance as a determinant of outcome	Schell, 1960
	Mouse (WEHI)	Footpad	25 virions	(LD)		
	Mouse (C57 B1)	Footpad	2×10^5 virions	(LD)		
Ectromelia (virulent strain)	Mouse (Bagg)	Footpad	1–2 virions	(ID)	Virus strain as a determinant of virulence	Roberts, 1963
			10–20 virions	(LD)		
Ectromelia (avirulent strain)	Mouse (Bagg)	Footpad	1–2 virions	(ID)		
			$>10^7$ virions	(LD)		
Yellow fever	Mosquito	By feeding on infected monkey	100 mouse LD_{50}	(ID)	Successful arbovirus infects mosquito with small dose	Kumm & Laemmert, 1950

infection can lead to a rapidly or uniformly lethal disease. Rabies is uniformly lethal in most vertebrate hosts including man once the disease becomes apparent.

Clearly then, the characteristics of the virus and of the host contribute to the outcome of an infection and either can exercise a determining influence. It is convenient to regard an infection as a race between the ability of the virus to multiply, spread and make its exit from the body, and the ability of the host to curtail and control these events. In most viral infections pathological change and illness is caused when there has been an adequate amount of viral replication in the target organs. The infection will be controlled before this stage if host defences are rapidly mobilised and the virus is not too virulent. The rate at which virus replicates *in vivo* and the speed with which host defences come into operation can be important determinants of virulence. They have not received the attention they deserve.

The severity (pathogenicity) of the infection therefore results from the interplay between virus virulence on the one hand, and host resistance on the other. They are the opposite sides of the coin. In this chapter the viral determinants of virulence and the host determinants of resistance will be discussed.

VIRAL DETERMINANTS OF VIRULENCE

Studies of viral genetics have given interesting results that increase our understanding of viral replication in cells and other *in vitro* phenomena, but disappointingly little that helps with our understanding of virulence in the infected host (reviews: Fenner and Sambrook, 1964; Joklik, 1980; Fields and Jaenisch, 1980; Fields and Greene, 1982). It is common knowledge that most viruses can be attenuated to cause less damage in the infected animal, often merely by prolonged *in vitro* culture. This might have been expected to give clues about the determinants of virulence. But things are not necessarily simple. The attenuated Sabin strain of poliovirus I for instance, has 57 separate nucleotide substitutions, any one of which might be responsible for the loss of virulence (Nomoto *et al.*, 1982). Work on *ts* mutants has given interesting results and, for respiratory viruses at least, *ts* mutants have generally been less virulent (Richman and Murphy, 1979). It may be noted that many naturally occurring viruses, such as enterovirus 70 (infecting the eye), alastrim (infecting skin) and various viruses infecting the upper respiratory tract, are temperature-sensitive. Unfortunately the studies of attenuated virus strains have given no clear leads as to the viral properties responsible for virulence (see Chapter 7). Indeed, apparent loss of virulence of viruses passed in cell culture does not always depend on genetic changes in the virus. Defective interfering (DI) particles (see Chapter 1) could theoretically be important (Huang, 1977), but other changes can play a part. Mouse CMV obtained from the salivary glands of infected mice is virulent, but becomes less virulent after as few as 1–2 passages in cell culture (Osborn and Walker, 1971). Virulence is equally rapidly regained by repassage in mice. It turns out that the virus particles in salivary gland preparations are coated with non-neutralising antibody from the infected mouse, and in any case are quite different in morphology and stability from those produced in cell culture (Chong *et al.*, 1981; Chong and Mims, 1981). These differences presumably play a large part in the so-called attenuation of mouse CMV.

Sometimes it has been possible to identify the pathogenic mechanisms by which a virus has become attenuated, as in the case of the behaviour of avirulent strains of ectromelia virus in mouse liver macrophages (Roberts, 1964b). At other times, although an attenuated virus may have been well studied epidemiologically, as with the evolution of myxoma virus in rabbits (Fenner *et al.*, 1974), almost nothing is known as to the reasons for its decreased virulence.

In the case of influenza virus all the gene products have been identified, but it has not been possible to associate virulence with any particular gene product (Rott, 1979). Indeed, our detailed understanding of influenza virus structure, chemistry and replication at the cellular level (Webster *et al.*, 1982) stands in striking contrast to our ignorance about its pathogenicity in the infected host (Sweet and Smith, 1980). Exchange of any of its eight RNA molecules can modify pathogenicity, and a 'certain constellation of genes' (Rott, 1979) is necessary for virulence. Thus, influenza virulence appears to be multifactorial. Rott has suggested that the susceptibility of the viral glycoproteins of avian influenza to cleavage is a possible mechanism for pathogenicity, cleavage of the molecule being essential for infectivity of the virion. In tissues in which cleavage readily occurs, more infectious virus is produced, the virus spreads more rapidly, and is more likely to overwhelm host defences (Rott, 1979; Rott *et al.*, 1980; Klenk *et al.*, 1982). A similar mechanism may operate in the virulence of Newcastle disease virus (Nagai *et al.*, 1976). Tashiro and Homma (1983) have shown that cleavage can be a determinant of virulence in a model system in the mouse lung. A mutant of Sendai virus that was activated (cleaved) by trypsin would replicate in the mouse lung and cause pulmonary disease. A strain cleaved by chymotrypsin in contrast, was not activated in the mouse lung and failed to cause disease even after pretreatment with chymotrypsin to enable it to infect an initial set of cells, because it failed to establish successive cycles of growth. Experimental observations on respiratory syncytial viral replication suggest host proteases as possible virulence determinants in human infection (Dubovi *et al.*, 1983).

Genetic engineering technology also makes it possible to assign virulence roles to known portions of the viral genome, but without necessarily clarifying the mechanisms of action. For instance, the ocular disease pattern induced by herpes simplex type 1 virus is determined by a sequence within a defined region of the genome, between map units 0.70 and 0.83 within the Bgl 11 F DNA fragment (Centifanto *et al.*, 1982).

Monoclonal antibodies can be used to identify antigenic determinants that are associated with virulence. Coulon *et al.* (1982) studied the neurovirulence of mutants of the CVS strain of rabies virus injected intracerebrally into adult mice. Of 39 strains that were no longer neutralised by monoclonal antibodies effective against the parent strain, two had lost their virulence for adult mice. They were not *ts* mutants, and they grew efficiently in neurone cultures and in the brains of suckling mice. The experiments show that loss of virulence was due to a change in a particular antigenic site on the viral glycoprotein that was recognised by the monoclonal antibodies. The mechanism of action of this virulence determinant is unknown.

There is one viral infection in which pathogenicity is successfully being elucidated at the genetic and molecular level. The reoviruses lend themselves to sophisticated genetic studies because their genome is segmented into ten discrete molecules which can readily be exchanged by reassortment. Each molecule is a separate gene and the product of each gene has been identified. In a series of imaginative studies (summarised in Fields, 1982, and Fields and Byers, 1983), Fields and his colleagues have shown that the neurotropism and neurovirulence of reovirus type 3 in suckling mice is attributable to the viral haemagglutinin, a minor capsid protein constituting only about 3% of the total protein on the surface of virus particles. The haemagglutinin, coded by the S1 RNA segment of the genome, binds the virus to neurones, whose sequential infection leads to fatal encephalitis (Weiner *et al.*, 1980). It also binds the virus to subsets of both T and B lymphocytes which are thereby infected. Studies with monoclonal antibodies have shown that the portion of the HA molecule responsible for these things is distinct from the portion that mediates haemagglutination (Nepom *et al.*, 1982). Furthermore, the same portion of the molecule (binding site Id3) is specifically recognised by both cytotoxic T cells and neutralising antibody (Finberg *et al.*, 1982). Reovirus 1, in contrast to reovirus 3, does not infect neurones. It infects the ependymal cells lining the ventricles of the brain and this leads to a different disease, hydrocephalus. But the specific tropism of reovirus 1, in this case for ependymal cells, is again determined by its haemagglutinin, which is quite distinct from that of reovirus 3.

In the above studies reovirus 3 was injected intracerebrally into mice. The virus is avirulent when given by mouth, partly because the M2 gene-product, a polypeptide in the outer capsid, is susceptible to inactivation by intestinal proteases such as chymotrypsin (Rubin and Fields,

1980). The M2 gene-product of reovirus type 1, in contrast, is resistant to these proteases, hence that virus successfully infects intestinal tissues when given by mouth. Furthermore, when a reovirus reassortant containing the M2 (intestinal infection) gene from reovirus 1 and the S1 (neurovirulence) gene from reovirus 3 is given by mouth there follows a fatal neurological disease. Under these circumstances, gene M2 is indirectly required for the expression of virulence by S1—a good example of the complexity of virulence phenomena in the intact host.

Reoviruses are not themselves responsible for serious infections in man or in domestic animals, but they provide an excellent model system. Indeed, reovirus 3, with its segmented genome and its band of devoted researchers, will probably be the first virus to give up the innermost secrets of its virulence at the molecular and genetic level.

HOST DETERMINANTS OF RESISTANCE

Introduction

Susceptibility to infection and disease, or its reciprocal, resistance, can be measured in experimental animals by determining the dose of virus required to cause infection, disease or death in 50% of the test group (see Table 5.1). The lethal dose is expressed in LD_{50}. Less commonly measured is susceptibility to infection, regardless of disease, as indicated for instance by seroconversion, and expressed in ID_{50}. Different strains of inbred mice may differ many thousand-fold in their susceptibility/resistance to a given virus. The outcome of an infection can be viewed as the product of viral virulence × host susceptibility. A highly virulent strain of virus is less lethal for a highly resistant strain of animal than for a susceptible one; conversely, a relatively avirulent strain of virus may be lethal for an unusually susceptible host. The determinants of susceptibility may be genetic or physiological.

Susceptibility to viral infection is always influenced and sometimes determined by the genetic constitution of the host. In man, of course, one cannot conduct a titration of the sort described above, yet an unusual opportunity to see the results of a viral infection when a standard dose is administered to large numbers of healthy young adults, occurred in 1942 when more than 45 000 United States military personnel were vaccinated against yellow fever. They were inadvertently injected at the same time with hepatitis B virus which was present as a contaminant in the human serum used to stabilise the vaccine. Each man received the same dose of hepatitis B virus but the course of the infection differed according to the individual (Sawyer *et al.*, 1944). Even with a given vaccine lot, the incubation period between vaccination and disease varied from 10 to 20 weeks. Of 914 cases, 580 were mild, 301 moderate and 33 severe. Serological tests were not available at this time and there were an unknown number of subclinical infections. Of course, a random population of humans is in no way analogous to a genetically inbred strain of mice, and it is impossible to assign the observed variations in response to genetic differences in susceptibility rather than physiological differences—both would have played a part. As another example there is the increased severity of influenza virus infection in smokers (Kark et al., 1982) but it is not known which of the various theoretically possible mechanisms are responsible.

Genetic differences in susceptibility are more obvious when different species are compared. Common virus infections tend to be less virulent in the natural host species than in previously unexposed species. For instance, yellow fever, which originated in Africa and did not arrive in the Americas until the 17th century, is more virulent in South American primates than in the original host, the African primate. In Africa, rinderpest virus causes a severe disease in Indian buffaloes or in European cattle but a relatively mild infection in native African (Zebu) cattle. When a mosquito carrying myxoma virus bites the South American rabbit (Sylvilagus brasiliensis) the virus causes no more than a local skin swelling, but the same virus in the European rabbit (Oryctolagus cuniculus) leads to a rapidly fatal disease.

In the above examples of differences in susceptibility between different species nothing is known about mechanisms. A better analysis is possible when susceptibility is studied in different individuals within a given species. Malaria in man provides a classic non-viral example. Carriers of the sickle cell gene are resistant to falciparum malaria. The sickle cell gene codes for an abnormal haemoglobulin molecule with a single amino acid substitution which happens to make erythrocytes less susceptible to this type of malaria. For viruses, the matter has been dissected out in some detail in laboratory mice but even here, with inbred strains available and considerable opportunity for experimental manipulation, our understanding is imperfect (Bang, 1978). Only rarely has it been possible to identify a host gene with a more or less defined role in determining susceptibility or resistance. It is generally true that increased replication and spread of viruses in the host leads to greater tissue damage and pathogenicity. On the other hand, a change in tissue tropism can also have a major effect.

Physiological factors, such as age, sex and hormones in the host often play a major role in influencing the outcome of an infection. Individuals from a given inbred strain of mice show marked differences in susceptibility. Even if a single animal could be repeatedly tested, it would doubtless suffer a different disease on different occasions, due to physiological changes in susceptibility. These physiological determinants will be discussed separately.

Cellular receptors for virus

The presence or absence of receptors for virus on the plasma membrane of a cell is a fundamental determinant of susceptibility, and has often been found to account for differences in susceptibility in the intact host. For instance, neuraminidase will destroy the cellular receptors for influenza virus, and it was shown many years ago (Stone, 1948) that pretreatment of mice with neuraminidase (in the form of receptor-destroying enzyme) intranasally confers substantial protection against subsequent intranasal challenge with influenza virus. The protection was short-lived (1–2 days) because there was rapid regeneration of receptors.

Primate neurones are susceptible to poliovirus infection and in man the structural gene for the poliovirus receptor is known to be on chromosome 19 (Miller *et al.*, 1974). Mice, in contrast, are insusceptible to infection with most strains of poliovirus because murine cells lack a receptor for this virus. If, however, they are injected intracerebrally with poliovirus RNA (Holland *et al.*, 1959) or with poliovirus genomes enclosed within the capsids of a mouse-pathogenic enterovirus such as coxsackievirus B1 (Cords and Holland, 1964) the cells are infected with poliovirus and support a single cycle of multiplication. But the progeny particles have the surface properties of normal poliovirions, and are therefore unable to attach to and produce infection of any more cells. The resistance of chickens to infection with certain strains of avian leukovirus is a direct consequence of the genetically determined absence of virus receptors on their cells (Weiss, 1982). A single pair of autosomal genes was shown to control the susceptibility of the chick chorio-allantoic membrane to Rous sarcoma virus, with susceptibility dominant to resistance (Bower *et al.*, 1965).

When an organ is taken from an intact animal and the cells dispersed with trypsin and cultivated *in vitro*, major changes in virus susceptibility are common. In monkeys infected with poliovirus for instance, the kidney is not involved, even when virus is injected directly into that organ. But trypsinised monkey kidney cells have long been the standard assay system and source of poliovirus *in vitro*. Poliovirus also shows little or no growth in intact sheets of human amnion nor in freshly trypsinised amnion cells. However, after maintenance in culture for about seven days, these cells acquire susceptibility to poliovirus (Gresser *et al.*, 1965). It is not known whether such changes in susceptibility are due to the generation (or possible unmasking) of cell receptors.

In a classic example of genetically determined resistance of laboratory mice to viral infection, receptors may be important, but the exact mechanism is still obscure. By selective breeding, Webster (1937) developed strains of mice which differed greatly in resistance to the flaviviruses, St Louis encephalitis and louping ill. He showed that resistance or susceptibility was correlated with the level of viral multi-plication both in the brain of the intact animal and in cultures of minced brain tissue. The resistance of PRI and susceptibility of C3H and BSVS mice to yellow fever was further analysed by Sabin (1954). From tests with F1 hybrids and with backcrosses to the parental strain, he showed that a single dominant gene conferred resistance. Subsequently it was shown with West Nile virus that this was associated with enhanced ability of the virus to multiply in many types of cell in susceptible strains of animals, including brain cells, macrophages and lung and kidney cells (Vainio, 1963a; 1963b). Interferon was brought into the picture when Hansen *et al.* (1969) showed that cells from both resistant and sus-ceptible strains of mice produced equal amounts of interferon, but inter-feron had a greater antiviral effect on cells of the resistant strain. The exact mechanism of action of the flavivirus resistance gene is still not clear.

Receptors sometimes determine the virus susceptibility of different types of cell in the host. EB virus for instance, infects human B cells because B cells have virus receptors, which are closely associated with but not identical to C3 receptors (Wells *et al.*, 1983). There is evidence that the receptor for rabies virus is the acetylcholine receptor (Lentz *et al.*, 1982) and this would help explain the pathogenesis of rabies. Although it is often assumed that a certain cell type is infected because it bears virus receptors, evidence for this is generally lacking. A cell might equally well escape infection because a virus fails to gain access to it. Thus, many strains of vaccinia virus never infect liver cells in mice because Kupffer cells prevent the access of circulating virus, but hepatic cells can be artificially infected from the biliary tract by retrograde injec-tion of virus up the bile duct (Mims, 1964). Again, influenza virus in ferrets is normally studied as a respiratory tract infection, but experi-mentally it is also capable of infecting the urinogenital tract (Toms *et al.*, 1974).

Surprisingly, the greater virulence of certain alphaviruses in mice has been correlated with decreased attachment to host cells (Marker and Jahrling, 1979). Viral strains that showed decreased attachment were less readily removed from the blood by reticuloendothelial cells, and were more virulent because they were more likely to establish infection in target organs. Similar suggestions have been made for encephalo-myocarditis virus, which binds to glycophorin on human erythrocytes, but does not bind to mouse erythrocytes. Erythrocyte-associated virus is less able to spread from the blood (see Chapter 2) and this is correlated with less effective dissemination of this virus in man than in mouse (McClintock *et al.*, 1980).

Host susceptibility can be determined not only by virus interactions with cell receptors, but also by other surface components of the virion. Recent work with Sindbis virus associates viraemia levels in different mice with the sialic acid content of the virion envelope, as determined by the sialic acid content of host cells. Decreased sialic acid in host cells means decreased levels on the virion, which in turn leads to greater activation of complement by the alternate pathway, and greater host control of the viraemia (Hirsch *et al.*, 1983).

If the presence of virus receptors in a target organ were under genetic control there would of course be important consequences for susceptibility. Individuals whose respiratory epithelial cells had a low density of influenza virus receptors might therefore be relatively resistant to influenza virus infection. This is theoretically possible, but differences in host susceptibility have generally not been shown to be due to differences in susceptibility of host cells or the yield of virus from cells. The susceptibility of various strains of mice to murine cytomegalovirus and to herpes simplex virus is correlated with the susceptibility and extent of viral replication in embryo fibroblasts (Harnett and Shellam, 1983; Collier *et al.*, 1983). In the case of MCMV the differences are too small to account for *in vivo* differences in susceptibility, and there are reasons for supposing that the *in vitro* result with herpes simplex is not a major factor in host susceptibility *in vivo*. The relative resistance of C57 B1 mice to mousepox was found to operate at the level of the immune response rather than cell susceptibility (Schell, 1960).

Cellular factors other than receptors may be important. These range from the genetically determined presence or absence of a cellular enzyme vital to the multiplication of the virus to differences in the physiological state of the cell. A single example suffices to make the point. The vulnerability of cells to parvovirus infection depends on their mitotic state (Johnson, 1980). Thus, in the adult cat feline panleukopenia virus infects mitotic cells in bone marrow and in intestinal epithelium to give leukopenia and diarrhoea, while in the cat foetus the mitotic germinal cells of the cerebellum are destroyed to give cerebellar aplasia (see Chapter 2).

Interferons

Since its discovery 26 years ago, interferon has looked as though it ought to be important in defence against viral infection. In recent years the different interferons have been cloned and purified, and much has been learnt about their antiviral, immunomodulatory, and other actions. There have been clinical trials of interferon in human virus infections and in human cancers. Although much remains to be learnt, interferons seem important enough for the subject to be treated at some length here in the context of determinants of host resistance. The possibility that interferons may also contribute to disease has been discussed in Chapter 4.

General features. In 1957 Isaacs and Lindenmann described a protein, 'interferon', which was secreted by virus-infected cells and could protect uninfected cells against infection with the same or unrelated viruses. Interferon was postulated, and subsequently proven, to be the principal mediator of the well known phenomenon of interference (see the following recent books: Gresser, 1979, 1980, 1981, 1982; Vilček *et al.*, 1980; de Maeyer *et al.*, 1981; de Maeyer and Schellekens, 1983; Merigan and Friedman, 1982; Pestka, 1981; Baron *et al.*, 1982; Burke and Morris, 1983; Tyrrell and Burke, 1982; Finter, 1983–4).

There are three antigenically and chemically distinct types of interferon (IFN), now known as α, β and γ (Table 5.2). In a spectacular demonstration of the power of modern molecular biology (Nagata *et al.*, 1980; Goeddel *et al.*, 1980; Derynck *et al.*, 1980; Taniguchi *et al.*, 1980) the last two or three years have seen the discovery and cloning by recombinant DNA technology of separate genes for at least a dozen subtypes of human interferon α (HuIFN-α) (Brack *et al.*, 1981; Goeddel *et al.*, 1981; Sehgal *et al.*, 1981; Weissmann, 1981); at least one β (Weissenbach *et al.*, 1980; Sagar *et al.*, 1981; 1982); and at least one γ (Yip *et al.*, 1982; Gray *et al.*, 1982; Gray and Goeddel, 1982). Most of these human genes have now been cloned in bacteria, yeasts and/or mammalian cells and the resulting protein products purified and sequenced (see Weissmann, 1981; Goeddel *et al.*, 1981; Gray and Goeddel, 1982; Mantei and Weiss-

Table 5.2. Physicochemical properties of human interferons.

Property	α	β	γ
Previous designations	Le-IFN Type I	F-IFN Type I	Immune IFN Type II
Subtypes	12	?5	1(?2)
Mr—major subtypes —cloned[b]	16–23 000 19 000	23 000 19 000	20(–25) 000 17 000
Glycosylation	No[a]	Yes	Yes
pH2 stability	Stable[a]	Stable	Labile
Induction	Viruses	Viruses	Mitogens
Principal source	Lymphocyte, etc.	Fibroblast	Lymphocyte
Activity in bovine cells	Yes	No	No
Introns in gene	No	No	Yes
Homology with HuIFN-α	80–95%	30–50%	<10%

[a]Most subtypes, but not all.
[b]Non-glycosylated.

man, 1982; Pestka *et al.*, 1982; Weissmann *et al.*, 1982; Pestka, 1983). IFNs-β and γ, but generally not α (Allen and Fantes, 1980; Pestka, 1983) are glycosylated (in mammalian cells). Most of the human interferons have molecular weights in the range 16 000–23 000 daltons, though some are larger. IFNs-α and β have the unusual property of being resistant to inactivation at pH 2 (see Finter, 1984), although some atypical acid-labile α-interferons have recently been described (Balkwill *et al.*, 1983; Grundy *et al.*, 1982; de Stefano *et al.*, 1982; Preble *et al.*, 1982).

Inteferon α and β are not made constitutively in significant amounts but are induced by any virus, multiplying in virtually any type of cell, in any species of vertebrate that has been tested, whether mammal, bird, amphibian, reptile or fish. IFN-γ is atypical in that it is made only by lymphocytes and only following antigen-specific or non-specific (e.g. mitogen) stimulation; it can be regarded as a lymphokine with immuno-regulatory functions (Epstein, 1981; Vilček *et al.*, 1981). Some IFNs (especially β and γ) display a degree of host species specificity; e.g. many murine interferons (MuIFNs) are ineffective in primates. There is no virus specificity, in the sense that IFN-α, β or γ induced by a para-myxovirus is effective against a togavirus; but certain cloned IFN sub-types may be much more effective against some viruses than against others in the same cell type (Weck *et al.*, 1981).

Antiviral action of interferons. The mechanism of antiviral action of IFN-α and β has recently been elucidated, in part at least (reviews: Baglioni, 1979; 1982; Revel, 1979; Cayley *et al.*, 1981; Lengyel, 1981; 1982; Pestka *et al.*, 1981; Sehgal *et al.*, 1982; Lebleu and Content, 1982).

Interferon binds to a specific receptor on the cell surface; there appears to be a common receptor for IFN-α and β (Aguet, 1980) and another for IFN-γ (Branca and Baglioni, 1981). Such binding triggers a cascade of biochemical events. No fewer than three new enzymes are induced: $(2'-5')$ $(A)_n$ synthetase (often abbreviated to 2-5A synthetase), RNase L (otherwise known as RNase F, or endoribonuclease), and a 73K protein kinase. Both the 2-5A synthetase and the protein kinase require for their activation double-stranded RNA (Kerr and Brown, 1978; Marcus, 1982), which is therefore assumed to be an intermediate or by-product in the replication of DNA as well as RNA viruses. Once activated, 2-5A synthetase catalyses the synthesis from ATP of an unusual family of short-lived oligonucleotides known as $(2'-5')$ $pppA(pA)_n$, or 2-5A for short (Kerr and Brown, 1978). In turn, 2-5A activates the latent endo-nuclease, RNase L, to destroy messenger RNA, hence to inhibit protein synthesis in interferon-treated virus-infected cells (see Baglioni, 1983; Lengyel, 1982). The 73K protein kinase, following activation by dsRNA, also inhibits protein synthesis, but in a completely different way, namely by inactivating (by phosphorylation) the peptide chain initiation factor, eIF-2 (see Lengyel, 1982).

Numerous other biochemical changes have been described following interferon treatment of cells, including, for example, inhibition of methylation of the 5'-terminal guanosine 'cap' of viral mRNA (see Baglioni, 1979; 1983; Revel, 1979; Lengyel, 1981; 1982). At the time of writing, it is not possible to assign any of these biochemical changes a critical role in the antiviral action of interferon. Indeed, recent data, while not disputing the reality of the several biochemical consequences of exposure to interferon, do throw into question the relevance of either the 2-5A synthetase/RNase L or the protein kinase pathway to the induction of the antiviral state (see Baglioni, 1983; Ball, 1982). Moreover, Baglioni and colleagues detected no dsRNA in cells infected with the exquisitely IFN-sensitive virus, VSV, therefore postulate that the critical mediator(s) of IFN action are not dependent on dsRNA and have yet to be discovered (see Baglioni, 1983).

Potentially, interferons would appear to be the ideal antiviral antibiotics: broad spectrum, of extremely high specific activity, relatively non-toxic (but see Chapter 4), and apparently incapable of generating resistant mutants. Clinical trials in man prior to 1982 were undertaken mainly with purified preparations of mixed human interferons produced in human leukocytes (Cantell et al., 1981), lymphoblastoid cells (Finter, 1982), or fibroblasts (Leong and Horoszewicz, 1981; van Damme and Billiau, 1981). They indicate that HuIFN-α and β, when inoculated early and in very large dosage (millions of units per day), can shorten the course of a number of viral diseases (Table 5.3; see also reviews: Dunnick and Galasso, 1979; 1980; Merigan, 1981; Came and Carter, 1983; Kono and Vilček, 1982; Münk and Kirchner, 1982; World Health Organization, 1982; Burke and Morris, 1983). Furthermore, there is some evidence that HuIFN can bring about temporary remission in a minority of cases of certain types of cancer (reviews: Gresser and Tovey, 1978; Dunnick and Galasso, 1979; 1980; de Maeyer et al., 1981; 1983; Merigan, 1981; Baron et al., 1982; Munk and Kirchner, 1982; Pollard, 1982; Burke and Morris, 1983). These exciting clinical successes, together with the breakthrough in recombinant DNA technology which facilitated and greatly reduced the cost of production of purified interferon, engendered a feeling of euphoria as we entered the 1980s. Full evaluation of the spectrum of biological activity and therapeutic potential of each individual HuIFN will now have to be undertaken separately with each cloned product. Already however, it is apparent that interferon is not a panacea for all ills, but rather, a valuable adjunct to antiviral and anticancer therapy. Fascinating as this topic may be, it is beyond the ambit of this book; the place of interferon and other agents in antiviral chemotherapy is reviewed elsewhere (White, 1984).

Interferons as hormones. Interferon was discovered as an antiviral agent, defined accordingly, and generally regarded as such by virologists for

Table 5.3. Antiviral activity of interferons in man.

Virus	Disease	Route
Rhinovirus	Common cold	Intranasal
Herpes simplex	Keratitis	Ocular
	Herpes facialis, genitalis	i.m.
Varicella-zoster	Herpes zoster	i.m.
	Varicella	
Cytomegalovirus	Activation in immunosuppressed	i.m.
Hepatitis B	Chronic hepatitis or carrier	i.m., i.v.
Papilloma	Laryngeal papilloma	Local
	Warts (common or genital)	
Adenovirus	Keratoconjunctivitis?	Ocular

Abbreviations:
i.m. = intramuscular; i.v. = intravenous; local = injected into lesion.

the next two decades. Yet, ever since about 1970, one voice in particular, that of Gresser, has been crying in the wilderness that interferon exerts a wide range of other effects on cells and that its antiviral effect may not necessarily be its principal function in nature (review: Gresser, 1977). It is now widely acknowledged that the interferons probably represent a family of hormones (Taylor-Papadimitriou, 1980; Inglot, 1983) which bind to specific receptors on the cell surface and initiate a cascade of biochemical events leading, perhaps under defined circumstances, not only to inhibition of viral replication, but also to inhibition of cell division, changes in the plasma membrane, modulation of the immune system, and several additional phenomena (see also, Balkwill, 1979; de Maeyer and de Maeyer-Guignard, 1979; Vilček *et al.*, 1980). Sceptical virologists, who had been inclined to attribute this plethora of apparently unrelated effects to contaminating proteins in crude interferon preparations, were finally won over by the report from Gresser *et al.* (1979) that purified IFN retained a wide spectrum of anti-cellular as well as anti-viral effects (Table 5.4). This observation has now been widely confirmed and extended to embrace individual subtypes of IFN, purified following production by recombinant DNA technology (Pestka *et al.*, 1982). All 'cloned' IFNs tested to date display antiproliferative as well as antiviral activity, though the ratio of the two differs, sometimes strikingly, from one subtype to another, with some being much more active as inhibitors of cell division or immunomodulators than of viral replication, and some more active against certain viruses or in certain cell types (Weck *et al.*, 1981; Lee *et al.*, 1982; Wallach *et al.*, 1982).

Table 5.4. Some biological effects of interferons.

Inhibition of multiplication of viruses

Inhibition of cell division
  In vitro: normal and malignant cells in culture
  In vivo: regenerating liver
         bone marrow
         neonatal mouse
         cancer in animals and man

Changes in plasma membrane
  Histocompatibility antigens increased
  β-microglobulin increased
  Fc receptors increased
  Lectin binding increased
  Negative charge increased
  Release of murine leukaemia virus decreased
  Cell motility decreased
  Organisation of microfilaments and fibronectin disturbed

Immunomodulation
B cell	antibody production decreased or increased
T cell	proliferation suppressed, lymphokine release enhanced
T_s cell	activated
T_d and/or T_{sd} cell	delayed hypersensitivity decreased or increased
T_c cell	cytotoxicity increased
NK cell	maturation, recycling and cytoxicity increased
Macrophage	activated

Inhibition of cell division. As long ago as 1962 Paucker *et al.* had reported that interferon inhibits the multiplication of cultured cells. The phenomenon was largely ignored until it was discovered that IFN also inhibits the growth of cancer cells (review: Gresser and Tovey, 1978). Now it is clear that normal cells of all types are just as susceptible to the growth-inhibitory effects of IFN as are their malignant counterparts (Balkwill, 1979). The inhibition takes the form of a lengthening of all phases of the cell cycle, especially G_1, and is fully reversible on removal of the drug, i.e. interferon is cytostatic, not cytocidal. Interferons α, β and γ differ in their relative efficacy as antiproliferative agents (Rubin and Gupta, 1980).

It is by no means clear whether the antiproliferative effects of interferon are mediated via the same induced enzymes as have been postulated to account for its antiviral activity. Mutant cell lines have been derived in which the two activities are dissociated. For example, whereas the human fibroblast cell line RSa is sensitive to interferon's antiviral and anticellular effects, the mutant IF^r is resistant to its anticellular action (Vandenbussche *et al.*, 1981). Yet, both lines produce comparable amounts of both 2-5A synthetase and the 73K phosphoprotein kinase on interferon treatment, suggesting that the anti-proliferative activity at least must be mediated by another mechanism.

Nor is it clear that IFN-γ acts via the same pathway(s) as α and β. For instance, both β and γ IFN induce the synthesis of both the dsRNA-dependent enzymes in the leukaemia cell line L1210^S, which is sensitive to the growth-inhibitory action of interferons, whereas only IFN-γ induces them in the resistant mutant L1210^R (Hovanessian et al., 1980). There is some evidence that interferons I and II potentiate one another in both their antiviral and their antiproliferative actions (see Fleischmann, 1982).

In vivo examples of the growth-inhibitory effects of IFN are also plentiful (reviews: Gresser, 1977; Balkwill, 1979; de Maeyer and de Maeyer-Guignard, 1979; Taylor-Papadimitriou, 1980). For instance, interferon blocks the regeneration of liver in partially hepatectomised mice, and also the multiplication of bone marrow cells in irradiated mice. The IFN levels attained during LCM virus replication in newborn mice are such as to inflict progressive organ damage, e.g. glomerulo-nephritis, and perhaps runting (Rivière et al., 1977); it should be added that such effects have not been seen in other animal species, e.g. monkeys. The anti-cancer effects of IFN, clearly demonstrable *in vivo* both in animals (review: Gresser and Tovey, 1978) and in man (see p. 170) may be principally attributable to another phenomenon, namely the immunomodulatory effects of IFN, particularly the activation of natural killer (NK) cells (Reid et al., 1981), macrophages and cytotoxic T (T_c) cells (see pp. 174–5).

Changes in the plasma membrane. Following binding to its specific receptor on the cell surface (Aguet, 1980; Branca and Baglioni, 1981), IFN induces a variety of changes referable to the plasma membrane (see Gresser, 1977; Balkwill, 1979; Taylor-Papadimitriou, 1980). These include increases in lectin binding and in net negative charge, as well as in the expression of histocompatibility antigens, β_2-microglobulin, Fc receptors (Fridman et al., 1980) and Ir gene-products (Nakamura et al., 1984). Wallach et al. (1982) found that IFN-γ induced increased synthesis of HLA-A, B, C and β_2-microglobulin mRNA and protein at IFN concentrations over 100 times lower than those needed to induce (2′–5′) oligo (A) synthetase and the antiviral state; this difference was not found with IFN-α or β. Cell motility is also decreased and the organisation of micro-filaments and fibronectin disturbed (Pfeffer et al., 1980). Effects of the hormone on the plasma membrane may explain the inhibition of budding of murine leukaemia virus from interferon-treated cells (Pitha et al., 1976).

Immunomodulation. The effects of interferons on the immune system are manifold and sometimes apparently contradictory (reviews: Epstein,

1981; Gresser, 1977; Johnson and Baron, 1977; Balkwill, 1979; de Maeyer and de Maeyer-Guignard, 1979; 1980; de Weck *et al.*, 1980; Mozes *et al.*, 1981; Moore, 1983).

Interferons α and γ are secreted by both T and B lymphocytes following binding of lectins or specific antigens. It is not yet clear whether certain T cell subsets are more efficient interferon producers than others. The observation that macrophages are essential for optimum interferon production by T cells on exposure to antigen may reflect the fact that T_h and T_d cells recognise antigen only in association with Ia antigen on macrophages (see Möller, 1981a; b; c). However, one would not expect macrophages to be required for interferon production by T_c cells, which recognise antigen in association with HLA antigen on the surface of any type of cell (Zinkernagel and Doherty, 1979); indeed, a T_c clone specifically recognising influenza A virus-infected H-2^d target cells was found to secrete IFN-γ, in the absence of macrophages, on exposure only to that particular target (Morris *et al.*, 1982).

Interferons, whether secreted by lymphocytes or by other types of cell, may inhibit the replication of lymphocytes as well as other cell types. Kadish *et al.* (1980) showed this to be the explanation of the well known 'anti-mitogenic effect' of interferon; interferon I and/or II secreted by lectin-treated lymphocytes suppresses the proliferation of the lectin-activated population as a whole. Indeed, 2-5A itself, or even its dephosphorylated 'core', blocks the mitogenic effect of concanavalin A on lymphocytes, principally by inhibiting the synthesis of histones and other proteins (Kimchi *et al.*, 1981). Furthermore, interferons α, β and γ in general seem to inhibit antibody synthesis when administered before or together with the immunogen, but to stimulate it if added some days later (see Johnson and Baron, 1977). The immunosuppression, by IFN-α and β at least, occurs with T-independent as well as T-dependent antigens, and with both primary and secondary response. Aune and Pierce (1982) presented evidence that suppression of antibody production by IFN-β is attributable to activation of suppressor T cells, which then secrete TsF. IFN-γ is considerably more potent than α and β as an inhibitor of B cells when given before the immunogen, and enhances the antibody response by stimulating T cells, when given after the immunogen (Sonnenfeld *et al.*, 1978). However, Nakamura *et al.* (1984) showed that cloned murine IFN-γ enhanced antibody production in mice when given together with antigen. Similarly, interferon 'type I' was found to inhibit the development of delayed hypersensitivity if administered before the immunogen, but to enhance it if given a few hours later (de Maeyer and de Maeyer-Guignard, 1980). This may be explicable by the subsequent observation of Knop *et al.* (1982) that interferons α and β inhibit the generation and function of the particular class of T_s cell that suppresses DTH.

On the other hand, interferon has been shown to enhance the cytotoxicity of T_c lymphocytes (Lindahl *et al.*, 1972), macrophages (Schultz *et al.*, 1978) and natural killer (NK) cells (Gidlund *et al.*, 1978; Trinchieri and Santoli, 1978). Indeed, IFN-γ appears to be the lymphokine known as MAF (macrophage-activating factor). Interferon, moreover, is the principal factor controlling the life cycle of NK cells—it triggers their maturation from pre-NK cells, enhances their recycling capacity, and augments their lytic potential (see Wigzell, in Mozes *et al.*, 1981). Furthermore, since NK cells also secrete interferon on contacting a virus-infected target cell, there exists a positive feed-back mechanism accelerating the elimination of virus from the body.

Overall, it appears that interferons may stimulate or inhibit various arms of the immune response, depending on the timing and dosage. One can think of interferons as lymphokines, induced principally by viral infection, and playing a key role in the regulation of the immunological response to that virus. Interferons secreted by virus-infected target cells, as well as by lymphocytes, macrophages and NK cells, activate T_c lymphocytes, macrophages and NK cells in the immediate vicinity to develop their cytotoxic potential. In turn, these effector cells not only destroy the target but produce more interferon following contact with viral antigen on its surface. The consequential cascade greatly amplifies the lytic arm of the immune response. Yet it is apparent that other important arms of the immune response are depressed by interferon, perhaps reflecting the propensity of interferon to inhibit the replication of lymphocytes. A full analysis of this complicated issue must await careful *in vitro* studies of the various actions of purified preparations of each cloned subtype of interferon on cloned populations of well characterised lymphocyte subtypes. Armed with that knowledge, it should then be feasible to go back to the whole animal to document the biological relevance of each of interferon's diverse effects.

By no means all of the immunomodulatory, growth-inhibitory and membrane effects listed in Table 5.4, let alone in the more comprehensive compilation given by Taylor-Papadimitriou (1980), have been demonstrated to occur with pure preparations of IFNs α, β and γ, and certainly not with the several cloned subtypes of each. Careful re-examination of the relative potency of each subtype in each of these and other previously untested activities now constitutes an important priority, because it may well emerge that particular subtypes are relatively specialised in their natural role as antiviral agent, hormone or lymphokine, and that these differences could be exploited in antiviral and anti-cancer therapy.

Genetic control of interferon production and susceptibility. The structural genes for most of the known human interferons (at least ten IFN-α and IFN-β_1) are clustered contiguously on chromosome 9 (Burke, 1980; Burke and Meager, 1980; Owerbach *et al.*, 1981; Sehgal *et al.*, 1981). A smaller number of others have been assigned to chromosomes 2 and 5 (Tan, 1977), and the gene for IFN-γ is on chromosome 12 (Naylor *et al.*, 1983).

Most of the genes for interferons contain no introns (Nagata *et al.*, 1980; Goeddel *et al.*, 1981; review: Weissmann, 1981)—an atypical circumstance in mammalian cells. This is fortunate indeed, for it has enabled HuIFN genes to be successfully cloned and expressed in bacteria and yeasts, neither of which possess the wherewithall for splicing. (The gene for HuIFN-γ does contain introns however; Gray and Goeddel, 1982.)

A genetic locus on human chromosome 21 is essential for the expression of antiviral activity by IFN-α, β and γ (Tan, 1977; Revel, 1979; Epstein *et al.*, 1980; Epstein, 1981). Some evidence suggests that this gene may code for the IFN receptor (Aguet, 1980).

The regulation of expression of the genes for IFN in mammalian cells is quite complex (Burke, 1983). It is a common observation of those groups assembling cDNA libraries for cloning purposes that there is differential expression of different IFN genes in different cell lines *in vitro*. Furthermore, various inbred strains of mouse differ in the amount of circulating interferon they produce following inoculation with different viruses; single but distinct autosomal loci were found to control IFN levels against each of several viruses tested by de Maeyer and de Maeyer-Guignard (1979; 1980). They have also presented evidence that several additional genes affect the interaction of interferons with cells of the immune system. Moreover, Haller *et al.* (1980; 1981a) have described a gene (Mx) which confers resistance to influenza virus in a certain strain of mouse by virtue of enhancing the sensitivity of influenza virus (but not of other viruses) to the antiviral action of interferon (Haller *et al.*, 1981b).

Production and distribution in vivo. It is difficult to determine which cell types, or even which tissues and organs, are responsible for most of the interferon production *in vivo*, but, extrapolating from the findings with cultured cells, one can probably safely assume that most cells in the body are capable of producing interferon in response to viral infection. Certainly, interferon can be found in the mucus bathing epithelial surfaces such as the respiratory tract, while 'fibroblast' (β) interferon is produced by most or all cells of mesenchymal derivation. Lymphocytes, especially T cells and 'null' leukocytes, presumably NK and K cells as well as macrophages produce large amounts of IFN-α and γ, and probably comprise the principal source of circulating IFN in viral infections characterised by a viraemic stage (de Maeyer and de Maeyer-Guignard, 1979).

Role in recovery from viral infection. Data supporting a central role for interferon in the recovery of experimental animals and man following viral infections have been reviewed by Sonnenfeld and Merigan (1979). The most telling evidence that interferon can indeed be instrumental in deciding the fate of the animal following natural viral infection has been provided by Gresser and his colleagues, who have shown that mice infected with any of several non-lethal viruses, or with sublethal doses of more virulent viruses, die if anti-IFN serum is administered (e.g. see Virelizier and Gresser, 1978). In an interesting recent example it was found that a large inoculum of herpes simplex virus induced more interferon and was less fatal than a smaller dose; under these conditions anti-interferon serum had a correspondingly more marked effect (Zawatsky et al., 1982). Further support is given by the genetic evidence of Haller et al. (1980; 1981a) and de Maeyer and de Maeyer-Guignard (1979; 1980), discussed above. The mechanism by which interferon protects against infection is usually not known. It is sometimes possible to distinguish between direct protection of susceptible cells and induction of NK cells (Chong et al., 1983). Immunomodulatory actions of interferon could be important when a disease is immunopathological in nature. An intriguing role for interferon in immunopathology has been suggested from work on LCM virus infection of mice (see above).

A mouse mutant lacking the structural genes for some, or preferably all of the interferons would make a useful experimental model. But, teleologically, one could argue that such an animal would not survive, if interferon does indeed play a crucial role in defence against viral infection or the regulation of growth or differentiation.

The recovery of any given individual will be influenced by the numerous genes encoding and regulating not only the amount of each species of interferon produced following infection, but also the efficacy of each interferon against that particular virus. Nothing is known of the extent of variation between individuals, or even between species, in the expression of these several genes, let alone of the causes or effects of such variation. Should prospective studies (or even *post hoc* tests during a particular illness) reveal a genetic or acquired deficiency in the production, regulation or action of some or all interferons in a particular individual, it may be feasible in the future to direct interferon therapy towards those most likely to benefit.

As might be expected, infants with certain congenital immunodeficiencies or infections, and patients otherwise immunosuppressed (e.g. for organ transplantation or as a consequence of malignancies of the lymphoid system) display diminished production of interferon α, and especially γ, when their lymphocytes are tested, e.g. by lectin stimulation *in vitro* (Stiehm et al., 1982). There are also some reports of diminished capacity to produce interferon by individuals who suffer from repeated or unusually severe infections, e.g. children with recurrent respiratory infections (Isaacs et al., 1981), or patients with acute fulminating viral hepatitis (Levin and Hahn, 1982). The serum interferon level may not necessarily represent the most reliable indicator of endogenous interferon production or the effectiveness of an individual's response. Schattner *et al.* (1981) developed an assay for 2-5A synthetase in peripheral leukocytes which could be useful, provided it can be shown to measure interferon responsiveness with the degree of specificity postulated.

While it is widely believed that interferon constitutes the first line of defence in the process of recovery from viral infections, it would be naive to believe that it is the only, or even the most important factor. If this were so, one might expect that a systemic infection with any virus, or indeed, immunisation with a live vaccine, might protect an individual, for a period at least, against challenge with an unrelated virus. While some data have been presented on this point, the phenomenon cannot be generally demonstrated. The evidence is somewhat stronger that infection of the upper respiratory tract with one virus will provide temporary protection against others. Perhaps this distinction provides the clue that the direct antiviral effect of interferon is limited in both time and space. Its main antiviral role may be to protect cells in the immediate vicinity of the initial focus of infection.

Macrophages

Macrophages play a central role as determinants of host resistance in many viral infections as discussed in Chapter 2. Macrophages are often considered as mere adjuncts to immune responses in viral infections. This is incorrect. They have their own intrinsic susceptibility to viral infection which is independent of antibodies or the action of lymphokines (see Chapter 3), although it is often influenced by these immune factors. The role of macrophages as determinants of host susceptibility/resistance (Mogensen, 1979) will now be discussed.

Many viruses multiply regularly in macrophages. In some instances macrophages appear to be the only susceptible cells in the body. e.g. to lactic dehydrogenase (LDH), equine infectious anaemia (EIA) and Aleutian disease (AD) viruses; the basis for this selective susceptibility is not known. In other instances macrophages are one of many types of cell that are susceptible. Often, however, the viral replication cycle in macrophages is abortive, with little or no yield of infectious progeny (see Table 5.5). Macrophage susceptibility appears to determine susceptibility of mice to murine hepatitis virus (MHV)-3, ectromelia and herpes simplex virus (HSV).

Bang and Warwick (1960) showed that PRI mice were more susceptible to infection with MHV than C_3H mice, and this was attributable to the destruction of PRI liver macrophages by the virus (Kantoch *et al.*, 1963). The virus adsorbed to and penetrated macrophages from each strain of mice, but it was not uncoated in the resistant C_3H macrophages.

Table 5.5. Macrophage susceptibility to virus infection.

Virus	Host	Type of macrophage[a]	Susceptibility insusceptible	Susceptibility defective growth cycle	Susceptibility susceptible
Feline peritonitis	cat	varied			+
Visna: fresh isolate	sheep	peritoneal, alveolar, colostral, blood[b]			+
laboratory strain				+	
K virus	mouse	liver, lung, spleen			+ +
LCM	mouse	most			+ +
Rubella	man	blood		?	
Mouse hepatitis (most strains)	mouse	peritoneal and liver			+
Lactic dehydrogenase	mouse	subset of macrophages[c]			+ +
Aleutian disease	mink	most			+ +
Equine infectious anaemia	horse	most			+
African swine fever	pig	liver and other macrophages		+	
Sendai	mouse	alveolar, peritoneal		+	
Ectromelia virulent	mouse	peritoneal and liver	±		±
avirulent				+	
Herpes simplex	mouse	peritoneal (adult)		+	
	man	blood		+	
Mouse CMV	mouse	peritoneal		+	
Pig CMV	pig	alveolar		+	+
Influenza A	mouse	peritoneal (subset)		+	
	mouse	alveolar		+	
	human	alveolar		+	

[a]Details differ according to type of macrophage and host genetic background. Tendency for lower susceptibility of activated macrophages or macrophages from adult animals.
[b]Narayan et al., 1982.
[c]Stueckemann et al., 1982.

The correlation of macrophage susceptibility with virulence is not seen with all strains of mouse hepatitis virus (Taguchi *et al.*, 1981), although it does hold for the neurotropic (JHM) strain of MHV (Stohlman *et al.*, 1982). Although the susceptibility of different strains of mice correlates with the *in vitro* susceptibility of macrophages, this is not the only factor. Studies with MHV3 showed that susceptibility also correlates with the *in vitro* susceptibility of hepatocytes (Arnheiter *et al.*, 1982). Hepatocytes from resistant strains of mice were infected by MHV3, but maturation was defective and virus yield reduced up to 1000-fold compared with hepatocytes from susceptible mice. It is possible that factors other than mere susceptibility of macrophages to infection play a part. Peripheral blood mononuclear cells from susceptible strains of mice show rapid and striking production of procoagulant activity following MHV3 infection when compared with cells from resistant strains of mice (Levy *et al.*, 1981). It is not known whether this plays a part in pathogenesis, but such phenomena have rarely been studied and could be important.

Roberts (1964a; 1964b) showed that a virulent strain of ectromelia virus could be distinguished from an avirulent strain by its behaviour in macrophages. The virulent strain killed mice as a result of extensive replication in the liver, made possible by productive infection of liver macrophages (see Chapter 2); the avirulent strain, in contrast, established infection in the liver macrophages only with difficulty and thus could not invade liver cells on a significant scale and lead to disease. The behaviour of the viruses in liver macrophages was paralleled by their behaviour in cultivated peritoneal macrophages. In this instance therefore the virulence of a virus for the host is determined by its ability to cause productive infection of macrophages.

The age-dependent resistance of mice to herpes simplex virus infection appears to be closely correlated with changes in the susceptibility of macrophages. Three-week-old mice are normally susceptible but, when transfused with peritoneal macrophages from (resistant) eight-week-old mice, they become resistant. Conversely eight-week-old mice become susceptible when their macrophages are damaged by treatment with silica (Mogensen, 1979).

More commonly, it turns out that differences in susceptibility of strains of mice, or differences in virulence of strains of virus, are not due to differences in the behaviour of macrophages. Macrophages may nevertheless be important in host defence. This would be so if the susceptible and resistant strains of mice being studied had equally good macrophage defences, or if a given strain of mice had equally good macrophage defences against the virulent and avirulent strains of virus being tested. The reader is referred once more to the classification of the interactions of macrophages with viruses or with virus-infected cells set out in Chapter 2.

Immune responses

Genetic determinants. General immune responsiveness is under genetic control, as illustrated by the immune defects in congenital agamma-globulinaemia and thymic aplasia (see below), but genetic control also operates at a more specific level because immune responses to individual antigens are under control of specific immune response (Ir) genes. There are thousands of these genes in mice and men, most of them situated in the I region of the H2 complex in the mouse (see Fig. 3.3) and the D/DR region of the HLA complex in man (reviews: Daussett and Svejgaard, 1977; Benacerraf and Germain, 1978; Zinkernagel, 1979; Klein, 1981). In the mouse, absence of a specific response is generally recessive. Individuals with a genetically determined poor immune response to a given viral antigen, especially the critical surface antigen, would theoretically have difficulty in controlling infection with that particular virus. The poor response could mean that antibody is produced too slowly, in small amounts, of the wrong class, of low avidity or to the wrong determinant on the viral antigen.

There is little direct evidence that genetically determined immune deficiencies of this type account for increased susceptibility. In the mouse, susceptibility to cytomegalovirus, leukaemia virus and LCM virus infections have been shown to be H2 associated, but most of the genetic determinants of virus susceptibility map outside the H2 region (Brinton and Nathanson, 1981; Lodmell, 1983). In man, HLA-CW3 is associated with poor CMI (lymphocyte transformation) responses but higher antibody responses to vaccinia virus (de Vries *et al.*, 1977), HLA-DRHO with low antibody titres in response to rubella vaccine (Kato *et al.*, 1982), and HLA-BW15 with higher incidence of antibodies to CMV but not herpes simplex, varicella-zoster, EB, measles and other viruses (Pereira *et al.*, 1978). In mice, susceptibility to herpes simplex and CMV infection has been associated with non-H2 loci as well as with H2 loci (Lopez, 1980; Grundy *et al.*, 1981).

H2 associations might be expected in infections where immuno-pathology plays a prominent part in pathogenesis (Oldstone *et al.*, 1973). There is a good example in mice of the independent control of immune responses to different viral antigens. Adult mice of most strains infected with LCM virus generally show severe pathological changes as a result of the cell-mediated response to the virus (see above). LCM virus multiplies in exactly the same way in mice of the C57 BL strain but they do not develop disease because they have a weak CMI response (as measured by delayed hypersensitivity) to the viral antigens (Tosolini and Mims, 1971). However, mice of the C57 BL strain are resistant to ectromelia (mousepox) virus, which grows in the liver and is often lethal in many other strains of mice. Genetic analysis shows that resistance is due to a single dominant autosomal gene (O'Neill and Blanden, 1983).

Schell (1960) correlated resistance to C57 BL mice with the development of a more rapid antibody response to infection with ectromelia virus. O'Neill and Blanden (1983), however, have shown that resistance, involving a radiosensitive block to the spread of infection, operates as early as 1–2 days after infection, and therefore seems unlikely to be due to a specific immune response. In both these examples C57 BL mice show a greater resistance to disease; resistance to LCM virus because of a weaker cell-mediated immune response, and resistance to the disease mousepox in association with, but not due to, a stronger antibody response.

Acquired immunodeficiencies. Persistent infections that are normally held in check by immune defences can be activated when immune defences are weakened (see Chapter 6). This occurs when patients with kidney or heart transplants are given immunosuppressive drugs, and in patients suffering from certain lymphoreticular tumours such as Hodgkin's disease. Cell-mediated immune defences in particular, are weakened, and cytomegalovirus, varicella-zoster, papovavirus and adenovirus infections are activated. Interestingly, there appears to be selective impairment of responses to varicella-zoster virus (Arvin *et al.*, 1978), as also reported in old age (see below). The acquired immuno-deficiencies that occur in childhood can make primary viral infections more severe. Children with leukaemia show depressed cell-mediated immune responses, and primary infection with varicella-zoster virus or measles virus can then be lifethreatening. Respiratory viral infections, such as those due to respiratory syncytial virus, are also more prolonged in children with disorders of cell-mediated immunity (Fishaut *et al.*, 1979).

Some mention must be made of AIDS (Acquired Immune Deficiency Syndrome), a major topic of conversation in 1983 (Cahill, 1983) and a disease which may exemplify some of the principles of immunovirology expounded in this book. AIDS is a severe immunosuppressive condition which is usually fatal, and is of unknown aetiology. It is characterised by skin test (delayed hypersensitivity) anergy, and a marked depletion of helper T cells, with normal or increased suppressor T cells, hence a striking reduction in the T4:T8 ratio. The patients are subject to repeated infections and usually die within two years. The commonest cause of death is pneumonia from *Pneumocystis carinii*. Other infections include tuberculosis, disseminated cryptococcosis, toxoplasmosis and candidiasis. Most of these infections under normal circumstances cause no illness. Persistent viruses such as cytomegalovirus, varicella-zoster virus and adenovirus are activated, as in immunosuppressed transplant patients (see Chapter 6). The AIDS patient may in addition develop an unusual type of Kaposi's sarcoma or malignant lymphoma; these are also seen in immunosuppressed renal transplant patients.

AIDS was first described in 1979, and the indications are that it is a new disease. Since then the number of reported cases has escalated rapidly, alarming the public, particularly the gay community. Most of the cases so far have occurred in promiscuous young male homosexuals in major U.S. cities, notably New York, San Francisco and Los Angeles (Gottlieb *et al.*, 1981; Masur *et al.*, 1981). The probability of acquiring the disease is proportional to the number of different sexual partners—the average is 60 per year in the reported cases and more than 1000 during a lifetime. Yet the incidence is not notably high in female prostitutes, indicating that some aspect of the sexual habits or life style of the male homosexual subculture is as relevant as promiscuity itself in the aetiology of AIDS. A clue as to what this may be is that the other minority groups (both male and female) conspicuously at risk are heroin addicts, haemophiliacs and Haitians (giving AIDS its popular pseudonym, the '4H disease').

Blood transmission is involved in the case of the haemophiliacs and drug addicts. There is no evidence for direct non-sexual person-to-person transmission, but conventional sexual transmission is probably the explanation in the cases now arising in female sexual partners of male AIDS patients. The relatively high incidence in Haitian immigrants to the U.S. who are not drug abusers and do not appear to be homosexuals is intriguing and may eventually provide the key to the puzzle; a focus of infection in central Africa is a possibility.

There is clear epidemiological evidence of case-to-case spread, for instance among male homosexuals, which strongly incriminates an infectious organism. The identity of that agent is still a mystery—it may well turn out to be a virus, not necessarily a new one, not necessarily of human origin. The target cell directly or indirectly involved appears to be a helper T cell. Known human viruses that could conceivably be responsible include novel strains of the T cell leukaemia/lymphoma virus, but there are probably new human viruses awaiting discovery; recent surprises include the human parvovirus which infects haemo-poietic cells in the bone marrow (Anderson, 1982). AIDS shares many epidemiological features with hepatitis B, including its transmission by blood and its frequency in the '4Hs'; most AIDS patients are also HBsAG positive.

It is possible that the epidemic will be controlled before the cause is identified. Male homosexuals and Haitians can be excluded as blood donors. Male homosexuals could wear condoms, avoid anal intercourse (which may be important in transmission) or become less promiscuous (which is already happening). If, however, the epidemic continues and involves increasing numbers of humans from outside the four Hs referred to previously, then it will be urgent for virologists and immunologists to identify the infectious agent and understand more clearly the immunological defect. Many apparently normal male homosexuals are found to have skin anergy, lymphadenopathy, reversed T4/T8 ratios (Editorial, 1981), and, if this should turn out to be 'prodromal AIDS', the magnitude of the epidemic will be greatly increased.

Fever

Fever so commonly accompanies viral infections that it is natural to suppose that it has some antiviral action (Lwoff, 1959; Roberts, 1979). There is a common mediator of the febrile response known as endogenous pyrogen. This is present in inflammatory exudates and in the plasma during fever, and it acts on the temperature-regulating centre in the anterior hypothalamus, resetting the body thermostat. Endogenous pyrogen is produced by macrophages, and appears to be identical with interleukin 1. It is induced by immunological mechanisms, being a common accompaniment of generalised antigen–antibody and cell-mediated immune reactions. Bodily functions are profoundly disturbed by fever, and the generally increased metabolic rate, by increasing the metabolic activity in phagocytic cells or increasing the rate at which inflammatory responses are induced, could theoretically produce antiviral effects. Recent *in vitro* studies have shown that both inter-leukin-1-induced T cell proliferation and antibody production are increased up to 20-fold when cells are cultured at 39°C rather than 37°C (Atkins, 1983). This sounds as if endogenous pyrogen (interleukin 1) provides a more optimal body temperature for the operation of host defence mechanisms.

   Is there any good evidence that fever does play a useful role in virus infections? Lwoff (1959) first suggested that fever constitutes a natural defence against viruses, and that virulent strains of virus have evolved with the ability to multiply in the host at temperatures achieved during fever. Temperature-sensitive (*ts*) virus mutants might therefore be expected to be less virulent. Fenner (1972) found this to be the case for single-step *ts* mutants of Semliki Forest and rabbitpox viruses in mice, and the correlation has since been observed with *ts* mutants of other viruses (Richman and Murphy, 1979).

   Much experimental work has concentrated on exposing infected animals to either abnormally low or abnormally high temperatures. Unfortunately under these circumstances complex physiological changes take place, including hormonally mediated stress responses and alterations in thyroid activity, which could have misleading indirect effects on the course of infection. For instance Thompson (1938) and Parker and Thompson (1942) showed that, when rabbits infected with myxoma virus were kept at high ambient temperatures so that their internal temperature was raised to 40°C, the rabbits survived an otherwise lethal infection. Marshall (1959) kept myxoma-infected rabbits at a low ambient temperature and greatly increased the severity of the disease and the mortality rate. However, he also showed that antibody production was affected in animals kept at the low temperature. He did not measure interferon production. Complex effects are also illustrated by the experiments of Roberts (1964c) who found that mice infected with ectromelia virus were about 100 times as susceptible when kept at 2°C rather than at 20°C. Mice kept in the cold showed an increased metabolic rate which appeared to predispose them to more severe liver damage without an increase in viral growth in the liver.

What happens to a viral infection when fever is prevented? Kirn et al. (1966) administered amidopyrine subcutaneously to rabbits infected intratracheally with vaccinia virus. Untreated infected animals became febrile and often died with pneumonia, but in those rendered afebrile by amidopyrine the mortality was more than doubled and the lungs contained 250 times more virus. A similar approach to the problem of fever was recently made by Husseini et al. (1982). They managed to reduce the febrile response of ferrets infected with influenza virus by shaving the animals and treating them with sodium salicylate, and showed that the treated animals shed more virus in nasal washings and that viral excretion continued for a longer period.

In one viral infection elevated body temperature actually promotes viral multiplication or at least its activation (see Chapter 6). This is the case in cold sores caused by recurrent herpes simplex in man. Fever induced by physical means, or occurring during the course of other infections, often precipitates a recurrence of herpes labialis ('cold sores') in carriers of herpes simplex virus.

Almost all severe viral infections in larger mammals are accompanied by fever (38–41°C). Therefore, it would be unwise to regard it as a purely accidental consequence of immune and inflammatory responses. Fever is costly in energy and is an ancient bodily response, quite probably of survival value. It may well have significance in antiviral defence. The fact that fever generally develops towards the end of the incubation period when viral multiplication is largely completed and pyrogenic antigen–antibody complexes are present, may argue somewhat against temperature-sensitivity of viral replication as the primary mechanism. But interleukin 1 (and perhaps interferon)—mediated enhancement of T lymphocyte-mediated immune responses may well be crucial.

Inflammation

Though inflammation is more obviously relevant as a source of immuno-pathology, it is difficult to imagine that this ancient response, any more than the febrile response, is of no value to the infected host. In a general sense, it is surely useful to deliver leukocytes and serum components, including antibody and complement, to the scene of infection by way of local inflammatory responses. Inflammation and oedema are produced as a result of the operation of several types of host defence. These include complement activation, whether by classical or alternate pathways, and the local release of lymphokines by T cells (see Chapter 3).

Are inflammation and oedema of any additional value in host defences against viruses? It has been suggested (Notkins, 1974) that cell-to-cell transfer of virus is impeded when there is local inflammation or oedema, especially if cells show a mild cytopathic effect with slight rounding up. With viruses that can spread directly from cell to cell this could be important, because the only method of spread would then be via extracellular fluids in which virus is exposed to antibody and complement. Also the increased blood supply and temperature in inflamed tissues favours maximal metabolic activity on the part of leukocytes, and the slight lowering of pH would tend to inactivate extracellular virions. Prostaglandins inhibit the *in vitro* replication of certain viruses, as in the case of prostaglandin A and vaccinia virus (Santoro *et al.*, 1982) but different prostaglandins have different effects and their *in vivo* role is unclear.

Nutrition

Malnutrition can interfere with any of the mechanisms that act as barriers to the multiplication or progress of viruses through the body. It has been repeatedly demonstrated that severe nutritional deficiencies will interfere with the generation of antibody and CMI responses, with the activity of phagocytes, and with the integrity of skin and mucous membranes (Chandra, 1979; 1983). Often, however, nutritional deficiencies are complex, and the identification of the important food factor is difficult. This is reflected in the use of inclusive terms such as 'protein-calorie malnutrition'. Also at times it is impossible to disentangle the nutritional effects from socio-economic effects such as poor housing, crowding, inadequate hygiene and microbial contamination of the environment. For reasons that are not clear, protein deficiency tends to depress the CMI response in particular, and this causes an increase in susceptibility to certain viral infections.

Children with protein deficiency (the extreme form being represented by the clinical condition called kwashiorkor) are uniquely susceptible to measles (Morley, 1969). This is partly the result of their weaker cell-mediated immune response to this infection, and also perhaps of the lowered resistance of mucosal surfaces of the body and greater susceptibility to the microorganisms that cause secondary infection. All the epithelial manifestations of measles are more severe (see Chapter 2). Lifethreatening bacterial infection of the lower respiratory tract is common, as well as otitis media, sinusitis, etc. Conjunctivitis at times progresses to cause severe eye damage and blindness, especially if there is associated vitamin A deficiency. The tiny ulcers of the mouth that constitute Koplik's spots in normally nourished children can enlarge to form massive ulcers or necrosis of the mouth (*cancrum oris*). The skin rash is worse, with numerous haemorrhages that give the condition referred to as 'black measles'. Instead of an occasional small focus of infection in the intestine, there is extensive intestinal involvement with severe diarrhoea which exacerbates the nutritional deficiency (Dossetor and Whittle, 1975; Koster *et al.*, 1981). Thus measles exacerbates malnutrition as well as vice versa, and this is not only because of diarrhoea but also because, during systemic febrile infections like measles, there is always a greatly increased breakdown and excretion of body nitrogen.

The scarcity of good medical care and antibiotic therapy adds to the serious outcome of the illness. Measles is about 300 times as lethal in developing countries as it is in the countries of northern Europe and North America. The case fatality approaches 10% and in severe famines may reach the tragic figure of 50%. The severe form of measles is seen in children in tropical Africa (Morley, 1969), in aboriginal children in certain parts of Australia, and it was also seen in children in European cities in the 19th century. Severe measles is seen especially in children aged 1–4 years, because this is the period when food intake is at its lowest, during the change from breast milk to an adult-type diet. A study of children in Guatemalan villages showed that measles and other respiratory and intestinal infections in infancy are responsible for periodic interruptions in weight gain (Mata, 1975). Body weights at two years of age were sometimes little more than half those of North American children and there was often almost no weight gain during the second and third year of life.

There are still puzzles in the interactions between measles infection and malnutrition. For instance, severely malnourished children in Asia do not appear to develop severe measles virus infections (Chandra, 1979). Also, recent immunological studies suggest that certain parameters of cell-mediated immunity, and also antibody production to measles virus are normal in malnourished children. However, immunosuppressive factors are present in the plasma and this contributes to the greater incidence of secondary bacterial infections (Whittle *et al.*, 1980).

Breast milk is an important determinant of resistance of infants to viral infections. Milk not only provides a uniquely balanced diet but also confers immunologically specific resistance to viral infection. This is largely mediated by the transfer of maternal antibodies. In human colostrum 97% of the protein is secretory IgA and in human milk about one gram of IgA is transferred to the infant each day. Milk or colostrum is especially important in species such as pigs, cattle, and horses where there is no transfer of antibodies via the placenta (see Chapter 2). When the antibodies are secretory IgA, they are not absorbed from the gut but can protect the infant against intestinal infections. In ruminants, colostrum also contains IgG antibodies, which are adsorbed from the intestine for a short period after birth, protecting the infant against a wider variety of viral infections (Newby *et al.*, 1982). In addition to specific antibodies milk contains maternal cells, including macrophages, and ill-defined antiviral lipids (Welsh *et al.*, 1978), but the antiviral role of these components *in vivo* is not known.

There have been a few experimental investigations of the impact of malnutrition on viral infections. Woodruff (1970) studied mice which, from the age of three weeks, had received one-quarter of the food intake necessary for optimal growth. They developed marked atrophy of lymphoid tissues, and were then much more susceptible than normal mice to coxsackievirus B3 infection. Malnourished mice developed severe and often fatal lesions in liver and heart, and a marked absence of cellular infiltration, suggesting an inadequate host immune response to the infection.

Interesting experimental observations have been made on the consequences of hyperalimentation (Campbell *et al.*, 1982). Mice rendered hypercholesterolaemic by a special diet (containing 18% lard) were more susceptible to coxsackievirus B5 infections, with up to 50% increase in mortality and increased virus titres in organs. Pathological changes were also more severe, but often without the inflammatory cells seen in control mice. It was suggested that the increased susceptibility to infection was due to impaired function of macrophages in the fatty, cholesterol-laden liver, and impaired mobilisation of monocytes from the blood.

Age

There are few viruses that cause exactly the same disease in infancy, adult life and old age. Susceptibility is generally greatest in the very young and very old. In the first place immune responses are generally weaker in immature and in ageing individuals, whether mice or men (Makinodan and Kay, 1980; Andersson *et al.*, 1981). Newborn animals are particularly susceptible. Newborn mice, for instance have been much used in experimental studies, and are notorious for their susceptibility to a very large number of different viruses. However, the newborn are normally protected from naturally occurring viral infections by a maternal umbrella of protective immunity, acquired transplacentally or via colostrum (see p. 187). Without this protection common viral infections can be very serious. Herpes simplex or varicella-zoster viruses can cause lethal disease in the rare human infant who is born without maternal antibodies. Polyomavirus causes an asymptomatic infection in infant mice born to immune mothers, but it causes a serious infection that leads to development of multiple tumours when antibody is not acquired from the mother (Rowe, 1961).

Viral infections in man. Most viral infections are milder in childhood, and more likely to be severe in adults. These include varicella, mumps, poliomyelitis, hepatitis A and EB virus infection. Varicella, a trivial disease in children, often causes pneumonia in adults, and mumps involves the testicle (also other glands such as the ovary and mammary gland) after puberty, giving a troublesome orchitis.

Infections with polioviruses tend to be asymptomatic in early childhood (Weinstein, 1957). When polioviruses arrived and caused a 'virgin soil' epidemic in certain isolated eskimo communities in the 1940s and on the island of St Helena in 1947, there was a strikingly high incidence of paralysis in adults, but mostly inapparent infections in childhood and old age. Therefore it might be expected that, in developing countries in Africa, central America, etc., where infection during early childhood is the rule, paralytic disease would be uncommon. In developed countries (U.S.A., Northern Europe, etc.), where there has been some interruption of the faecal-oral spread of infection, poliovirus infection was, in the prevaccine era, more likely to be delayed until later in childhood or adult life (Nathanson and Martin, 1979) and more likely to cause paralysis. Surveys from rural Ghana show that paralytic poliomyelitis is quite common in children (Ofosu-Amah *et al.*, 1977), although there have been suggestions that this is associated with injections of antibiotics, vaccines, etc. which are known to predispose to paralysis of the injected limb. In developed countries another enterovirus, hepatitis A, appears to be developing epidemiological features that parallel the behaviour of poliovirus in earlier times; primary infection has become commoner in adults, who suffer more severe disease.

EB virus is excreted in saliva, and in developing countries most individuals are infected as young children, most of them undergoing at that age only an inapparent infection (Epstein and Achong, 1977; 1979). In developed countries where childhood infection is less common, primary infection often occurs in adolescence or early adult life following the extensive salivary exchanges that take place during kissing. In this age group, and in these countries, EB virus causes the more serious disease, glandular fever (infectious mononucleosis). This results from immunological warfare in the host, the antiviral activity of T_c lymphocytes being directed against infected B lymphocytes. In the course of this conflict lymphoid tissues become enlarged and swollen and tender. In adolescents and young adults the immune responses are more vigorous, the lymphoproliferative features more marked, and the disease more severe than in children. In other viral infections also, a less powerful immunological contribution to pathology and disease might be expected in young children.

The 1918–19 pandemic of influenza showed a unique age-specific mortality curve with a peak in young adult life (Fig. 5.1). This is not a general characteristic of influenza, because all previous and subsequent epidemics displayed peaks of mortality in the very young and very old. The reason for this 'young adult' peak of mortality is obscure, but an increased immunopathological or inflammatory response in the lungs of this age group seems likely, as originally postulated by Burnet (1952; 1955).

Age-related differences in susceptibility are at times attributable to physical or physiological differences. The increased susceptibility of old people to respiratory infections is partly due to things like the loss of elastic tissue around alveoli, weaker respiratory muscles and a poorer cough reflex. Both old people and infants sometimes fail to show the usual signs of infection such as fever. The lungs of infants are particularly susceptible to bronchiolitis and pneumonia partly because the airways are narrow and more readily blocked by secretion and exudate. Infants are also the first to suffer the effects of fluid and electrolyte loss, so that infections characterised by fever, vomiting or diarrhoea tend to be more severe at this time of life. But often the reason for increased susceptibility in infancy is not clear. Respiratory syncytial virus for instance, causes more severe illness in infancy and early childhood, with croup, bronchitis, bronchiolitis or bronchopneumonia. There is a peak of severity in the two-month-old infant. In adults the same virus causes a minor upper respiratory infection, but in early life there is invasion and growth of virus in the lower respiratory tract. It is not

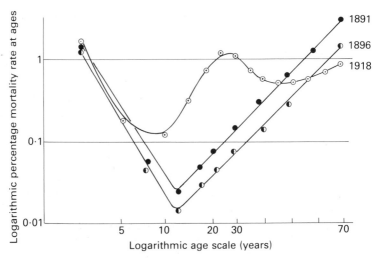

Fig. 5.1. Mortality by age from respiratory infections in England and Wales in the influenza years 1891 and 1918 and a non-influenza year 1896. Time scale for age changes from logarithmic to linear at 25 years. Courtesy of Burnet (1952).

known whether this is because respiratory epithelium or alveolar macrophages are more vulnerable to infection in infants, or because host defences are less effective, or because maternally derived immunity gives an immunopathologically mediated disease (McIntosh and Fishaut, 1980; Welliver *et al.*, 1981).

The susceptibility of aged individuals to reactivation of latent viral infections is discussed in Chapter 6, and is attributable to their waning immune defences. Cell-mediated immune responses (lymphocyte transformation) to varicella-zoster virus appear to be selectively depressed in the elderly, with the response to other antigens unaffected (Miller, 1980). A similar selective impairment of lymphocyte reactivity to varicella-zoster virus is seen in patients with lymphoma (Arvin *et al.*, 1978), in whom zoster is common following reactivation of this virus.

Viral infections in experimental animals. Newborn animals are more susceptible to many viral infections. Indeed the coxsackieviruses were first discovered as a result of the use of suckling mice (Dalldorf and Sickles, 1948) and the newborn mouse is still a sensitive host for the isolation of arboviruses. A classic experimental example of age-related differences in susceptibility is the susceptibility of suckling but not of adult mice to encephalitis after peripheral inoculation with a variety of viruses. Both age groups are susceptible following intracerebral inoculation. Viruses used include herpesviruses, most of the toga-viruses, vesicular stomatitis virus, coxsackieviruses, etc. The immaturity of immune responsiveness in infant mice plays a part but other factors, many of which have been referred to in Chapter 2, do also. For instance, invasion of the central nervous system from the periphery depends on the development of a viraemia of adequate size and duration. This depends on the extraneural growth of virus in tissues such as liver, muscle, brown fat, etc. The host factors that determine increased extraneural growth of these viruses in infant mice are not known. For the maintenance of viraemia, the behaviour of viruses in macrophages may be very important (see Chapter 2) and differences in the suscepti-bility of macrophages from newborn and adult mice have often been described. For instance, Johnson (1964b) found that newborn and adult mouse peritoneal macrophages were equally susceptible to infection with herpes simplex virus *in vitro*, but with adult macrophages the virus failed to spread to other cells whether these were Hela cells or adult macrophages, whereas spreading infection always occurred when suckling macrophages were primarily infected. In later studies (Hirsch *et al.*, 1970) it was shown that adult macrophages produced more inter-feron than suckling mouse macrophages. But suckling mice also show defective antibody-dependent cell-mediated cytotoxicity (ADCC). Kohl and Loo (1980) found that leukocytes from newborn mice failed to lyse herpes simplex virus infected cells in the presence of antibody, and the development of resistance to infection on ageing paralleled the development of ADCC capacity. Infected suckling mice could be protected when transfused with ADCC-effective human mononuclear cells as long as specific antiviral antibody, even at dilutions of 10^{-8}, was also given (Kohl and Loo, 1982).

Physiological factors could play a part in age-related susceptibility to neural infection. Virus-sized particles pass more readily across capillary walls in suckling animals (Suter and Majno, 1965), and this would favour the passage of infection from the blood into the brain (or other susceptible organs) of suckling animals. Adult mice are more susceptible that suckling mice to paralysis by intracerebrally injected type 2 poliovirus. Jubelt et al. (1980) produced evidence that this was because, in adult mice, the virus spreads more rapidly down neural pathways to reach the spinal cord which in turn is attributable to a faster axonal transport system in adults.

The age-dependent resistance of mice to mouse hepatitis virus and its neurotropic variant JHM has also been analysed. With a low-virulence strain of MHV, one-week-old C_3H mice were killed when 10^3 pfu of virus were injected intraperitoneally, whereas it took more than 10^6 pfu intraperitoneally to kill four-week-old mice (Taguchi et al., 1979). Peritoneal macrophages from one-week-old mice produced 10–1000 times as much virus, whether infected in vitro or in vivo. Also, there was less interferon in the serum of one-week-old mice twelve hours after infection and, although this difference had disappeared by 24 hours, interferon may have contributed to the differences in susceptibility. In this, as in other examples of age-dependent resistance, immunological factors are likely to play a part (Levy-Leblond and Dupuy, 1977).

More often than not we can describe age-dependent differences in the pathogenesis of a viral infection in mice without being able to explain them. Possible factors include virus receptors, susceptibility of key cells such as macrophages, body temperature, immune responses, interferon production, and so on. For instance, suckling mice are much more susceptible than adults to intranasal infection with Sendai (parainfluenza 1) virus. In sucklings the virus spreads from initially infected respiratory epithelium to give extensive infection of interstitial cells in the lungs, whereas in adult mice the infection is largely restricted to the respiratory epithelium of the airways (Mims and Murphy, 1973). The basis for this difference is unknown. Infection with K virus (a papovavirus) is also more lethal in suckling mice. This virus multiplies in vascular endothelial cells, especially in alveolar capillaries in the lungs, and mice less than one-week-old develop fatal interstitial pneumonia after infection by the intraperitoneal, intracerebral or oral route (Greenlee, 1979; 1981). This virus, unlike Sendai virus, does not replicate in respiratory epithelial cells. Factors that localise the endothelial infection to the lung have been investigated, and Margolis et al. (1976)

found no evidence that oxygen tension was involved. In older mice the infection is more limited in extent, and is not lethal.

It may be noted that the weak immune responsiveness that helps make infant mice more susceptible to most virus infections, renders them less susceptible to virus infections in which immunopathology plays a large part. Thus newborn mice, unlike adult mice, fail to develop an acute disease when infected intracerebrally with LCM virus. Instead they undergo a persistent infection (see Chapter 6).

Sex, hormones, pregnancy and lactation

There are small but significant differences between sexes in the severity of many viral infections. These are distinct from differences in the incidence of infection, which are often due to differences in exposure. Almost nothing is known about mechanisms. Sex differences in susceptibility can have an obvious anatomical basis. A virus that grows in mammary tissues is more likely to do so in females just as tropism for the testis (mumps in adults) can only be expressed in males.

Hormones presumably play a large part and also differences in immune responsiveness. For instance, an experimental analysis of sex differences in the susceptibility of mice to coxsackievirus B3 infection (Wong et al., 1977) showed that males generated an earlier and more powerful cytotoxic T cell response but a lower antibody response than females. The more severe disease suffered by infected males was attributed to the immunopathology mediated by a more vigorous T cell response.

During pregnancy and lactation the differences are often more striking. Pregnant women are more likely to suffer severe infection with smallpox, poliomyelitis, hepatitis B, hepatitis A (Christie et al., 1976), nonA-nonB hepatitis (Khuroo et al., 1981) and herpes simplex type 2 (Young et al., 1976). The picture can be confused because of a poorer nutritional state of pregnant women in developing countries. But changes in the level of hormones such as corticosteroids, oestrogens and progesterone are important, and in pregnant individuals it is often possible to demonstrate a decrease in immune responsiveness. Certain persistent latent viruses often reactivate in pregnancy. This is true for human papovaviruses (Coleman et al., 1980), CMV (Stagno et al., 1975), and possibly herpes simplex type 2 (Ng et al., 1970; Corey et al., 1983). Pregnancy reactivation of mouse CMV occurs in association with depressed CMI (delayed hypersensitivity) responses to the virus (Chong and Mims, 1982), and the same is true of human CMV (Gehrz et al., 1981). Quite separately, the pregnant female is the site of development of a novel set of tissues, including the foetus, placenta and lactating mammary glands, each providing a new and possibly susceptible target for viral infection. The viral infections of lactating mammary glands, and of the placenta and foetus have been referred to in Chapter 2.

Baker and Plotkin (1978) tried to find out why pregnant mice are more susceptible to intravaginal inoculation with herpes simplex type 1. They showed that non-pregnant females treated with progesterone suffered as high a mortality as seven-day-pregnant females. Differences in vaginal virus titres were not marked, and progesterone may have acted by altering immune responses or by local effects that promoted the spread of virus from the vaginal wall. Herpes simplex type 2, when inoculated intraperitoneally or intranasally, is not more severe in pregnant mice (Young and Gomez, 1979), so that local rather than general effects seem more likely.

Corticosteroid hormones are known to have deleterious effects on resistance to viral infections in the intact host. This was shown for experimental infections more than 30 years ago (Kilbourne and Horsfall, 1951; Shwartzman and Aronson, 1953), and clinically, infections due to herpes simplex, varicella, vaccinia, etc. are often exacerbated in patients given corticosteroids. Corticosteroids act partly by reducing antiviral inflammatory and immune responses (Kass and Finland, 1958) and partly by depressing interferon responses (Rytel and Kilbourne, 1966; Reinicke, 1965). When a hormone enhances replication in individual cells, it may mean that the tissue that produces this hormone is particularly vulnerable. For instance, the adrenal cortex is severely affected in rabbits infected with rabbitpox virus (Boulter et al., 1961).

Very little work has been done on the potentially important topic of the influence of hormones, including oestrogens, protesterone, insulin, growth hormone, etc. on the replication of viruses in vitro. They often have a dramatic effect on experimental viral infections in vivo (e.g. Hurst et al., 1960), but little is known of mechanisms. In vitro studies show that the plaque count and yield of mouse CMV is significantly increased by physiological concentrations of oestrogen, progesterone and corticosteroids (Chong and Mims, 1983) and this could be important in the susceptibility of pregnant mice to reactivating CMV, but nothing is known about the mechanisms of hormone action. With rubella virus, on the other hand, oestrogen-responsive human cells showed a 70% reduction of virus yield after treatment with 17β-oestradiol (Roehrig et al., 1979). The pathogenicity of mouse mammary tumour virus has been studied in some detail at the cellular level. There are strong host genetic determinants, but, in some strains of mice at least, virus grows in the mammary glands and is shed in milk. Primary cultures of infected mouse mammary tumour cells show a three-fold increase in viral production in the presence of physiological concentrations of glucocorticoid hormones (Shyamala and Dickson, 1976). Also, when infected mammary carcinoma cells are treated with glucocorticoid, there is an increase in virus-specific mRNA within 15 minutes (Ringold *et al.*, 1975), following binding of the hormone to its receptor on the cell. The molecular basis for these effects is not known.

It should be noted that, although the administration of excess corticosteroid hormones enhances the severity of viral infection and may depress immune responses, adequate production of these hormones in the body is vital for normal resistance to infection. During an infectious disease, there is an increase in the rate of tissue utilisation of corticosteroids, which prevent inflammatory expression of the immune response, partly by blocking the movement of plasma and leukocytes from blood vessels. This ensures that continued bodily function and homeostasis is maintained—excessive or widespread inflammatory responses being harmful, and the increased corticosteroid levels are essential for a successful host response to infection. When endogenous corticosteroid production is depressed in Addison's disease in man, or abolished by bilateral adrenalectomy in experimental animals, viral infections often show much greater severity.

Dual infections

Simultaneous infections with two different viruses would be expected to occur at times merely by chance, especially in children. One infection could interfere with the other by competing for susceptible cells or by producing interferon. Especially in tropical countries, where inapparent infections with enteroviruses are exceedingly common, these can interfere with the multiplication of oral polio vaccine. Furthermore, this vaccine contains the three types of poliovirus, which tend to interfere with each other's growth in the intestinal tract. The vaccine is therefore given on at least three occasions to ensure that each strain of virus replicates and generates an adequate response (see Chapter 7).

It might be expected that when interferon is produced during a systemic viral infection, the host would be more resistant at that time to a separate viral infection, but there is little evidence for this. Live virus vaccines for rubella, measles and mumps are routinely administered as a mixture to children, apparently without mutual interference (Weibel *et al.*, 1979). There are isolated reports of local interference of one virus with another in skin lesions, such as the absence of a measles rash round chickenpox lesions in a dually infected child (Knight *et al.*, 1964), but nothing is known of the mechanisms.

Dual infections are more important when one of them is bacterial. For instance, when local defences are damaged by an initial viral invasion secondary bacterial infection can cause severe illness or death. The destruction of ciliated epithelium in the lung by viruses such as influenza or measles allows normally non-pathogenic resident bacteria of the nose and throat, such as the pneumococcus or *Haemophilus influenzae*, to invade the lung and cause secondary pneumonia. If these bacteria enter the lung under normal circumstances, they are removed by the mucociliary escalator or destroyed by alveolar macrophages. Specialised respiratory pathogens such as influenza, measles, parainfluenza or rhinoviruses also damage the mucosa in the nasopharynx and sinuses leading to secondary bacterial infection with purulent nasal discharge, sinusitis, otitis media or mastoiditis. Otitis media in children is commonly associated with viral infections. Generally the mechanism is assumed to be by a loss of epithelial integrity and of normal cleansing mechanisms, but defects in polymorph function are seen in mice infected with influenza virus and have been associated with the development of pneumococcal otitis media (Abramson et al., 1982b). Addition of certain strains of influenza A virus to human polymorphs in vitro is reported to cause defects in polymorph function. (Abramson et al., 1982a). Effects on macrophages are also reported, although there are many difficulties in the interpretation of experiments (Couch, 1981). Mice infected with parainfluenza 1 (Sendai) virus show greatly increased susceptibility to infection with Haemophilus influenzae and Pasteurella pneumotropica (Jacab and Dick, 1973) and this is largely due to the fact that alveolar macrophages infected with the virus show a poor ability to phagocytose and kill the bacteria. An interesting alternative mechanism for susceptibility to secondary bacterial infection has been proposed (Sanford et al., 1978). It was found that cells infected with influenza virus had an enhanced capacity to bind certain bacteria, a fact which might increase the ease with which such bacteria cause secondary infection. Unfortunately the bacteria were group B streptococci rather than those usually responsible for secondary infection in patients with influenza.

The phenomenon of one infection enhancing susceptibility to another is not restricted to superficial viral infections. The pathogenicity of mouse hepatitis virus is greatly enhanced by concurrent infection of mice with a normally harmless blood parasite, Eperythrozoon coccoides (Gledhill, 1956). It is probably caused by an effect on reticuloendothelial macrophages. Freund's adjuvant, BCG, bacterial endotoxin and other agents have notable effects on immune and reticuloendothelial functions including macrophage activation, and this is often correlated with changes in susceptibility to viral and other infections (Allison, 1978). Bale et al. (1982) showed that intranasally inoculated E. coli strain K1 was more lethal for mice infected with CMV. This was associated with reduced clearance of E. coli from the blood, lungs, liver and spleen, and with a decreased inflammatory response to the bacteria when introduced subcutaneously in a sponge. This could be an effect mediated by macrophages. During many acute viral infections there is a temporary depression in immune response to unrelated antigens (see Chapter 6) and increased susceptibility to other microorganisms or parasitic infections might be expected. For instance, the depressed CMI and antibody responses seen in adult mice during acute infection with LCM virus are associated with increased susceptibility to ectromelia virus (Mims and Wainwright, 1968). Viruses that depress immune responses can exacerbate other chronic infections. In measles there is a temporary depression of cell-mediated immunity so that tuberculin-positive individuals become temporarily tuberculin-negative on the first day or two of the measles rash (Starr and Berkovich, 1964). More importantly, studies in Greenland showed that tuberculosis can be made more severe as a result of measles (Christensen *et al.*, 1953).

SUMMARY

Virulence provides a measure of the pathogenicity of a virus—its capacity to produce tissue damage and physiological dysfunction (disease). The outcome of infection is also affected by a variety of host factors which in combination provide a measure of the resistance/ susceptibility of that host. The interaction between these two determines the severity of the disease resulting from any given virus–host combination. In mice, for instance, the spectrum ranges from a completely harmless yet lifelong infection (lactic dehydrogenase virus) to one than can lead to death within hours (Rift Valley fever virus).

In spite of extensive developments in our knowledge of viral replication at the cellular level, little is known of viral determinants of virulence *in vivo*. Nevertheless, the recent application of biochemical and genetic techniques to the pathogenesis of reovirus infection in mice has opened up a new era of 'molecular pathogenesis'. Virulence can not usually be attributed to a single viral gene. Rather, a number of genes can be assigned particular biological functions, each of which contributes to the total pathogenetic picture. For instance, one reovirus protein determines the capacity of the virus to grow in the intestine, another its neurovirulence.

Host factors influencing the course of an infection may be genetic or physiological. Genetic determinants of immunity, such as immune response (Ir) genes, are important, but numerous additional factors unrelated to the immune response also contribute to host resistance. These include the presence or absence of cell receptors for particular viruses in particular hosts or tissues, and other more subtle (generally unknown) differences between cells in their capacity to support the multiplication of individual viruses. In this and other respects macrophages may play a determining role in host resistance/susceptibility. Inflammation, despite its contribution to immunopathology, presumably also facilitates recovery.

Interferons comprise a family of hormones and lymphokines which are induced by viral infection. Interferons of all three types (α, β, γ) have been shown to inhibit the replication of virtually all viruses in cultured cells and are beginning to be used as antiviral chemotherapeutic agents in man. Moreover, they exert a remarkable range of effects on the immune system, including activation of NK cells, macrophages and T_c cells, but suppression of certain other arms of the immune response. As anti-interferon antibodies have been shown to exacerbate some viral infections in experimental animals, it can be assumed that interferons play a significant role in recovery from infections in man.

Fever presumably serves a purpose in recovery from infection. Temperature-sensitive mutants are generally less virulent than the wild-type virus. Interleukin 1-induced fever may accelerate and augment immune responses. Malnutrition, particularly protein deficiency seen after weaning in tropical countries, can predispose to infection and greatly increase the mortality from diseases such as measles. Hormonal changes during pregnancy and other forms of stress can also render people more vulnerable to infection. The age of the host often has a decisive influence on susceptibility. The very young and the old are generally more vulnerable, but maternal antibody protects infants, and infections in children are usually mild. Concurrent or supervening infection with bacteria often complicates viral infection.

SELECTED READING

Bang, F. B. (1978). Genetics of resistance of animals to viruses. I Introduction and studies in mice. *Adv. Virus Res.* **23**, 269.

Brinton, M. A. and Nathanson, N. (1981). Genetic determinants of virus susceptibility: epidemiologic implications of murine models. *Epidemiol. Rev.* **3**, 115.

Buchmeier, M. J., Welsh, R. M., Dukto, F. J., and Oldstone, M. B. A. (1980). The virology and immunobiology of lymphocytic choriomeningitis virus infection. *Adv. Immunol.* **30**, 275.

Chandra, R. K. (1979). Nutritional deficiency and susceptibility to infection. *Bull. WHO* **57**, 167.

Choppin, P. W. and Scheid, A. (1980). The role of viral glycoproteins in adsorption, penetration and pathogenicity of viruses. *Rev. Infect. Dis.* **2**, 40.

Fields, B. N. (1981). Genetics of reovirus. *Curr. Top. Microbiol. Immunol.* **91**, 1.

Fields, B. N. and Byers, K. (1983). The genetic basis of viral virulence. *Phil. Trans. R. Soc. Lond. B* **303**, 209.

Fields, B. N. and Greene, M. I. (1982). Genetic and molecular mechanisms of viral pathogenesis: implications for prevention and treatment. *Nature* **300**, 19.

Fields, B. N. and Jaenisch, R. (1980). *Animal Virus Genetics*. Academic Press, New York.

Finter, N. B. (ed.) (1983–4). *Interferons*, 3rd edn, vols. 1–4. Elsevier North-Holland, Amsterdam.

Gresser, I. (ed.) (1979, 1980, 1981, 1982). *Interferons*, vols. 1, 2, 3, 4. Academic Press, New York.

Huang, A. S. (1977). Viral pathogenesis and molecular biology. *Bact. Rev.* **41**, 811.

Klenk, H. D., Garten, W., Bosch, F. X., and Rott, R. (1982). Viral glycoproteins as determinants of pathogenicity. *Med. Microbiol. Immunol.* **170**, 145.

Lonberg-Holm, K. and Philipson, L. (1981). *Animal Virus Receptors. Series B: Receptors and Recognition*. Chapman and Hall, London.

Palese, P. and Roizman, B. (eds.) (1980). Genetic Variation of Viruses. *Annals N.Y. Acad. Sci.* **354**.

Rosenstreich, D. L., Weinblatt, A. C., and O'Brien, A. D. (1982). Genetic control of resistance to infection in mice. *CRC Critical Reviews in Immunol.* **3**, 263.

Smith, H. (1980). The little-known determinants of virus pathogenicity. *Scand. J. Inf. Dis. Suppl.* **24**, 119.

Smith, H. Skehel, J. H., and Turner, M. J. (eds.) (1980). *The Molecular Basis of Microbial Pathogenicity*, report on the Dahlem Workshop on The Molecular Basis of the Infective Process, Berlin, October 1979. Verlag Chemie, Basel.

White, D. O. (1984). *Antiviral chemotherapy, interferons and vaccines——a status report.* Monographs in Virology, vol. 16. Karger, Basel.

Chapter Six
Persistent Infections

There are many infections in which the virus is not eliminated from the body but persists in the host for months, years or a lifetime. This is in contrast to acute infections such as influenza, poliomyelitis, yellow fever or smallpox, in which the virus is eliminated from the body within a few weeks. In a persistent infection the virus either continues to multiply, hence remains demonstrable (chronic infection), or may survive in some non-infectious form (latent infection) with the potential to be reactivated later. In the latter case the viral genome can be detected in particular cells or tissues by a suitable radiolabelled nucleic acid probe. Sometimes certain viral genes may continue to be expressed and some virus-coded proteins may be detected serologically, e.g. by immunofluorescence. Full expression of the viral genome is restricted by cellular or general host factors. Cells from the persistently infected host can sometimes be induced to produce infectious virus when cultured *in vitro* or when co-cultivated or fused with permissive cells of a different type.

Persistent infections, by definition, cannot be acutely lethal; in fact they tend to cause only mild tissue damage or disease in the host. Some of the persistent infections, however, can reactivate, usually with increased expression of the viral genome and production of infectious virus. This may be associated with an acute disease episode (e.g. herpes simplex coldsore, or shingles), the 'latent' virus having become 'patent'. The word 'latency', therefore, refers to persistent viruses that can become manifest and cause disease following reactivation.

'Slow virus' is a catchy and often loosely used term. It was originally introduced by Sigurdsson (1954) to refer to infections with a long drawn-out incubation period, a protracted course of disease, and a restricted host and organ susceptibility. The most important feature is that the incubation period often lasts a large portion of the life span. Persistent infections in this category include SSPE, infections with agents of the scrapie group, and infection with the lentivirus visna (it may be noted that lentivirus = slow virus).

In some persistent infections (e.g. adenoviruses) small amounts of infectious virus are produced steadily in the host, while in others there is large-scale and continuous formation of infectious virus, often with shedding of virus to the outside world. These are 'chronic' infections, e.g. infection of mice with LCM virus or of man with hepatitis B virus.

Examples of persistent viral infections are given in Table 6.1. It is difficult to draw sharp distinctions between the several types of persistent infection, but it is helpful to have a simple classification. Fig. 6.1 is an attempt to clarify our thinking on this difficult subject. Persistent viral infections are particularly important for four reasons:

1 They can be activated to cause acute episodes of disease.

2 They are sometimes associated with immunopathological disease, as described in Chapter 4, or with other chronic diseases, especially of the central nervous system.

3 They are sometimes associated with neoplasms.

4 They enable the virus to persist in the community.

One way of looking at persistent infections is to regard them as failures of the host defence mechanisms which are designed to eliminate invading viruses from tissues. In this chapter many of the most important persistent infections are described in detail, and this is followed by an analysis of the various ways in which host defence mechanisms can fail. We shall also take the virus' point of view, and consider the methods by which persistent viruses bypass or evade host defences.

PERSISTENT INFECTIONS OF CULTURED CELLS

Persistent viral infections pose great practical problems to the physician and veterinarian. They also pose problems to the scientist who wishes to understand them. A great deal has been learnt from persistent viral infections of cultured cells, where events can be controlled and manipu-

Table 6.1. Examples of persistent viral infections (mainly human).

Virus	Site of persistence	Infectiousness of persistent virus	Consequence	Shedding of virus to exterior
Herpes simplex	Dorsal root ganglia	−	Activation, cold sore	+
	Salivary glands	+	None known	+
Varicella-zoster	Dorsal root ganglia	−	Activation, zoster	+
Cytomegalovirus	Lymphoid tissue[a]	−	Activation ± disease	+
EB virus	Lymphoid tissue	−	Lymphoid tumour? (Burkitt's lymphoma)	−
Hepatitis B	Salivary glands	+	None known	+
	Liver (virus shed into blood)	+	Blood remains infectious[b]	+
Adenoviruses	Lymphoid tissue	−	None known	+
Polyoma (mice)	Kidney tubules	+	None known	+
Polyomaviruses BK and JC (man)	Kidney	−	Activation (pregnancy, immunosuppression)	+
Leukaemia (mice)	Lymphoid and other tissues	±	Late leukaemia	−
Measles	Brain (rarely)	±	Subacute sclerosing panencephalitis	−
LCM (mice)	Widespread	+	Late glomerulonephritis	+
LDH (mice)	Macrophages	+	None	+
Lassa fever (the rat, Mastomys natalensis)	Kidney	+	None known	+
Mouse thymic virus	Salivary glands	+	None known	+
Visna (sheep)	Brain; macrophages	±	Chronic disease	?

[a]CMV may also cause persistent infection in kidney tubules, with continuous shedding of virus in urine.
[b]Hepatocellular carcinoma is a possible consequence.

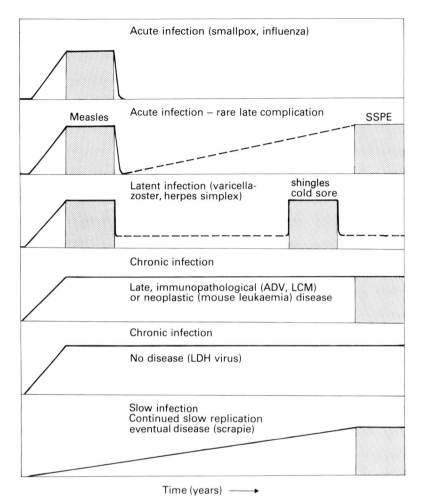

Fig. 6.1. Types of persistent infection. Box = disease; solid line = infectious virus; dotted line = virus not demonstrable.

lated and observations made with greater facility than in the intact host. Unfortunately, as with other aspects of pathogenesis, some aspects of persistence phenomena can be studied only in the intact host.

Persistent viral infections of cultured cells can be conveniently, but not rigidly, divided into three types:

Steady state infections

In steady state infections most or all of the cells in the culture are infected, and the virus is slowly but continuously released. This type of infection was described for the paramyxovirus, SV5, a common contaminant of primary cultures of rhesus monkey kidney cells. This is a relatively non-cytocidal infection (Compans *et al.*, 1966), and the infected cells survive and multiply. Similar infections have been described with other paramyxoviruses, togaviruses, rhabdoviruses, arenaviruses, and retroviruses. The cultures cannot generally be 'cured' with antibody, because the dividing infected cells transmit the virus to progeny cells. Rubella virus infection of cultured human embryo cells provides an interesting example, which is referred to in Chapter 2. Persistent infection of mouse cells with LCM virus has been studied *in vitro* in attempts to understand persistence in the mouse. Cultures often show a cyclic pattern of production of infectious virus, and the part played by slow-growing virus variants, defective interfering particles, etc. has been investigated (Hotchin 1974).

Simian vacuolating virus 40 (SV40) causes a classic persistent infection in rhesus or cynomolgus monkey kidney cells *in vitro* (Sweet and Hilleman, 1960). The infected cells grew well in culture and cytopathic effects, although subsequently demonstrated (Easton, 1964), were not obvious. These persistently infected cells were widely used for the cultivation of other viruses, including the polioviruses used for the Salk vaccine (see Chapter 7). The persistent SV40 virus was detected only when culture fluids were tested in African green monkey kidney cells in which characteristic cytopathic effects were produced, with vacuolation of the cytoplasm.

Shope fibroma virus provides another example. This causes a relatively non-cytocidal infection in cultured rabbit kidney cells (Hinze and Walker, 1971). Infected cells multiply at a slightly slower rate than control cells, show altered morphology and loss of contact inhibition, and cellular and viral DNA synthesis alternate.

Measles virus establishes a persistent infection in the Daudi lymphoblastoid cell line. The non-infectious virions that are produced are characterised by an uncleaved F protein (Fujinami and Oldstone, 1981). As cleavage of the fusion protein is necessary for continuing infection, it has been postulated that the persistence of measles in normal lymphoid cells *in vivo* may be attributable to the absence of a suitable cleavage protease in these cells.

Carrier cultures

In these cultures, although infectious virus often, but not always, continues to be produced, virus-free cells are always present and can be recovered by cloning. The culture is a balanced system in which fresh cells are constantly produced, but not all of them are being infected. In some cases, e.g. coxsackievirus A9 in Hela cells, the virus-free cells are genetically resistant, the infection being perpetuated in a minority of susceptible cells (Takemoto and Habel, 1959). In others the virus-free cells are susceptible but are protected by antibody (herpes simplex in Hela cells; Wheeler, 1960), by interferon (NDV in L cells; Henle, 1963), or by defective interfering (DI) virus particles. The virus in such cultures is often temperature-sensitive (Kimura et al., 1975). Even when antibody is not present, it is often difficult to assess the relative importance of the temperature-sensitive (ts) mutation, DI particles, and interferon (Youngner et al., 1978; Workshop, 1976). In these, as in other types of persistently infected cultures, changes occur over long periods, including an accumulation of viral mutations (Holland et al., 1979; Rowlands et al., 1980). Temperature-sensitive mutants sometimes show a striking ability to persist in vivo (Knobler et al., 1982) but generally neither ts mutants nor DI particles have been shown to be important in the persistently infected host.

Transformation

In these cultures all cells are persistently infected, but little or no infectious virus is produced, and the viral nucleic acid is integrated with host nucleic acid. Tumour viruses establish this type of persistent infection (reviews: Tooze, 1980; Weiss et al., 1982).

Many DNA viruses transform infected cells, causing morphological and physiological alterations, often including loss of growth control, but infectious viral particles are not formed. Viral DNA remains in the infected cells, either integrated into the cell genome or in episomal form, and is replicated and passed on to the daughter cells. Examples include the papovaviruses, polyomavirus and SV40 (Sambrook, 1981), some herpesviruses (Klein, 1982–4) and many adenoviruses (Sambrook, 1981). Retroviruses (Weiss et al., 1982) can establish the same type of persistent infection in culture, when a DNA copy of the viral RNA is inserted into the host genome.

PERSISTENT INFECTIONS IN THE INTACT HOST

Examples of persistent viral infections are given in Table 6.1. These will now be discussed in detail.

RNA tumour viruses

The retroviruses include the viruses cause leukaemia in mammals and leukoses in birds. When a ds DNA copy of the viral RNA is present in the host genome, this puts the virus in a special category, obviously protected from host defences as long as viral antigens are not expressed on the cell surface. Retrovirus DNA sequences are common in the genome of most vertebrates. For instance, endogenous retrovirus sequences are said to account for 0.04% of the total genome in mice

(Todaro *et al.*, 1978), and the genome of white leghorn chickens contains 16 separate endogenous virus elements, stably inherited as Mendelian loci (Weiss, 1982). Retrovirus sequences are regularly present in human chromosomal DNA (Repaske *et al.*, 1983), and a human retrovirus causing T cell leukaemias has been isolated (Reitz *et al.*, 1983). Following infection, T cells express receptors for T cell growth factor (interleukin 2), and thus acquire a growth advantage (Lando *et al.*, 1983).

Much remains to be learnt about the control of gene expression in retroviruses (Varmus, 1982). If the viral genome is partially or fully expressed in cells, with antigens or infectious virus produced, or if virus is transmitted horizontally from individual to individual, many of the mechanisms of persistence referred to at the end of this chapter will be relevant. CMI responses may be generated but they fail to control the infection. The viruses are generally sensitive to interferon, which depresses the production of virus particles without affecting viral RNA and protein synthesis (Friedman, 1977), but interferon is not detectable in the persistently infected animal. Antibody responses may occur, but they are ineffective. Neutralising antibodies are produced in some of the horizontally transmitted RNA tumour virus infections and antigenic variation, possibly in a given infected animal (see p. 249) may contribute to persistence. With the endogenous RNA tumour viruses, in contrast, the genes coding for the envelope antigens are well preserved and show remarkably little variation.

Complexes of leukaemia virus antigen with antibody are deposited in glomeruli of many strains of mice, but there are no pathogenic consequences (see Chapter 4). Autoimmune responses are seen under certain circumstances, such as the aplastic or haemolytic anaemia sometimes produced in cats by the subgroup C serotype of feline leukaemia virus (Jarrett, 1980) and the autoimmune disease of NZB mice which is either caused by or exacerbated by mouse leukaemia virus (Talal and Steinberg, 1974).

Herpes simplex

Primary infection with herpes simplex virus normally occurs during infancy or early childhood, and causes a mild illness with stomatitis and slight fever (Burnet and Williams, 1939). The infection is often not noticed. Virus replicates in mucosal and submucosal tissues, enters peripheral nerve endings and travels up the sensory nerve to the trigeminal ganglion which supplies the mouth and related parts. After apparent recovery from the initial infection the virus remains in a non-infectious state (latent) in the ganglion. At least 50% of normal adults, whether or not they suffer from coldsores, have herpes simplex virus DNA present in the trigeminal ganglion (Baringer and Swoveland, 1973). The virus can often be rendered infectious and thus detected by explantation of ganglion cells or co-cultivation with cells that are suscep-tible to herpes simplex virus infection (Stevens and Cook, 1973). At intervals later in life the virus can be activated in the ganglion, then travel down the nerve and cause a vesicular eruption, usually round the lip or nostrils (Fig. 6.2). This is called a coldsore, and virus from a cold-sore can infect a susceptible individual. Coldsores occur particularly in certain individuals and the factors that activate virus in the ganglion include colds, certain fevers, sunlight, menstruation and possibly psychological factors. Their mode of action is not understood. The eruption is restricted to the area supplied by the particular sensory ganglion that was involved during the original childhood infection. The venereally transmitted variety of herpes simplex (herpes simplex type 2) causes a primary infection of parts such as the penis or the cervix with latent infection of the corresponding sacral ganglia. It causes recurrent lesions in these areas if reactivated later in life.

In coldsores, infectious virus (up to 10^6 pfu per ml) is present in the vesicle (Spruance et al., 1977), often in the form of infectious immune complexes (Daniels et al., 1975) and interferon is generally present (Spruance et al., 1982). Pain or other sensations at the site of the eruption may precede the visible lesion. This is perhaps to be expected if the reactivation is taking place specifically in those neurones whose axons carry sensation from the affected area (see p. 208). Virus cannot be recovered between attacks from skin biopsies at the site of the recurrent eruptions (Rustigian et al., 1966), but virus is often recovered from saliva in the absence of a clinical coldsore. This is possibly a result of a sub-clinical reactivation involving a local mucosal surface or salivary gland.

The trigeminal ganglion had been identified as a possible source of virus for coldsores many years go. Harvey Cushing, the great American surgeon, had noticed that coldsores appear 3–4 days after severing the sensory nerve root to the spinal cord from the trigeminal ganglion (Fig. 6.2) and mere exposure without direct manipulation of the ganglion at operation can have the same effect (Pazin et al., 1978). But this does not occur if there has been preceding interruption of the sensory nerve supply to the affected area (Carton, 1953). Also in the 1920s histological lesions were observed in the ganglia of experimentally infected animals (Friedenwald, 1923). As studied in cell culture, herpes simplex virus invariably causes a cytolytic infection, and the state in which the virus exists in the ganglion is not understood.

Various model systems have been developed in attempts to investigate herpes simplex latency and reactivation. In mice and rabbits inoculated in the ear, tongue, lip or eye, the virus multiplies locally and then spreads to the dorsal root ganglia via peripheral nerves. It appears to be transported up the nerve in axons at the rate of 2–10 mm per hour (Kristensson et al., 1971; Kristensson et al., 1978). After recovery from the acute infection, virus disappears from the body surface; reports

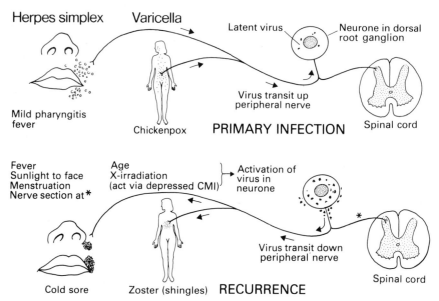

Fig. 6.2. Mechanisms of herpes simplex and varicella-zoster virus latency and reactivation in man.

(Hill *et al.*, 1980) of its presence in skin during latency are of uncertain status because of the possibility of spontaneous reactivation (see p. 212). The virus is no longer detectable by routine methods in the ganglion, but there is clear evidence it is dormant there (Stevens and Cook, 1973). Reactivation is induced by anaphylaxis or by injecting adrenalin (in the rabbit), by local burning with solid CO_2 (Openshaw *et al.*, 1979), by hair plucking (Hurd and Robinson, 1976) or by X-irradiation and cyclo-phosphamide treatment (Sekizawa *et al.*, 1980). In the experimental system described by Hill *et al.* (1975) reactivation can be induced by more physiological methods. Mice are inoculated in the ear, and after recovery from the initial infection, spontaneous reactivations take place, with virus once again present in the inoculated ear which often becomes red and develops vesicles. These reactivations can also be induced by causing erythema in the ear by repeated applications of cellophane tape or by exposure to ultraviolet light (Hill *et al.*, 1978); also by treatments with chemicals such as xylene and retinoic acid (Harbour *et al.*, 1983). As well as causing immediate inflammation, the stimuli generally lead to a rise in local levels of prostaglandins E and F, which could enhance the virus spread (Harbour *et al.*, 1978) and reduce local immune responses. A slender thread linking these varied reactivation stimuli is that they could all cause changes in the metabolism of latently infected neurones.

It now seems firmly established that the neurone is the site of latent herpes simplex virus in the ganglion. This has been done by following the course of reactivation in ganglia either implanted in millipore chambers *in vivo* (Cook *et al*., 1974) or explanted *in vitro* (McLennan and Darby, 1980). In each case the first cells to produce virus or viral antigens as detected by immunofluorescence or other methods were neurones.

What is the evidence as to the state of herpes simplex virus in the latently infected neurone? Low level viral replication in ganglia seems unlikely because latent infection can be established by temperature-sensitive mutants for which body temperatures are non-permissive (McLennan and Darby, 1980). It also seems unlikely that significant amounts of viral antigen are present, because McLennan (Wildy *et al*., 1982) found none with fluorescent antibody staining when examining serial sections of entire ganglia from 50 latently infected mice. Herpes simplex virus DNA has been detected in latently infected neurones, and Puga *et al*. (1978) found that ganglia in chronically infected mice contained a very low proportion of herpes simplex mRNA in relation to herpes simplex DNA as compared with ganglia during the acute infection. This suggests that there is a block in transcription in the latently infected ganglia. One of the problems with the interpretation of these experiments is that, if spontaneous reactivations are constantly occurring, the state of affairs at a given time may partly reflect reactivation events. There are indications from the work of Rock and Fraser (1983) that, although all of the viral genome appears to be present in sensory ganglia and brain (see p. 210) of latently infected mice, it is not in the form of unit-length linear DNA. The terminal repeated sequences, which are present in the acute stage of the infection, are not detected in latently infected brain or ganglia. In another study, paravertebral ganglia from 40 human beings were examined for herpes simplex type 2 RNA by *in situ* hybridisation (Galloway *et al*., 1982). Ganglia from 14 were positive, and all of these had the RNA sequences representing the left hand 30% of the virus genome. This contains a number of genes, including that for viral thymidine kinase. Other left hand regions were present less frequently, and sequences from the S component of the genome were never detected. Evidently there is regular transcription of specific portions of the viral genome in latently infected ganglia. In sensory neurones of latently infected rabbits, Green *et al*. (1981) detected an immediate early polypeptide of HSV by fluorescent antibody staining, but this is not coded for by the transcripts detected in human ganglia by Galloway *et al*. These matters will doubtless be resolved in the near future.

So far there are no really good *in vitro* models for herpes simplex latency (Levine *et al*., 1980; Wigdahl *et al*., 1982; Hammer *et al*., 1981), although these are becoming more promising (Wigdahl *et al*., 1983). But Youssoufian *et al*. (1982) studied herpes simplex latency in a lymphoid cell line and found an intriguing association between latency and methylation of the viral genome. Non-producing, unstimulated cells contained 1–2 extensively methylated HSV genome copies per cell, whereas PHA-stimulated producer cultures contained 40–80 genome copies per cell, none of them methylated.

Following reactivation in the ganglion, the virus must spread down the peripheral nerve to the skin surface, exit from the nerve, then infect dermal and finally epidermal cells to produce the lesion. From their mouse model studies, Hill and Blyth (1976) have suggested that viral reactivation in the ganglion is constantly occurring, but the infection is usually aborted before the local lesion has been established. If this were so, the question of what induces a coldsore would not only be what induces reactivation in the ganglion, but also what allows the reactivated virus to spread down the peripheral nerve, generating a whole series of pathogenic events which culminate in the local lesion. Another problem concerns the virological axiom that herpes simplex virus, during productive infection of the cell, destroys that cell. If this is the case, then virus reactivating in neurones will destroy those particular neurones and ultimately the supply of latently infected neurones would be exhausted. Therefore, it has been suggested that, during each coldsore attack, there is retrograde infection up the peripheral nerve, as in the original infection. Latency is thus re-established in new sets of neurones by a 'round trip' mechanism.

From the diagram of herpes simplex latency (Fig. 6.2) it can be seen that virus from the reactivated neurone could spread centrally to the spinal cord as well as peripherally to the skin. This is known to occur with other viruses such as varicella-zoster that reactivate from ganglion cells. In mice with latent ganglion infections it has been shown that 30% have herpes simplex DNA sequences in the brain and in the ganglia (Cabrera et al., 1980). But this (brain) virus is not easily reactivated in vitro, in contrast to the virus latent in sensory ganglia, although immunosuppression may lead to viral expression in the brain (Kastroff et al., 1981). There are reports that herpes simplex virus DNA has been detected in the human brain (Brown et al., 1979; Sequera et al., 1979), and Davis and Johnson (1979) have suggested that herpes simplex encephalitis in adults could result from activation and central spread of virus from the trigeminal ganglion. The situation may be more complex because restriction enzyme analysis of virus isolates from brain and orolabial region showed that, in three of eight patients, strains from the two sites were different, suggesting reinfection with a second virus or dual infection (Whitley et al., 1982).

Immunological factors are likely to be important in the control of herpes simplex virus latency, especially during the period of spread of the virus from reactivating neurones and production of the skin lesions. It has been shown that patients undergoing recrudescence of herpes simplex skin lesions have impaired cell-mediated immunity (Shillitoe et al., 1977). Their T lymphocytes showed defective MIF production in response to herpes antigens although lymphoproliferative responses were raised or normal and responses to unrelated antigens such as Candida and PPD were normal. Cunningham and Merigan (1983) showed that cells spontaneously producing interferon γ appear in peripheral blood 1–3 weeks after a cold sore. The next attack was longer delayed in those whose cells produced higher levels of interferon. This could mean interferon protects against recurrences, or alternatively that spontaneous interferon production merely reflects the operation of other more important immune events. Also, in the week preceding the attack, there is a striking fall in the activity of NK-like cells, rising to higher-than-normal levels during and for a few weeks after the coldsore (Rola-Pleszczynski and Lieu, 1983). Perhaps these cytotoxic cells produce the interferon, which in turn sustains their activity.

Experimental evidence suggests that antibodies are of limited importance in maintaining latency, which may be maintained in the absence of detectable neutralising antibodies (Sekizawa et al., 1980). Antibody levels may rise after the appearance of a coldsore, but the levels in patients who are about to develop coldsores do not differ from normal controls. However, tests with defined viral antigens have not been made and it is too early to assign relative importance to humoral and cell-mediated immunity in the control of latency, and, in any case, NK-like cells and interferon may also be important. In the mouse system more is being discovered about the role of immune mechanisms in recovery from primary infections than in the control of latency. Also, one must distinguish between factors that control the latent infection in the neurone from the factors that might control the post-reactivation events leading up to the formation of the local skin lesion. Good surveys of the present position have been given by Wildy et al. (1982b), by Klein (1982), and by Hill (1983).

Although herpes simplex virus has been considered here in some detail because of its human importance and the voluminous literature, there are a number of herpesvirus infections of animals, including pseudorabies virus infection of swine and B virus infection of rhesus monkeys in which similar episodes of reactivation from infected ganglia occur. Interestingly, when pseudorabies reactivates in sensory neurones in pigs, the sensory changes referred to above in herpes simplex are prominent enough to give rise to the clinical condition called 'mad itch'.

Varicella-zoster

Primary infection with this virus causes the disease chickenpox, a systemic infection in which vesicular skin lesions are formed after a complex and poorly understood series of events in pathogenesis (see Chapter 2). The virus in skin lesions then ascends in sensory nerve axons, as with herpes simplex, to infect dorsal root ganglion cells. Latency is established as the child recovers from the initial infection and develops antiviral humoral and cell-mediated immune responses. Many years later, with increasing probability after the age of 55, attacks of zoster (shingles) are seen. The virus reactivates randomly in a ganglion and then spreads down the peripheral nerve to give vesicular skin lesions at the site supplied by the affected neurones (Fig. 6.2). A classic description of the disease was given in 1900 by Head and Campbell. Preceding malaise and fever, together with sensory phenomena (especially itching and pain), are common, and indeed may occur without the infection progressing far enough to produce skin lesions. Pain may persist for long periods after recovery from zoster, but the basis is not known. Infectious virus is produced in the vesicles, and causes chickenpox when it spreads to infect susceptible children.

The annual rate of attack with zoster is 3–5 per 1000 and the patient is equally at risk for a future attack. There are notable histological changes in the dorsal root ganglia during zoster, with neuronal destruction. The virus has been isolated from ganglia (Bastian *et al.*, 1974) but in patients with zoster rather than from normal individuals. Basic knowledge of this virus is in a backward state, but all the epidemiological, virological and serological evidence, although indirect, shows that the above series of events is the correct one. Recently Hyman *et al.* (1983), using *in situ* hybridisation, detected varicella-zoster specific RNA in a small proportion of neurones in trigeminal ganglia from subjects with no history of zoster.

The spontaneous reactivations in old age are associated with defects in cell-mediated immunity specifically to varicella-zoster that occur on ageing (Miller, 1980). This selective decline in control of the infection is probably why zoster is more painful and protracted when it occurs in elderly rather than in younger patients. Reactivation also occurs when CMI responses are impaired in Hodgkin's disease and in other lympho-reticular neoplasms, in artificially immunosuppressed patients, and after X-irradiation of the spine. Antibodies are not known to be important in the control of varicella-zoster latency, but there are interesting differences in the response to primary versus reactivated infection. Sundquist *et al.* (1983) found that the antibody response in zoster was mainly IgG_1, whereas in varicella it was mainly IgG_3.

If herpes simplex and varicella-zoster viruses are initially seeded into dorsal root ganglia neurones from localised lesions, it may be asked why reactivated varicella-zoster virus affects a large area of skin (often the whole of the dermatone served by the ganglion) whereas reactivated herpes simplex virus causes a relatively localised lesion. Possibly this is because varicella-zoster virus more readily spreads to uninfected neurones in the dorsal root ganglion, so that a larger area of skin is, therefore, involved. In any case the differences are not absolute. In experimental animals locally inoculated herpes simplex virus can cause zoster-like lesions in the acute stage of the disease (Dillard *et al.*, 1972) and there are reports of a similar phenomenon in infants and young children infected with herpes simplex virus (Mok, 1971).

Cytomegaloviruses

Human CMV (Ho, 1982), like mouse CMV or pig CMV, causes a ubiquitous and persistent infection in the host species, and is not normally pathogenic. Cytomegaloviruses are generally species-specific, although often less exclusively so at the level of cell susceptibility *in vitro*. Infection occurs in childhood, with little or no accompanying illness, and virus is shed in the throat and urine. In London on any given day, about 10% of children under the age of five years are excreting CMV in urine. The acute infection subsides gradually over the course of months as antibodies and CMI develop, and the virus becomes persistent. Later in life, especially during the immunosuppression of kidney or bone marrow transplant patients, the infection may reactivate, giving viraemia, fever and sometimes hepatitis or pneumonitis (Glenn, 1981). The only other times CMV causes damage is when primary infection in adults gives a mild disease with mononucleosis, or when primary infection occurs during pregnancy. CMV can then infect the placenta and thus the foetus, causing abnormalities of development in the brain and ear (see Chapter 2). Infection of the foetus is also known to occur as a result of pregnancy reactivation of the virus (see below), but is then less likely to cause damage (Stagno *et al.*, 1982). When pregnancy reactivation leads to foetal infection, this presumably involves the spread of bloodborne virus to placenta and foetus. Antibodies are already present, and the virus must be leukocyte-associated. There seems no reason why the foetus should not be infected again in subsequent pregnancies, a phenomenon which is described for human CMV (Stagno *et al.*, 1977) and which is also reported for mice persistently infected with Japanese encephalitis virus (Mathur *et al.*, 1982).

CMV reactivates in pregnancy, both in man and the mouse (Gould and Mims, 1980) in association with depressed CMI responses specifically to CMV antigens (Gehrz *et al.*, 1981; Chong and Mims, 1982). In man there are increased rates of recovery of virus from the cervix during pregnancy, and virus is present in milk from about one-third of nursing mothers (Stagno *et al.*, 1980). Hormonal changes during pregnancy could also play a part in pregnancy reactivation. Serum from pregnant mice, or physiological concentrations of progesterone, oestrogen and corticosteroid are known to increase the replication of mouse CMV *in vitro* (Chong and Mims, 1984).

During the acute infection CMV is excreted in saliva, urine, milk and semen and may continue to be present in these fluids for many months (Embil *et al.*, 1982; Lang and Kummer, 1975). It is not certain which cells are the site of persistent infection. In the persistently infected mouse, CMV-specific DNA sequences have been reported to be present in macrophages (Brautigam *et al.*, 1979), but other evidence suggests that B cells rather than macrophages are infected (Jordan and Mar, 1982). B and T lymphocytes appear to be involved during the acute infection (Wu and Ho, 1979) but the picture is less clear during persistent infection. In man there have been conflicting reports (Jordan, 1983) about the infectivity of blood, but it seems that CMV can be transmitted by transfusions of blood from a small proportion of apparently normal persistently infected individuals. Virus is thought to be present in leukocytes in non-infectious form and is perhaps reactivated during immune interactions between transfused and host lymphocytes. Unfortunately there is no good evidence for infection of human lympho-cytes or monocytes—indeed one recent study suggests that polymorphs are the source of CMV in transfused blood. Perhaps a study of granu-lopoietic cells in bone marrow would throw light on this.

A fuller understanding of persistent CMV infections will come from studies on mouse CMV where the interplay of virus with lymphocytes and macrophages (see pp. 241–2) is being studied in some detail (Hudson, 1979; Ho, 1982).

Epstein-Barr virus

EB virus causes an almost universal persistent human infection. Initially virus is shed in the saliva, often for many months. The site of persistent infection is known to be B lymphocytes which have EB virus receptors (closely associated with C3d receptors; Wells *et al.*, 1983) on their surface. Epithelial cells adjacent to the oropharynx are probably also involved in the acute stages, although acute cytolytic infection may occur in these cells in contrast to the lymphocyte. The virus probably replicates in salivary glands because fluid from the parotid gland duct contains more virus than does buccal fluid (Morgan *et al.*, 1979).

EB virus persists in B cells, mostly in episomal but partly in inte-grated form. It is difficult to obtain EB viral genome-containing cells from the circulation in normal, persistently infected individuals, because these occur with a frequency of about 1 in 10^7 mononuclear cells (Rocchi *et al.*, 1977), hence most studies have been made with EBV-transformed lymphoblastoid cell lines where the state of the viral genome and the number of EB DNA genome equivalents per cell can be calculated. Infectious virus is not detectable in lymphocytes freshly removed from EBV carriers, and is revealed only when they are cultivated *in vitro* with uninfected lymphocytes, which become transformed (Pope *et al.*, 1968). The transformed cells form small clusters, which can be counted.

Virus-specific T cells are present in persistently infected individuals, and will inhibit the development of the clusters of transformed cells (Rickinson *et al.*, 1981). Epithelial cells are probably infected (Shapiro and Volsky, 1983) but little is known of persistence in these cells, although such information could provide a basis for our understanding of the role of EB virus in nasopharyngeal carcinoma (NPC).

When infection takes place in childhood it is commonly symptomless, but in adolescence and in young adults it causes the disease glandular fever (infectious mononucleosis). Lymphoid tissues are swollen because they are the site of viral growth and of a proliferative immune response. The throat, a possible site of necrotic infected epithelial cells, is inflamed and sore. Thus the patient has fever, pharyngitis, lymphadenopathy and often an enlarged spleen. Virus isolation is not easy, and may require that throat washings are added to cultures of uninfected human lymphocytes obtained from the umbilical cord of infants at birth.

During the acute infection, the immune system is in a turmoil (Sugden, 1982). Infected B cells differentiate, and produce antibody (Robinson *et al.*, 1981), but only 0.2–1.0% of blood B lymphocytes are susceptible to this transformation (Yarchoan *et al.*, 1983). Antibody is produced, not only against EB virus antigens, but also against irrelevant antigens; an example is the heterophile antibody reacting with the surface of sheep or horse erythrocytes, which has for many years been used to diagnose glandular fever. The virus causes polyclonal activation of B cells. Immunoregulatory disturbances are known to occur, with increases in the number of suppressor T cells (Crawford *et al.*, 1981), but they are not understood.

EB virus is reactivated in immunosuppressed renal transplant patients, but without causing illness. Its main claim to long-term harmful effects is in the aetiology of Burkitt's lymphoma and nasopharyngeal carcinoma (NPC) (Epstein and Achong, 1979; Epstein and Morgan, 1983). In each condition a co-factor is required—possibly malaria in Burkitt's lymphoma, and possibly a chemical carcinogen in NPC—together with predisposing host genetic factors. EB virus causes lymphomas in monkeys, and the evidence for its involvement in these human tumours is very strong indeed. It will not be feasible to reproduce the tumours in human volunteers, but if the tumours can be prevented by preventing EB virus infection with a vaccine (see Chapter 7) this would constitute equally powerful evidence of an aetiological relationship.

EB virus infects man, but there are other so-called lymphotropic persistent herpesviruses that cause similar diseases in other species. *Herpesvirus gorilla*, *H. pan* and *H. papio* are B lymphotropic viruses like EB virus. These viruses have been isolated from lymphoid cell lines established from respectively, gorillas, chimpanzees and baboons, and from oral secretions from immunosuppressed chimpanzees. They are closely related to EB virus, sharing 20–45% homology in DNA sequences and cross-reacting serologically. Almost nothing is known of the diseases they cause in their natural hosts. *H. saimiri* is a T lymphotropic virus which is non-pathogenic in its natural host, the squirrel monkey. However, it causes lymphomas when it infects other types of monkeys. A survey of these non-human primate lymphotropic herpesviruses is given by Wolfe (1979).

Marek's disease virus is a lymphotropic virus that causes a persistent infection in chickens. It infects both T and B cells causing a lympho-proliferative condition in young chickens, and lesions in peripheral nerves in older birds. Viral replication is generally abortive both in lymphoid cells and the Schwann cells that are involved in peripheral nerve tumours. The virus spreads from chicken to chicken as a result of a productive infection and shedding of infectious virus from epithelial cells in feather follicles (Calnek and Hitchner, 1969; Payne *et al.*, 1976).

Visna

Visna is a lentivirus, one of the group of non-oncogenic retroviruses that cause chronic demyelinating diseases, chronic pneumonitis (maedi) and chronic arthritis in sheep and goats (Haase, 1975; Narayan *et al.*, 1980). Visna causes a fatal paralytic disease in sheep when inoculated intracerebrally, with an incubation period ranging from months to years, during which time the infected animal remains well. There is a prompt CMI response with a mononuclear infiltration into the meninges and around blood vessels, but neutralising antibody is not formed until after 1–3 months. Large numbers of macrophages are seen in the brain and spinal cord lesions, and also in the lung alveoli when this virus causes chronic pneumonitis.

Extracellular virus is generally recoverable from infected brains, but viral antigens are not readily demonstrable. Most of the virus is present in cells as proviral DNA, demonstrable by *in situ* hybridisation (Brahic *et al.*, 1981a). Productive infection is not seen in choroid plexuses in infected animals, yet choroid plexus cells from uninfected sheep are the standard cells used to isolate virus, for instance from spleen cells or peripheral blood leukocytes, by co-cultivation. Productive viral replication then occurs, with giant cell formation and cell death. Evidently there are *in vivo* restraints on the expression of the viral genome. The restraints are not necessarily immunological, because in one study sheep were neonatally thymectomised and treated with antilymphocyte serum, but viral replication was still restricted (Narayan *et al.*, 1977).

The mechanism of production of the late demyelinating lesions is not understood, and the role of primary viral as opposed to secondary immunological effects is not clear (Nathanson *et al.*, 1983), but a number of studies have helped explain virus persistence. It has been shown that antigenic mutants of visna virus develop in the persistently infected sheep. Viruses recovered from circulating leukocytes are not neutralised by antibody directed against the original infecting virus. The mutations accumulate in that portion of the viral genome coding for the surface glycoprotein that elicits neutralising antibody (Clements *et al.*, 1980). Antigenic drift of virus in a single infected host has also been shown for another persistent infection, equine infectious anaemia in horses (Kono *et al.*, 1973).

If the immune response restricts viral growth, the generation of these mutants would enable the virus to escape from immune restraint and would favour persistence. However, recent work (Narayan *et al.*, 1983b; Lutley *et al.*, 1983; Thormar *et al.*, 1983) shows that the antigenic mutants may be present from a very early stage after initial infection, do not necessarily replace the original strain, and are not necessarily associated with persistence.

One difficulty in the interpretation of the studies on visna is that most of them have been carried out with strains of virus that have been used and adapted in the laboratory for 20–30 years. When freshly isolated or field strains of virus are used, fresh features of the infection appear that may be important for persistence. For one thing infected animals now fail to develop neutralising antibodies (Sheffield *et al.*, 1980), which argues against the role of antigenic drift in enabling virus to escape from antibody control (Narayan *et al.*, 1983b). Also, macrophages are now infected, with budding of visna virus particles into intracellular vacuoles (Narayan *et al.*, 1982).

Subacute sclerosing panencephalitis (SSPE)

This is a rare disease with an incidence of about 1 case per million children per year. The average age of onset is 7–8 years and it begins 1–10 years after recovery from uncomplicated measles virus infection. Pathological changes are confined to the central nervous system and there is a progressive encephalitis, with measles virus antigens present in neurones and glial cells. But the virus is highly cell-associated and no infectious virus is directly demonstrable. Isolations can be made in about half the cases by co-cultivation of brain cells with susceptible non-neural cells. There is no doubt that the disease is due to measles, and there has been a decline in frequency since the introduction of the measles vaccine. High levels of measles antibody are present both in serum and in cerebrospinal fluid, and antibody is produced by plasma cells in the infected brain. A good survey of SSPE, and the similar condition caused by distemper virus in dogs is given by ter Meulen and Carter (1982).

The mechanism of localisation of measles virus in the brain is not clear, but increased lymphocyte levels in the cerebrospinal fluid and abnormal electroencephalogram recordings have been described in uncomplicated measles (Hanninen *et al.*, 1980), suggesting that silent invasion of the brain is a fairly common event. If so, why does this only very rarely lead to disease? Could these effects be due to the toxicity of interferon produced during the acute infection? Administration of large doses of purified interferon are known to cause neurological side-effects and electroencephalogram abnormalities (Rohatiner *et al.*, 1983). So far there have been no immune deficits described in affected children, either in antibody or cell-mediated immunity.

Many studies have been made of encephalitis induced in experimental animals by SSPE strains of measles virus, but these have given few indications as to the pathogenesis of the condition in man. There is no evidence for a special SSPE strain of measles virus. Many of the SSPE strains produce little or no M (matrix) protein (see p. 219), and certain other strains produce H (haemagglutinin) and F (fusion) proteins in reduced amounts (Rima, 1983). SSPE strains also differ among themselves in growth rate, plaque size, neuropathogenicity, etc. and there is no single, stable property that clearly distinguishes them from wild measles viruses (ter Meulen and Carter, 1982). It seems likely that strains with SSPE features are selected out in the individual patients, probably during growth in the brain. SSPE strains of measles virus tend to be defective and also more neurotropic than regular wild measles virus.

An interesting phenomenon which is likely to be important in this persistent infection was discovered by Oldstone and his colleagues and is surveyed in Oldstone *et al.* (1980) and Oldstone and Fujinami (1982). This is antibody-induced modulation of viral antigens on the infected cell. Patients with SSPE produce very high titres of antibodies to measles virus envelope glycoproteins, and as studied *in vitro* these antibodies combine with viral antigens on the surface of infected cells to form immune complexes. The complexes then move in the fluid matrix that comprises the cell membrane and reach the end of the cell (so-called 'capping'), where they are either shed (exocytosis) or ingested (endocytosis). The stripping of viral envelope antigens from the cell surface interferes with the budding process and results in a retention of nucleocapsids and other viral antigens in the cell. Cell-to-cell spread of the infection via free virus particles is therefore not possible. Also, surprisingly, the synthesis of viral products within the cell is inhibited (Oldstone and Tishon, 1978; Fujinami and Oldstone, 1980). If antibodies are removed after a few hours, viral antigens are soon re-expressed on the cell surface, but if antibodies remain present for several days before being removed, viral antigens do not reappear until after a much longer time interval (Joseph and Oldstone, 1975). It seems likely that this is a powerful mechanism that may operate *in vivo*. Measles antibody removes antigen from cells, renders them insusceptible to immune lysis and at the same time interferes with extracellular spread of the virus, thus promoting the persistent infection.

There is one other mechanism for this particular persistent infection. SSPE strains of virus fail to synthesise the measles M protein in neural cells, and affected patients have very low levels of antibody to this antigen. The M protein normally anchors the viral nucleocapsids to the underside of the plasma membrane prior to budding, and this sequence is blocked in infected cells (Choppin *et al.*, 1981). The gene coding for the M protein is present in SSPE virus strains but there is a block in its translation (Carter *et al.*, 1983).

It is also possible that measles infection is readily converted into an 'indolent' state in neural cells as a result of their metabolic state. Mouse and human neural cells infected with regular measles virus and treated with papaverine to affect cyclic nucleotide metabolism showed decreased production of infectious virus, accumulation of nucleocapsids in the cytoplasm, and disappearance of intracellular M protein. This was not seen in similarly treated non-neural cells (Miller and Carrigan, 1982).

Our understanding of this persistent infection is still incomplete, but it is clear that the M protein defect, coupled with antibody-mediated stripping of viral antigen from infected cells, would help account for:

1 the progress of the infection in spite of adequate immune responses in the host;

2 the very slow evolution of the infection, because only direct cell-to-cell spread by means of the fusion protein would be possible (Choppin *et al.*, 1981), and even this would not be possible if the fusion protein is removed from the cell surface by antibody.

Aleutian disease

Aleutian disease virus is an autonomous parvovirus that causes early death in the type of mink that are homozygous for a recessive gene conferring the Aleutian coat colour. These animals are extensively farmed in the U.S.A. and infection with Aleutian disease virus is economically important as well as of great intrinsic interest.

After experimental infection (Porter and Larsen, 1974) there is extensive replication of virus, mainly in macrophages, and after ten days there are up to 10^9 ID_{50}/g in spleen, liver and lymph nodes. Titres fall to about 10^5 ID_{50}/g after a few months, as the infection becomes persistent. Virus excretion in saliva, urine and faeces continues for at least seven years. Very large numbers of plasma cells are present in organs and very large amounts of IgG antibody are produced. Specific antiviral antibody titres are as high as 100 000 by complement fixation or by immunofluorescence, and the total gammaglobulin level in serum rises from 0.74 g/100 ml to 3.5 g/100 ml. This represents a maximum immune response by the infected animal. During the first few months of the infection the response to other antigens, which have to compete immunologically with the response to the infecting virus, is depressed. The antiviral antibody produced, however, does not neutralise the virus, although it binds to virus particles so that the infectivity of serum is reduced by treatment with antiglobulin. Later on there is an increase in anti-DNA antibodies (Hahn and Hahn, 1983), but the mechanism is not known. Immune complexes are present in the blood. These are progressively deposited in glomeruli, blood vessels, etc. (see Chapter 4), and give rise to glomerulonephritis and arteritis.

The usual cause of death, typically 3–5 months after infection, is glomerulonephritis, and mink sometimes die when one of the larger affected arteries bursts. The viral infection is not in itself pathogenic, and lesions can be prevented when antibody production is inhibited by treatment with cyclophosphamide. All strains of mink, and also ferrets, are susceptible to infection, but mink with the Aleutian genotype develop a much more severe disease. Non-Aleutian mink show a mild disease and rarely die before five months after infection.

The virus infects macrophages almost exclusively and, like LDH virus (see p. 244) 'buds' into cytoplasmic vacuoles. Nothing is known of the basis for macrophage susceptibility, nor of the significance of virus–antibody complexes in the infection of macrophages. The antibody attached to virus particles might increase infection of macrophages if the enhancement phenomenon (see Chapter 4) operates in this system. As isolated from persistently infected mink, the virus, in feline kidney cells, is temperature-sensitive and replicates at 32°C but not at 37–39°C (Porter et al., 1980). This also could be important in the maintenance of the persistent infection.

The key to this disease is immunological, and its severity is determined by the genetic control in the host of the quantity and quality of antibody produced against the infecting virus.

Hepatitis B

Human viral hepatitis is caused by hepatitis A (once called 'infectious' or 'epidemic' hepatitis), hepatitis B ('serum' hepatitis) and at least two viruses responsible for nonA-nonB hepatitis (Szmuness et al., 1982). Hepatitis A does not persist in the host, but hepatitis B and nonA-nonB hepatitis (Robinson, 1982) can lead to persistent infections.

During human infection with hepatitis B virus (Ganem, 1982), the infectious virus particles (Dane particles), together with a large excess (up to 10^{13}/ml) of viral surface antigen particles (HB$_s$ or 'Australia' antigen) appear in the plasma. These reflect viral replication in hepatic cells and HB$_s$Ag is detected before the onset of liver dysfunction or illness. The virus cannot be routinely cultivated, but it is assumed to be present when HB$_s$Ag (readily detected serologically) is present. In most individuals both HB$_s$Ag and the infectious virus particles are cleared from the circulation and from the liver as antibodies to HB$_s$Ag appear during convalescence. It occasionally takes as long as a year to clear HB$_s$Ag from the circulation. In some individuals, however, the virus is not eliminated and a persistent infection is established. This can extend over 20 years (Zuckerman, 1982), and in some individuals may be life long. On the other hand, the carrier state is sometimes terminated. More importantly from a practical point of view, carriers, while remaining HB$_s$Ag-positive, may produce fewer and fewer Dane particles, so that their blood becomes less important as a source of infection. Persistent infection is sometimes accompanied by progressive immunopathological damage to the liver but it is commonly symptomless.

Approximately 5–10% of infections become persistent, but the proportion is much higher when infection is acquired during childhood. Transmission from carrier mothers to babies during the perinatal period gives very high rates of persistence. In studies from Taiwan (Beasley et al., 1982) 90–95% of perinatally infected infants developed persistent infection, compared with 23% of children infected at a mean age of 29 months, and only 3% of individuals infected while university students. Hence, in countries where childhood infection is common, there are more carriers. In Asia, 3–5% of the population are carriers and in several tropical countries 15–20%, whereas in Western Europe, North America and Australia the figure is 0.1%. It is not exactly clear why childhood infection is commoner in developing countries, except is so far as transmission would be favoured by the high carriage rates in mothers. The virus is present in blood and, although it can be spread by contaminated syringes and the needle of the tattooist, acupuncturist, or ear piercer, there are also other important mechanisms for its transmission. Infection is commoner in male homosexuals, and the virus has been detected in saliva and semen of carriers. Presumably this represents 'leakage' of virus from blood, because hepatitis B has not been thought to replicate in sites other than the liver. On the other hand, except for the immunopathological features (see Chapter 4), the extrahepatic manifestations have been poorly investigated, and there is evidence suggesting viral replication in the pancreas (see pp. 222–3). Mosquitoes or other biting arthropods could transmit the infection when the virus, which is fairly stable, contaminates their mouth parts, and this would help account for transmission early in life in tropical and subtropical countries.

Host immune responses directed against HB$_s$Ag are thought to be responsible for recovery from infection and for the elimination of the virus. Interestingly, the same immune responses appear to be the cause of much of the liver pathology. Children (or immunodeficient individuals) develop less vigorous immune responses and are therefore less likely to suffer severe disease, but more likely to become carriers.

The carrier state is characterised by persistence of HB_sAg in the blood, generally with no antibody to HB_sAg, and the presence of infectious virus (Hoofnagle, 1981). Dane particles are detectable by electron microscopy. Antibody to the core antigen (HB_cAg) is present. Some carriers appear to be more infectious than others, with HB_e antigen in the blood and presumably larger numbers of infectious virus particles. The e antigen is located in the core of the virion and correlates closely with the number of virus particles and with infectivity. Males are more likely to become carriers than females. Among patients infected by haemodialysis with contaminated blood, 68% of males became carriers whereas more of the females developed HB_s antibodies and only 33% become carriers (London et al., 1977). Presumably the sex differences are based on differences in the immune response to virus. Patients with high serum ferritin levels before infection are more likely to become carriers (Lustbader et al., 1983). This is not easy to explain but suggests biochemical features influencing the response of liver cells to hepatitis B virus.

Hepatitis B virus carriage is closely linked with development of primary hepatocellular carcinoma. In a study of 22 297 civil servants in Taiwan, 1.2% of hepatitis B carriers developed liver cancer compared with 0.005% of non-carriers (Beasley et al., 1981). This represents a relative risk of 223/1. The mechanism is not clear, but there are integrated hepatitis B virus DNA sequences in the tumour cells (Brechot et al., 1980). Now that the viral genome has been cloned and sequenced, and the genes for HB_sAg and HB_cAg defined, it will not be long before we elucidate the state of the virus in the chronically infected liver cells of carriers (Deinhardt and Gust, 1982). Hepatitis B carriers in Africa, Asia, etc. are more likely to develop hepatocellular carcinoma than carriers in Western Europe or North America, and it is possible that a co-carcinogen such as aflatoxin from contaminated nuts is involved.

Viruses related to hepatitis B have been found in the eastern woodchuck and in Beechey ground squirrels. They are all circular double stranded DNA-containing viruses with similar morphology, now classified as hepadnaviruses, and cause persistent infection with excess HB_s-like particles present in the blood. The woodchuck virus, at least, is associated with chronic hepatitis and with primary hepatocellular carcinoma. A similar virus has been detected in domestic ducks, and the virus is present in the embryo (O'Connell et al., 1983). Advances in our understanding of human infection with hepatitis B virus may come from studies on these related viruses in animals. For instance, infected Pekin ducks show extrahepatic sites of virus growth, including the liver, pancreas and kidney (Halpern et al., 1983). In human infection HB_sAg has been detected in pancreatic juice and in the cytoplasm of pancreatic acinar cells (Shimoda *et al.*, 1981), and the report of infection of cultured human lymphoblastoid cells (Romet-Lemonne *et al.*, 1983) raised the question of infection of lymphoreticular tissues (see Table 6.4) by this virus (Mims, 1982).

When infected blood is a source of infection of susceptible individuals, either by contact or by arthropod transmission, the virus can be said to have been 'shed' into the blood (see Chapter 2). A person persistently infected with hepatitis B virus remains a source of infection for many years, which enables this virus to maintain itself in small or isolated populations. This is also true for many other persistent viruses.

NonA-nonB hepatitis is now being recognised increasingly throughout the world, in both its epidemic (e.g. water-borne) and its sporadic forms (Alter *et al.*, 1982). With the sharp decline in incidence of post-transfusion hepatitis B following the widespread screening of donated blood by radioimmunoassay (Hoofnagle, 1981), nonA-nonB hepatitis has emerged as by far the commonest form of post-transfusion hepatitis in Western countries. It is a particular problem in haemophiliacs, as many batches of Factor VIII are contaminated with the putative virus(es). Intravenous drug users are also especially vulnerable. Though clinically milder than hepatitis B, nonA-nonB far more frequently (approx. 65%) progresses to chronic hepatitis, and virus, antigen and immune-complexes circulate in the blood in high titre for a considerable time. Despite the fact that the viruses have not yet been cultured, epidemiological evidence as well as electron microscopic examination of the livers of chimpanzees and marmosets to which the agents have been transmitted has established the existence of at least two distinct nonA-nonB viruses, yet to be positively identified.

Simian haemorrhagic fever virus is another virus that persists in serum. It is so-called because it gives rise to a fatal haemorrhagic disease in rhesus monkeys. In patas monkeys, however, there are no symptoms and the virus persists, probably for life, in the serum (London, 1977). Very little is known of the pathogenesis and natural transmission in patas monkeys of this togavirus.

Lymphocytic choriomeningitis virus

Infection of mice *in utero* or neonatally with LCM virus results in a high degree of immune tolerance to viral antigens. There are no detectable complement fixing or neutralising antibodies in the plasma, but immune complexes are present. The complexes are deposited in kidney glomeruli (see Chapter 4) from which small amounts of antiviral antibody can be eluted (Oldstone and Dixon, 1967). There are no cell-mediated responses to the infecting virus. Immune responses to unrelated antigens are normal. All tissues of the body are infected and large

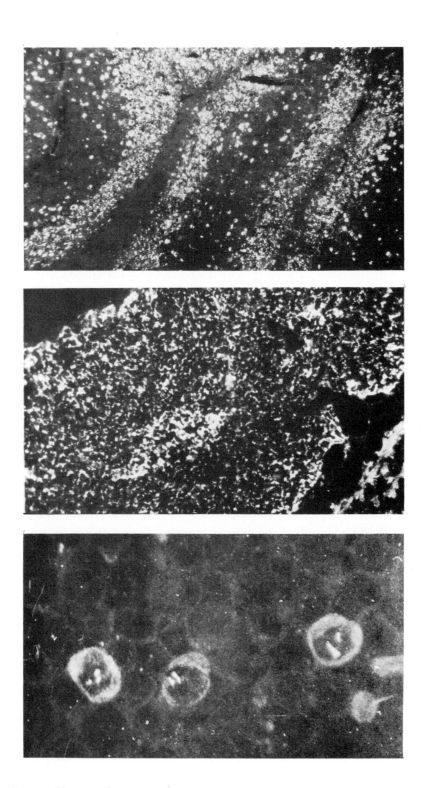

amounts of viral antigen are produced, but the infected cells show no obvious sign of dysfunction and no pathological changes.

In one carrier colony studied (Mims, 1966), intestinal epithelial cells, tubular epithelial cells in the kidney, salivary gland and respiratory epithelial cells were infected, so that infectious virus was continuously shed into faeces, urine, saliva and respiratory secretions. Lymphoid cells also were infected (Fig. 6.3). Almost all cells in tissues such as the cerebellum (Fig. 6.3) and retina were infected, and presumably synthesise virus and viral antigen from birth to death. Mice, nevertheless, remain well and only suffer delayed tissue damage, dying rather earlier in life than controls, mostly from chronic glomerulonephritis as a result of their own immune responses to the infection (see immune complex diseases, Chapter 4). There are indications that persistently infected cells can show subtle and not dramatically harmful defects in 'luxury' functions. For instance, abnormalities in the behaviour of carrier mice (Hotchin and Seegal, 1977) have been demonstrated, and this might be associated with alterations in neurotransmitter synthesis seen in persistenly infected neuroblastoma cells (Oldstone *et al.*, 1977). Indeed, the caged carrier mouse could be mentally defective, in spite of its healthy appearance, because it has no need for the complex behaviour pattern that is vital in wild animals. It has long been known that LCM carrier mice are runted (Mims, 1970), and Oldstone *et al.* (1982) have provided an interesting explanation for this phenomenon. The cells in the anterior pituitary that produce growth hormone are infected and appear to have impaired 'luxury functions'; the blood contains half the normal amount of growth hormone, and if suckling carrier mice are transplanted with growth hormone-producing cells, the runting is prevented (Oldstone *et al.*, 1983).

Immune responses to LCM virus are genetically determined, and the immunopathological consequences of persistent infection differ in severity according to the strain of mouse. Wild house mice carrying the virus appear to be unaffected by immune complex disease (Lehmann-Grube, 1982), indicating a less vigorous pathogenic immune response than in laboratory mice. On the other hand, reproductive inefficiency, with fewer and smaller litters, which has been reported in LCM carrier colonies of laboratory mice (Mims, 1970) is also seen in carrier colonies of wild house mice. Evidently LCM virus exists in almost, but by no means perfect, harmony with wild mice.

Fig. 6.3. Tissue sections or smears from LCM virus carrier mice stained for LCM viral antigen by immunofluorescence. *Top* Cerebellum from an old mouse. Infection of most Purkinje cells and nearly all cells in granular layer. × 100. *Middle* Thymus from newborn mouse. Large numbers of antigen-containing cells in cortex and medulla. × 200. *Bottom* Smear from spleen of an adult mouse. LCM antigen in cytoplasm and nucleus of small lymphocytes. × 800.

The mechanism of persistent infection with LCM virus is still not understood, either at the immunological or the virological level. Certainly the absence of an effective immune response, of the sort that in primarily infected adult mice restrains the spread of infection yet can also kill the infected animal when expressed in vulnerable organs (see Chapter 4), enables the virus to persist. It seems unlikely that this is a result of antigen-specific suppression of these responses in carrier mice (Dunlop and Blanden, 1977; Lehmann-Grube et al., 1982a). One interesting possibility is that it is due to clonal deletion of reactive cells. This would be ensured if T cells specifically reactive with LCM viral antigens were preferentially infected, their immunological receptors for viral antigen acting as receptors for infectious virus. Small numbers of T cells are known to be infected in carrier mice (Popescu et al., 1979). Mere dysfunction of these cells would then lead to their effective clonal deletion (Lehmann-Grube et al., 1982b). It is known that hybridoma cells make less antibody when they are persistently infected with LCM virus (Oldstone and Fujinami, 1982).

At the virological level, many cells in the carrier do not contain detectable viral antigen, but nevertheless resist infection with LCM virus (Mims and Subrahmanyan, 1966). The infectivity titres of organs are low in relation to the number of infected (antigen-containing) cells visible by immunofluorescence (Mims, 1970), and defective interfering particles are possibly involved in persistence in vivo (Buchmeier et al., 1980). Various possibilities have been raised by in vitro studies (Weber et al., 1983). In persistently infected L cell cultures infectious virus eventually ceased to be produced, although many cells contained viral antigen. When antibody was added, antigen-containing cells decreased in number (Lehmann-Grube et al., 1969). If antibody formed in carrier mice reacted with viral antigens on carrier cells, capping and shedding of complexes could not only remove viral antigen from cells but conceivably depress production of infectious virus, as described for measles (Oldstone and Fujinami, 1982). Immune peroxidase studies show that, in neurones of persistently infected mice, viral antigens are exclusively associated with ribosomes, and are not detectable on the cell surface (Rodriguez et al., 1983a). Interferon is a possible factor, because carrier mice have type I (alpha, beta) interferon in the blood (Saron et al., 1982), and LCM virus is very sensitive to interferon. This would help account for the variable and perhaps fluctuating level of infection in individual cells in the carrier mice. Persistent infection of mice with LCM virus has been surveyed by Buchmeier et al. (1980) and by Lehmann-Grube et al. (1982b).

Fundamental studies by Lehmann-Grube and his colleagues are fast bringing LCM virus into a state where the classic immuno-virological phenomena can be investigated at the molecular level (Bruns and Lehmann-Grube, 1983; Bruns et al., 1983).

Lactic dehydrogenase virus

Lactic dehydrogenase virus (LDH) in mice provides one of the most fascinating examples of persistence (Riley, 1974). After infection of adult mice, the virus replicates and reaches levels of up to 10^{11} ID_{50}/ml of plasma within 24 hours. This astounding acute infection causes no ill effects, and after a few weeks the viraemia subsides to about 10^5 ID_{50}/ml of plasma and there is a life long carrier state. No pathological effects are detectable. After a month or two antibodies are produced. They become attached to circulating virus particles as indicated by a fall in virus titre after treatment of infected plasma with anti-mouse immunoglobulin (Notkins et al., 1966), but fail to neutralise the virus. Immune complexes are deposited in glomeruli (Chapter 4) but do not cause significant glomerulonephritis.

It appears that macrophages are the only cells that are infected (Porter et al., 1969). Certain macrophage functions are affected, including their ability to remove from the plasma a variety of endogenous host enzymes such as asparaginase and lactic dehydrogenase. In the assay system for this virus, mice are injected with serial ten-fold dilutions of virus, their sera tested 3–4 days later for raised levels of lactic dehydrogenase, and a mouse infectivity titre thus determined. There is no satisfactory or easy assay in cultured cells. The in vivo assay system gives the virus its name, and although it is simple and accurate, it appals rather than appeals to the average virologist. This helps account for the unwillingness of many virologists to tackle the fascinating research problems posed by this virus. The demonstration that in certain strains of mice LDH virus can cause a paralytic disease with growth of the virus in anterior horn cells (Nawrocki et al., 1980) has stimulated fresh research.

As well as the effects on enzyme clearance, there are immunological perturbations in infected mice. When sheep erythrocytes are injected during the first few days of the infection increased numbers of antibody-producing spleen cells are formed. This may be due to increased trapping of the injected sheep erythrocytes in the spleen (Isakov et al., 1982). Later on, although some immune responses are elevated, responsiveness to sheep erythrocytes is lowered. This is associated with impaired antigen-presenting capacity of macrophages for sheep erythrocytes and for other antigens (Isakov et al., 1980). LDH virus has ill-defined actions on the thymus (Santisteran et al., 1972) and we have a poor understanding of the interactions of this virus with lymphoid cells. Perhaps the immunological effects are secondary to the infection of macrophages, and certainly the most promising recent studies of this virus have concentrated on macrophages. Stueckemann and his colleagues (Stueckemann et al., 1981) have shown that less than 20% of peritoneal macrophages are susceptible to infection in vitro, and that infected cells subsequently disappear from cultures. It is suggested that persistent infection in mice results from the steady generation of fresh macrophages of the susceptible subclass (Stueckemann et al., 1982). Future work will perhaps answer intriguing questions about the cellular basis for the exclusive vulnerability of macrophages.

Polyomaviruses

Classical studies (Rowe, 1961) showed that, after infection of infant mice with polyomavirus, the virus persists in salivary glands and kidneys and is shed in saliva and urine for very long periods, thus maintaining itself in colonies of mice. Infection of tubular epithelial cells in the kidney was demonstrated (Levinthal et al., 1962). Unfortunately almost all work on pathogenesis halted when virologists, hungry for cancer viruses, discovered that this virus transformed cells. Now we understand a great deal of the basic virology and the complete genome of the virus has been mapped, but persistence in the host is poorly understood. In carrier colonies, infant mice encounter the virus when partially protected by maternal immunity. Under these circumstances the infection is completely subclinical. When unprotected infant mice or when immunosuppressed adult mice are infected multiple tumours are formed consisting of virus-transformed tumour cells, but the virus does not cause tumours under natural circumstances in mice.

Renewed interest in persistent infection of mice with polyomavirus arose from the discovery of two human polyomaviruses, BK and JC (Gardner, 1977; Norkin, 1982). These infect most human beings in childhood, as determined by antibody surveys, causing unrecognised mild or inapparent disease. Virus is shed from urine and probably the throat. The infection would remain unnoticed except that reactivation may occur later in life and cause trouble. The immunosuppressive drugs given to renal transplant patients allow either of these viruses to reactivate and appear in urine, being shed from tubular epithelial cells. This is very common in renal transplant patients but is usually symptomless except in occasional individuals where infection of epithelial cells lining the ureter results in interference with the flow of urine. The viruses also reactivate and appear in the urine during normal pregnancy (Coleman et al., 1980), but with no harmful effects. The mechanism of reactivation in pregnancy is not known, and the immunological control of persistent infection is not understood.

Less commonly, reactivated virus is not only excreted in urine but also causes large scale infection of oligodendrocytes in the brain, which finally leads to a lethal demyelinating disease called progressive multifocal leukoencephalopathy (PML). Affected patients are generally immunosuppressed as a result of lymphoreticular malignancy or kidney transplantation. Virus-specific DNA sequences are present in lymph nodes, spleen, liver, lung, and in larger amounts in the brain (Grinnell *et al.*, 1983). By electron microscopy the nuclei of oligodendrocytes are full of papovavirus particles, with 10^{10} particles per gram of brain. Infectious virus can at times be demonstrated by growth in human foetal brain cell cultures. Oligodendrocytes are destroyed as a result of the infection and areas of demyelination are produced. The virus was called JC, the initials of the first patient from whom an isolation was made. BK virus in contrast, is recovered from urine but not the brain, and was also named after the first patient. JC virus in particular has been difficult to study because of its very long (several weeks) and unpredictable growth in a specialised type of cell. But viral DNA can be cloned, and there are reports of satisfactory growth in urinary epithelial cells (Beckmann and Shah, 1983). The discovery that both JC and BK DNA sequences are present in normal human kidney (Heritage *et al.*, 1981) gives a rationale for their reactivation, but the pathogenesis of progressive multifocal leukoencephalopathy is still obscure. We do not know for instance how often virus reaches the brain or whether subclinical neural infection can occur.

These viruses are closely related to SV40, another 'tumour virus'. SV40 does not cause tumours under natural circumstances but gives rise to a persistent asymptomatic infection in rhesus monkeys, with shedding of virus in urine. It can also cause progressive multifocal leukoencephalopathy in monkeys (Holmberg *et al.*, 1977). All these papovaviruses transform cells *in vitro* and can be induced to cause tumours in experimental animals. It is conceivable that they are involved in human cancer in the brain or urinary tract, but so far the evidence has been negative.

Studies on persistent polyomavirus infection in mice show that this virus, like the human viruses, is reactivated during pregnancy (McCance and Mims, 1979) and can cause a neurological disease with paralysis in immunodeficient animals (McCance *et al.*, 1983). In the latter disease neural cells are infected, but paralysis could also be due to pressure effects by the very small tumours of bone that are seen in vertebrae.

The scrapie group

Probably the most difficult and challenging 'slow virus' infections are scrapie, transmissible mink encephalopathy, kuru and Creutzfeldt–Jakob disease (Kimberlin, 1976; Hadlow and Prusiner, 1979). They are included in this book on viruses although they are caused by transmissible replicating agents of unknown nature. They challenge our concepts of replicating agents (Prusiner, 1982) because so far they have not been shown to contain either DNA or RNA. They have been compared to viroids (Diener, 1982) but are different from them.

Scrapie is a neurological disease of sheep that has been known in Europe for hundreds of years, affected animals scraping themselves on posts and other objects to relieve the pruritis associated with the disease. It has been known for about 50 years that the condition is transmissible from sheep to sheep, but our understanding of both the infectious agent and the disease remained in a primitive state until the discovery (Chandler, 1961) that scrapie was also transmissible to mice. The use of a relatively inexpensive animal with inbred strains available has been of tremendous importance. Furthermore, the incubation period in mice may be as little as four months, compared with years in sheep, and as a result the rate of research progress has accelerated markedly. Laboratory work is still very slow because the infectious agent grows only in the intact animal and merely to determine the amount present in a specimen takes about a year. It is a formidable research area, attracting scientists with patience and intellectual stamina.

The scrapie agent is known to be unusually resistant to physical and chemical agents. For instance, it is stable between pH 2 and 10. The infectivity titre is unaffected at 80°C for 60 minutes, and a small proportion remains after boiling. The infectious material is still present after the immersion of infected tissue for two years in formol saline, and there is a striking resistance to ionising and UV-irradiation. Radiation studies indicate a nucleic acid target of less than 10^5 daltons (Gibbs *et al.*, 1978) which is too little to code for a single protein. Filtration experiments indicate that the agent has a diameter of 20–30 nm, but virus-like particles have never been seen by electron microscopy. Replication in the fastest system known, the mouse brain, is slow, with an average doubling time of about one week. After extraneural infection there is a preliminary phase of growth in the spleen before the agent localises, perhaps via peripheral nerves (Kimberlin and Walker, 1980), and grows in the central nervous system (Fraser and Dickinson, 1978). Replication proceeds inexorably, the brain finally containing up to 10^9 LD_{50}/g, and the mouse sickens and dies. It is an impressive feature of the pathogenesis of scrapie that there is no evidence for the slightest flicker of an immune response. Careful tests have been made for antibodies and for sensitised immune cells but these have been negative. The histological picture, moreover, has none of the features of immunological activity. Interferon is not induced in infected animals, and scrapie in any case is insensitive to its action (Gresser *et al.*, 1983). The agent replicates in the brain apparently without interruption by host defence mechanisms. Transmissible mink encephalopathy is a similar disease seen in mink, and it probably originated on mink farms when animals were fed the heads of scrapie-infected sheep (Hartsough and Burger, 1965).

Kuru is a progressive fatal neurological disease of man, affecting people of the Fore tribe in the highlands of New Guinea. It can be transmitted from the brains of patients to chimpanzees and other primates after an incubation period of $1\frac{1}{2}$–3 years. Transmission of human disease apparently took place during the cannibalistic consumption of relatives dying of the disease. After 1957 cannibalism in this part of the world declined abruptly, and there have been no new cases of kuru reported in those born since then (Gajdusek, 1977). There have been a total of approximately 3700 cases, all of whom died, which were in a small area of New Guinea with a total population of 35 000.

Creutzfeldt–Jakob disease is a rare condition (although perhaps commoner than human rabies, for example) with about 200 cases recorded so far, but it has been reported in most continents of the world (Brown, 1980; Masters *et al.*, 1980). It too has been transmitted to chimpanzees, the incubation period being about 13 months. The natural route of human infection is unknown but there have been instances of transmission from man to man via imperfectly sterilised stereotactic electrodes used in brain surgery and also via a corneal graft. The most likely origin of kuru is that a sporadic case of Creutzfeldt–Jakob disease occurred in New Guinea and during cannibalistic consumption of the corpse by relatives the infection was spread among the Fore people and a rather different strain of the agent emerged.

All the indications are that the kuru and Creutzfeldt–Jakob agents have the same properties as scrapie, and a common ancestry is possible. They all produce characteristic vacuoles (spongiform change) in the infected brain. Creutzfeldt–Jakob disease has been transmitted to mice and experiments in mice constitute the moving edge of research into these infectious agents. *In vitro* methods of study and assay are not available, but careful quantitative studies of histopathological profiles in infected mouse brains have made it clear that there are as many as 15 strains of scrapie. Also the genotype of the host exercises a decisive influence on the disease process (Dickinson, 1975). An appropriate combination of mouse strain, scrapie strain and dose administered can give an interesting result in which scrapie replicates progressively in the brain but fails to cause disease before the mouse dies of old age. In other words, the incubation period exceeds the life span (Dickinson *et al.*, 1975).

Scrapie replicates in lymphoid tissues such as the spleen and in salivary glands as well in the brain (Eklund *et al.*, 1967; Hadlow *et al.*, 1982). The extraneural sites of growth are important because the infectious agent would be unlikely to spread effectively from animal to animal under natural circumstances if the sole site of growth was in the central nervous system. If it is assumed that infection with Creutzfeldt–Jakob agent is common in man but nearly always subclinical, the neurological disease being a very rare manifestation, then the same remarks can be made about the need for a natural route of transmission. It would thus seem to be very important to have a better understanding of the behaviour of these agents in extraneural tissues.

MECHANISMS OF PERSISTENT INFECTION

As mentioned earlier in this chapter, virus persistence means that the host antiviral forces have failed to eliminate the foreign invader. Since the host defences have evolved in order to combat infection, it might be expected that the most desirable end result of their operation would be complete elimination of the infectious agent. There are many infectious agents, viral and non-viral, that have developed strategies for by-passing, avoiding or actively interfering with host defences. The primary significance of this is that the virus stays in the host, and at a later stage can be shed to the exterior and infect other individuals. This enables such viruses to maintain themselves in small communities. Viruses, e.g. measles, poliomyelitis and influenza, do not persist in the host in a form that enables them to be re-shed to the exterior and in most cases the immune response both controls the infection and eliminates virus from the body. These viruses are not very stable in the environ-ment, and they therefore cannot persist in the community unless at all times some individuals are being infected. Studies of island communities (Black, 1966) have shown that the minimum sized population needed to maintain measles without introduction from the outside is about 500 000. Chickenpox, in contrast, causes a persistent infection. When susceptible children have been infected, the disease chickenpox disappears from the community but the virus re-emerges many years later as older individuals suffer attacks of zoster. Fresh crops of suscep-tible children can now be infected. In this way, chickenpox maintains itself indefinitely even in communities of less than 1000. The same argument applies to other persistent infections. Antibody surveys showed that the viruses maintained in completely isolated Indian communities in the Amazon basin were the persistent viruses and also arthropod-borne viruses with alternative vertebrate hosts, but not measles, polioviruses, influenza viruses and other non-persistent viruses (Black et al., 1974).

Quite separately, evasion of or interference with host defences may facilitate the process of primary infection of the host. This is especially so when the incubation period is measured in weeks or months, and the infection might otherwise be controlled before the steps in pathogenesis have been completed and virus has been shed to the exterior (Mims, 1982c). Infections in this category include rabies and hepatitis B in man, with incubation periods of more than a month, but the same remark might also apply to rubella with an incubation period of 2–3 weeks.

There have been few studies that suggest how, or indeed whether, host defences are evaded or interfered with during primary infection with these viruses, but on general principles it might well occur.

As far as is known, persistent viral infections confer no actual benefit on the host. However well balanced the virus–host association, it is still clearly parasitism rather than symbiosis. Damage to the host occurs in some (herpes simplex, varicella-zoster) although not in other (adenovirus, polyomavirus) persistent infections. It probably takes many thousands of years for a persistent virus to reach a completely balanced and non-pathogenic state in its host species, and many infections have not yet reached this stage. Many of the most lethal and interesting persistent infections, such as SSPE, PML (see p. 217) occur as very rare complications of infection. If one individual in a thousand develops serious disease or dies as a result of a persistent viral infection, this may be of great importance for physicians and of course for relatives, but in terms of its effect on the balance between virus and host species it is irrelevant. Although a very small disadvantage expressed in most infected individuals is often significant on an evolutionary time scale, a serious disease occurring only in a rare individual is less likely to matter. In the latter case, there would be no selective advantage to be gained by the host in developing novel defence mechanisms to deal with the persistent virus. In any case viruses evolve very rapidly com-pared with their hosts, and from an evolutionary point of view can be assumed to be one step ahead of the host.

The mechanisms by which viruses become persistent will now be surveyed in terms of the methods by which they evade or interfere with host defences. Many, but not all, host defences are immunological in nature, and these were surveyed in Chapter 3. A general summary of mechanisms of interference with immune defences is given in Table 6.2. Many of the suggested mechanisms are no more than possibilities. As we learn more about the interactions of viruses with immune cells, and as immunology itself advances and throws light on these things, the picture will be modified.

Persistent viruses often exist in a state of balance with host immune defences. When these are weakened, the persistent virus may reactivate, sometimes causing clinical disease. Reactivation during pregnancy (e.g. JC, BK viruses) and old age (varicella-zoster virus) have been referred to (see p. 212; p. 193). Patients immunosuppressed after transplant opera-tions (Ho, 1977) or immunodeficient as a result of lymphomas or leukaemias, are also subject to reactivation. Reactivation of persistent viruses in man is summarised in Table 6.3. Herpesviruses and papova-viruses are especially prominent. Adenoviruses are not generally de-tected, although in the acquired immunodeficiency syndrome (AIDS; see Chapter 5) adenovirus is commonly isolated from urine (de Jong *et*

Table 6.2. Persistent viral infections—immune responses ineffective or viral interference with immune responses.

Phenomenon[a]		Mechanisms	Examples	In vivo status
Antibody production	Ineffective antibody	Antibody in small amounts, of poor specificity, or low affinity, fails to neutralise	Thymic necrosis virus (mice), LCM virus, Aleutian disease virus	+
	Late antibody	Antibody produced too late to prevent initiation of persistence	CMV (man), Visna (sheep)	?
	Blocking antibody	Non-neutralising antibody bound to virus blocks action of neutralising antibody or immune lymphocytes	LCM virus	+
	Enhancing antibody	Antibody bound to virus enhances infection of phagocyte	CMV, LDH virus	+
	No antibody	No detectable antibody	Scrapie	++
General interference with effective immune response		Infection of lymphocytes; 'swamping' of lymphoid tissues with viral antigens	Many examples (see Table 6.4)	?
Viral interference with antigen processing or presentation		Infection of macrophages	LDH virus	+
Viral induction of antigen-specific immune suppression		Viral invasion of lymphoid tissue leads to suppressor T cell induction or clonal deletion of T cells	LCM virus Herpes simplex virus	+ ?
'Silent' infection of host cell without making it vulnerable to immune lysis		Failure to display viral antigen on infected cell surface[b]	Herpes simplex in ganglion cell, EB virus in B lymphocyte	+
		Loss of viral antigen by capping	Measles	+

Table 6.2. *continued*.

Phenomenon[a]	Mechanisms	Examples	*In vivo* status
	Budding of virus into intracellular vacuoles	Flaviviruses, Coronaviruses	?
Fc receptor induced on infected host cell	IgG nonspecifically binds to infected cell and blocks immune lysis	Herpes simplex Cytomegalovirus	?
Specific antibodies or immune cells 'inactivated' by soluble viral antigens	Viral surface antigens in extracellular fluids combine with and 'divert' antibodies or immune cells	Hepatitis B	?
Infection in bodily site inaccessible to antibody or immune cells	Persistent infection of glands, etc. inaccessible to circulating antibody or immune cells	Cytomegalovirus Rabies virus Marek's disease virus	+ +
Antigenic variation	Viral antigens change within individual host	Visna, Equine infectious anaemia virus	+
	Viral antigens evolve within host population	Influenza virus	+ +

[a]These phenomena are not restricted to persistent viral infections, e.g. enhancing antibody in dengue virus infections.
[b]Or viral antigens produced in very low density on cell surface.

al., 1983). Surprisingly, all the 13 adenoviruses isolated in this study from ten patients appeared to be type 35.

When latent viruses reactivate, there must first be a change in control at the cellular level as a result of which infectious virus is produced, and second the reactivated virus must undergo further replication and spread in the host. This distinction was mentioned in the discussion of herpes simplex virus reactivation. It is easy to see that replication and spread in the host would be favoured when antiviral immune responses are depressed, but there are likely to be additional factors accounting for the initial reactivation in the cell. These factors include hormones and body temperature, as discussed above for CMV and herpes simplex viruses. Cell differentiation or other metabolic changes in the cell may be important. If resting lymphocytes are infected with measles or vesicular

Table 6.3. Reactivation of persistent viral infections of man.

Circumstance	Virus	Features	Clinical severity
Old age	Varicella-zoster	Rash	+
Pregnancy	JC, BK	Viruria	−
	CMV	Virus replication cervix	−
	Herpes simplex type 2	Virus replication cervix	−
Immunosuppression e.g. for transplant[a]	Herpes simplex	Lesion. Can be severe	+
	Varicella-zoster	Rash. Less common than in Hodgkin's disease	+
	CMV	Fever, occasional hepatitis, pneumonitis can be lethal	+ or −
	EBV	Increased shedding of virus in throat	−
	BK, JC	Very common, viruria	−[b]
	Wart	Appearance of skin warts	−
	Hepatitis B	Viraemia	−
Lymphoreticular tumours, e.g. Hodgkin's disease	Varicella-zoster	Rash. Common	+
	JC	Progressive multifocal leukoencephalopathy	+ +

[a]Also following the use of cytotoxic drugs for malignancies.
[b]Rarely ureteric obstruction.

stomatitis virus, the infection remains non-productive, but infectious virus is produced when cell differentiation and division is induced by mitogens (Lucas *et al.*, 1978). Also, Dutko and Oldstone (1981) showed that mouse CMV in undifferentiated teratocarcinoma cells was converted from a non-productive to productive form when cell differentiation was induced. Viral DNA entered the undifferentiated cells but there was a block in transcription, and viral RNA, viral antigens and infectious virus were not produced until the cells differentiated. Goats infected with the caprine arthritis-encephalitis virus have non-productively infected blood monocytes that act as infectious centres. Infectious virus is produced when monocytes differentiate into macrophages (Narayan *et al.*, 1983a). As a final example, differentiation of mouse B cells to produce immunoglobulin leads also to synthesis of leukaemia virus protein (Alberto *et al.*, 1982).

The possible persistence of viral antigens in the absence of the viral genome is referred to in Chapter 3. It may explain, at least in part, the maintenance of very long lasting antibody responses after systemic viral infections, but is a separate phenomenon from persistent infection.

Tolerance

Tolerance is an immunologically specific reduction in the immune response to a given antigen. If there is a feeble host immune response to the relevant viral antigens, the process of infection may be facilitated and the possibility of persistence increased. This does not involve a general failure of immune responses, but a weakness in relation to a particular antigen. This can be stated by referring to this antigen as a 'poor antigen'. If infection and persistence is to be favoured then the immunological weakness must be in relation to the viral antigens that are important for infectivity, invasiveness or persistence. Also, because in a given infection either antibody or CMI may be the most important antiviral force (see Chapter 3) there must be a weakness in that arm of the immune response to which the virus is most susceptible. Tolerance can involve either antibody or CMI to some extent independently. If CMI tolerance makes the host more susceptible to infections in which the CMI response is critical, then a strong antibody response may be irrelevant. At times, however, it is harmful, causing immunopathology. At other times, specific antibody is ineffective and, by coating virions or infected cells, protects them from the action of immune forces.

Tolerance is often exerted at the level of the T cell, whether by failure of T inducer cells (T_h) to respond, or alternatively following the generation of suppressor T (T_s) cells as reviewed by Germain and Benacerraf (1981). B cells are known to be susceptible to 'tolerisation' during their differentiation (e.g. Rajewsky and Brenig, 1974; Diener and Feldman, 1972). There is recent evidence that T cells can be 'tolerised' independently of suppressor T cells. Lamb *et al.* (1983) showed that, when cloned human T cells with reactivity for a defined synthetic peptide were incubated with moderately high concentrations of the specific peptide, they became unresponsive (tolerant), in spite of the fact that they continued to multiply. The mechanisms are not known, but this is the sort of thing that could happen when viruses invade and multiply in lymphoid tissues, locally releasing viral antigens, as discussed below under Immunosuppression.

Tolerance is rarely absolute, with no trace of an immune response to an antigen, but even slight specific weaknesses may favour the viral infection. The weakness may be that only a low level of antibodies are produced to relevant viral components, or these antibodies may be of poor affinity (LDH and Aleutian disease virus, see p. 219). Also, the rapidity with which they are produced can be of major importance. Each infection can be regarded as a race between growth and spread of the virus and the generation of an effective immune response. An important immune response appearing a day or two late may make all the difference, permitting viral invasion of a key tissue and the initiation of a persistent infection. Although the speed with which immune responses are generated is of great importance, few studies have considered this aspect of infection. It is referred to here to draw attention to the fact that the rate of generation as well as the final level of the response can be critical.

Specific immune responses are undoubtedly controlled by genetic factors, and in several instances the genetic locus responsible for the immune response to a given antigen has been identified. Many of the genes controlling these specific immune responses are linked to those controlling the major histocompatibility antigens. This is so in the mouse, guinea pig, rat and man. For instance there are genes in mice that control the immune response to the relevant antigens of mouse leukaemia virus. Strains of mice with RfV-1 ('recovery from Friend virus') gene are resistant to Friend virus leukaemia. The gene, which is located in the D region of the H2 complex (see Chapter 3), appears to confer resistance by causing a rapid onset of the specific cytotoxic T cell response to cells carrying viral antigen (Britt and Cheseboro, 1983). Another gene, RgV-1 ('recovery from Gross virus') also gives resistance to viral leukaemia which is probably mediated by T_c responses, and this gene is located in the K region of the H2 locus. In mice persistently infected with LCM virus the severity of the glomerulonephritis depends on the strain of mouse, and wild mice show minimal harmful effects (Lehmann-Grube, 1982). Other examples are referred to in Chapter 5.

There is commonly a degree of tolerance to a virus when infection occurs during foetal or early postnatal life. At one time it was thought that any antigen present in the foetus during development of the immune system was regarded as 'self', and as a result of this there was no immune response to it, either then or throughout postnatal life. But immune responses do occur under these circumstances, although often they are weak or inappropriate, perhaps reacting with only a few antigenic determinants, and they fail to control the infection. For instance, rubella virus infects the foetus, causing congenital malformation (see Chapter 2). The foetus receives rubella IgG antibodies from the mother and makes its own IgM antibodies, but the CMI response is particularly poor and this enables the virus to persist during foetal life and for long periods after birth. In mouse colonies carrying LCM virus, the virus is present in the foetus from the earliest stages of development. The congenitally infected mouse makes a feeble antibody response to the virus (Oldstone and Dixon, 1967), there is no CMI response, and virus persists in most parts of the body for the entire life of the animal. Hepatitis B in man occasionally infects the foetus and establishes persistent infection. More importantly, it often induces persistence after infecting infants and children, presumably because immune responses are less vigorous at this age.

If a viral antigen is very similar to a normal host antigen, the immune response to this antigen might for this reason be weak, giving a degree of tolerance. Strong immune responses to normal host antigens are potentially harmful. The mimicking of host antigens by viral antigens ('molecular mimicry') is not known to occur in viral infections although it is theoretically possible.

Immunosuppression

Primary unresponsiveness to viral antigens depends on genetic defects in the host. The persistent virus can take advantage of these immunological 'blind spots'. There is also the possibility that tolerance results from specific suppression of immune responses, which have been induced by the infection. This leads to the question of immunosuppression.

A large variety of viruses cause general immunosuppression in the infected host. This means that the host shows depressed immune responses to antigens unrelated to those of the infecting virus. For instance, during the acute stage of measles infection a patient with a positive tuberculin skin test becomes temporarily tuberculin-negative, and there is a reduction in cutaneous sensitivity to poison ivy and other antigens lasting for several weeks. Depressed CMI or antibody responses to unrelated antigens have been described in a great variety of viral infections (Notkins *et al.*, 1970). These include mumps, EB virus and cytomegalovirus infections in man, LCM, murine leukaemia virus and cytomegalovirus in mice, and rinderpest virus in cattle. General immunosuppression of this type does not necessarily favour persistence but generally reflects invasion of lymphoid tissues (Denman *et al.*, 1983), with infection in either lymphocytes or macrophages (see Table 6.4). The acquired immunodeficiency disease syndrome (AIDS) in humans is a particularly severe example of general immunosuppression and seems likely to be virus-induced with an incubation period which may be as long as 1–2 years. AIDS in macaques shows similar features (Letvin *et al.*, 1983). In humans skin test anergy and T cell abnormalities are seen, and the disease is commonly fatal either as a result of opportunist infections or following the development of unusual tumours (Gottlieb *et al.*, 1983; Editorial, 1983). Different subclasses of macrophages may show different susceptibility to infection (see LDH virus p. 219, and Chapter 5) and the same is probably true for lymphocytes (e.g. Isaak and Caerny, 1983), so that a variety of immunomodulatory effects are theoretically possible. The physiological state of the cell is also important. Viruses such as measles and VSV infect resting lymphocytes *in vitro* but replication does not proceed until phytohaemagglutinin is added to induce DNA synthesis and mitosis (Lucas *et al.*, 1978). Lymphoid cells also show changes in virus receptors and thus in susceptibility during the course of these physiological changes (Morishima *et al.*, 1982). Replication of parvoviruses depends on cell functions

Table 6.4. Infection of lymphoreticular tissues by viruses exhibiting systemic infection or persistence[a].

Virus	Host
Adenoviruses (L)	Man
EB virus (L)	Man
Cytomegalovirus (LM)	Man, mouse, pig
Leukaemia virus (LM)	Mouse, man, etc.
Visna virus (LM)	Sheep
LCM virus (LM)	Mouse
Varicella-zoster virus (L)	Man
Thymic necrosis virus (L)	Mouse
Measles virus (L)	Man
Rubella virus (LM)	Man
Lactic dehydrogenase virus (M)	Mouse
Aleutian disease virus (M)	Mink
Equine infectious anaemia virus (M)	Horse
African swine fever virus (M)	Pig
Infectious bursal disease virus (L)	Chicken
Mumps virus (L)	Man
Dengue virus (M)	Man
Marek's disease virus (L)	Chicken
Reovirus 3 (L)	Mouse
Mouse hepatitis virus (LM)	Mouse
Scapie (?)	Mouse

L = lymphocytes known to be infected; M = macrophages known to be infected.
[a]Infection of lymphoreticular tissues is not only seen with these viruses; influenza, for instance infects human lymphocytes, at least *in vitro* (Brownson *et al.*, 1979), but in man it is not a systemic infection.

expressed during the S phase of the cell cycle, and tropism for actively dividing cells accounts for developmental abnormalities induced by these viruses in the foetus (see Table 2.4). Similar dependence on the phase of the cell cycle may underlie the immunosuppressive effect of MVM(1), a strain of minute virus of mice which infects T cells (Tattersall and Bratton, 1983).

Mechanisms of general immunosuppression have been studied with CMV, for instance, and macrophages have been suggested as mediators of suppression both in human (Carney and Hirsch, 1981) and in mouse (Bixler and Booss, 1981; Loh and Hudson, 1982) CMV infections. An alternative mechanism has been suggested for the immunosuppression seen in acute LCM virus infection in mice, where immune dysfunction may be part of a general depression of stem cells in the bone marrow (Thomsen *et al.*, 1982). The immunosuppression seen in mice persistently infected with LDH virus involves macrophages, at least partly (Isakov *et al.*, 1982; Isakov *et al.*, 1980), although effects on other types of cell have not been excluded. *In vitro* analysis of virus-induced immunosuppression, as tested by inhibition of Con A or PHA driven mitogenesis in mouse spleen cells, has been reported (Israel *et al.*, 1980).

Invasion of lymphoid tissues may be a general rule for persistent viruses, and would enable the infecting virus to manipulate host immune responses to its own advantage, as suggested below. On the other hand, certain non-persistent viruses can infect macrophages or lymphocytes, so that the phenomenon does not always have this significance. For instance, influenza and vesicular stomatitis viruses, which are not known to persist, can infect host lymphocytes. It is not always easy to exclude persistence, which has been described in unexpected infections such as foot-and-mouth disease in cattle (Burrows, 1966). Also in mouse enteroviruses, which appear to exist as latent infections in certain mouse colonies and become activated by infections and other stimuli (Melnick and Riordan, 1947), or cause chronic disease of the central nervous system (Lipton, 1975). During the chronic stage of the disease, at a time when virus particles cannot be detected, viral RNA is demonstrable in glial cells by *in situ* hybridisation (Brahic *et al.*, 1981b). Immunopathology appears to be important in the genesis of this disease, and viral antigens remain demonstrable in oligodendrocytes for up to one year after initial infection (Rodriguez *et al.*, 1983).

Virus persistence would be effectively promoted if the infecting virus suppressed responses to its own antigens. This is antigen-specific immunosuppression or 'autoimmunosuppression' (Mims, 1974). There are several possible mechanisms for antigen-specific immunosuppression. During a normal response there is careful control over the distribution and concentration of antigen in lymphoid tissues. Antigens are delivered to lymphocytes only in minute quantities and in an appropriate setting after processing and handling by macrophages. If large amounts of antigen are liberated locally in these tissues by an invading virus, a disordered response might be expected, for example by tolerisation of T cells or B cells as described (p. 237). Alternatively, the invading viruses might generate antigen-specific suppressor cells or other suppressor factors. Another mechanism would be for the invading virus to preferentially infect the T or B cells that responded specifically to its own surface antigens—the antigen-binding receptors on the lymphocyte acting as specific receptors for the virus. If the infected T or B cells were functionally impaired or destroyed, there would be elimination of clones of cells that might otherwise have generated specific antiviral responses. There is increasing evidence for this mechanism in the generation of tolerance to LCM virus in persistently infected mice (Lehmann-Grube *et al.*, 1982).

So far the evidence for antigen-specific immunosuppression by viruses is not exactly overwhelming. But it seems such a logical, powerful and specific strategy that viruses, with their almost unique capacity to invade lymphoid tissues without destroying them, might be expected to have developed it. Antigen-specific suppressor T cells are induced during infection of mice with reovirus (Greene and Weiner, 1980), influenza virus (Liew and Russell, 1980), herpes simplex virus (Nash *et al.*, 1981), mouse CMV (Chong and Mims, 1983) and Japanese encephalitis virus (Mathur *et al.*, 1983). So far, for reasons that are not clear, the suppression, which is virus strain-specific, almost always involves only delayed hypersensitivity responses (see Chapter 3), while antibody and other immune responses are unaffected. With reovirus the effect is seen only after the intravenous injection of large doses of inactivated virus. Antigen-specific suppression of delayed hyper-sensitivity responses is also seen after intravenous injection of large amounts of non-viral antigens such as sheep erythrocytes. However, smaller doses (10^4 pfu) of live virus by more physiological routes (intradermally) are effective in the case of herpes simplex. The phenom-enon itself is of theoretical interest, and it could also have a major significance for a persistent viral infection if suppression was generated by natural sized doses of virus, administered by a physiological route. In the case of influenza virus, harmful DTH responses can be reduced by antigen-specific suppression, with benefit to the infected host (Liew and Russell, 1983). On the other hand, one can go too far in the search for significance. Doubtless some of the immunosuppressive phenomena seen in viral infections are due to the operation of normal immuno-regulatory mechanisms.

Ineffective antibody responses

There are many persistent viral infections in which antibody responses are ineffective (Table 6.2). The antibody response is sometimes ineffec-tive because neutralising antibodies are produced only in low titres. For instance, mice infected as infants with mouse thymic virus undergo a life long infection and never form detectable antibodies (Cross *et al.*, 1979) and, in mice persistently infected with cytomegalovirus, neutral-ising antibodies are present only in very low titres. This would theoretically favour persistence. Other viral infections in which little if any neutralising antibody is produced include Ebola and Marburg infections in man, and Lassa fever, Pichinde and Junin viruses in their rodent hosts. It is not known whether this is due to a primary defect in neutralising antibody production or whether there is also the production of large amounts of non-neutralising interfering viral antibody. Perhaps more importantly the protective antibody response, as mentioned above, evolves sluggishly in persistent viral infections such as visna in sheep and CMV in mice or in man. Sheep infected with visna virus do not develop detectable neutralising antibodies for $1\frac{1}{2}$–3 months, slowly reaching a peak by two years. In human infection with CMV neutralising antibodies are not detectable in the serum until seven weeks after the onset of illness (Stalder and Ehrensberger, 1980). If a key antibody is produced a day or two late it may give a decisive advantage to the infecting virus enabling it to spread through the body, replicate and persist in a way that would not otherwise have been possible.

In some cases the mechanisms are fairly well understood. For instance, the non-neutralising antibodies induced by LDH or Aleutian disease virus infections (see above) are well recognised. The antibodies may be of low affinity or more probably, as shown by monoclonal antibody studies (Massey and Schochetman, 1981), they bind to non-critical sites on the surface of the virus particle. When such antibodies are attached to virus particles they are known to block the binding of otherwise effective neutralising antibodies. In Aleutian disease of mink, host genetic factors influence the production of these ineffective (yet in this case pathogenic) antibodies (see pp. 219–20).

Non-neutralising antibodies that combine with virions and block the attachment of neutralising antibodies are not an exclusive feature of persistent viral infections. They have been shown to be present, for instance, in regular rabbit antiserum to Sindbis virus (Symington et al., 1977). We know that any antiserum contains a mixture of large numbers of individual antibodies produced by many distinct clones of B cells, and monoclonal antibody studies are now unravelling the complexity of these antibody responses. Curious effects may be seen in neutralisation tests as a given antiviral antiserum is diluted. Neutralisation by high affinity antibody seen at high serum concentrations can disappear on dilution as blocking antibodies become more important, only to reappear at higher dilutions where the blocking antibodies are no longer present but high-titre low-affinity neutralising antibodies are (Symington et al., 1977).

Another way in which antibody responses are rendered ineffective is when viruses fail to produce antigen on the surface of an infected cell. In persistent viral infections caused by EB virus in lymphocytes, herpes simplex virus in dorsal root ganglion cells, and polyomavirus in epithelial cells in the kidney, the virus remains in the cell in a latent form without expressing antigens on the cell surface, which is therefore insusceptible to immune attack. The same result could be achieved if the density of viral antigens expressed on the cell surface was too low for T cell lysis or for antibody-dependent lysis by complement or by K cells.

A few enveloped viruses produce antigen on the membranes of intracellular vacuoles and are released from the cell after budding into these vacuoles. Flaviviruses and coronaviruses mature in this fashion and also visna and LDH viruses in macrophages (Narayan *et al.*, 1982; Stueckemann *et al.*, 1981). There have been very few investigations of viral antigens on the outer cell membrane in these cases but, if they were absent or present only in low density, a degree of insusceptibility to immune defences might be predicted.

Antibodies can be the mechanism by which viral antigens are removed from the cell surface. After antibodies have reacted with viral components on the cell surface the complex moves to the edge of the cell and is shed or taken into the cell. This renders the cell insusceptible to immune lysis. The phenomenon occurs with various mouse leukaemia viruses and with mouse mammary tumour virus (Joachim and Sabbath, 1979; Calafat *et al.*, 1976). In the case of measles virus in SSPE (see pp. 217–19) it also perhaps restricts viral replication in the cell and thus further promotes persistence. Capping and stripping of antigen from infected cells by antibody presumably occurs also during primary infection with measles, but it is not known whether it significantly interferes with immune defences under these circumstances. The same phenomenon could theoretically be important in other persistent viral infections, such as those due to LCM virus (see pp. 223–6). Antibody-induced modulation of infection with reduction in viral maturation and release, has been demonstrated for VSV infection in neurone cultures (Dubois-Dalcq *et al.*, 1980).

Antibodies are made to look even more ridiculous when, instead of neutralising infectivity, they enhance it. Enhancing antibodies act only when cells bearing Fc receptors, such as macrophages, are susceptible to infection. Infectivity is neutralised when the virus particles are coated with larger amounts of antibody, but as the antibody density is reduced or when only non-neutralising antibodies are bound, the probability of infection is actually increased due to the fact that the virion–antibody complex binds (via the Fc end of the non-neutralising antibody) to the Fc receptor on the macrophage. In this way virus uptake into macrophages is promoted rather than prevented. Monoclonal antibody studies show that, although some antibodies both neutralise and enhance, others neutralise without enhancing or vice versa, suggesting that the outcome depends on the particular antigenic site on the virion to which the antibody binds. The enhancement phenomenon, described classically for dengue and other presumably non-persistent togaviruses (Halstead, 1979; Peiris and Porterfield, 1979), and for feline infectious peritonitis virus, a coronavirus (Weiss and Scott, 1981) is now known to occur in LDH (Cafruny and Plagemann, 1982) and reovirus (Burstin *et al.*, 1983) infections. It may be important, especially in LDH infection, because the unique susceptibility of macrophages is then enhanced as a result of the antibody response. A comparable phenomenon has been recorded when cells susceptible to infection bear complement receptors; the latter mediate binding and uptake of the virus–antibody–complement complex. Infection of macrophages by West Nile virus is enhanced in the presence of antiviral IgM antibody plus complement, and this is prevented by monoclonal antibody to the complement receptor but not by monoclonal antibody to the Fc receptor (Cardosa *et al.*, 1983).

Many persistent viruses spread directly from cell to cell without entering extracellular fluid so that virus spread is not restricted by neutralising antibodies. This is characteristic of herpes simplex, cytomegalovirus, mumps and foamy virus infections (Hooks *et al.*, 1976) and has been intensively analysed for measles (Merz *et al.*, 1980), where anti-F (fusion protein) antibody prevents cell-to-cell spread but neutralising antibody (anti-HN) does not. In a cell monolayer, neutralising antibodies will prevent extracellular virus infecting the first set of cells, but, if this has already occurred, addition of antibodies fails to inhibit the subsequent spread of the infection and the development of plaques. This is most likely to be important *in vivo* if the infected cells are relatively insusceptible to immune destruction, either because of a low density of viral antigen on the cell surface or, for instance, because of a local shortage of complement, as appears to be the case in the central nervous system (Albrecht, 1978).

An interference with antibody action that looks very much like a virus strategy is seen in certain herpesvirus infections. Cells infected with herpes simplex, varicella-zoster or cytomegalovirus develop Fc receptors on their surface (Westmoreland and Watkins, 1974; Furukawa *et al.*, 1975). The Fc receptors bind IgG non-specifically; they are virus-coded (Para *et al.*, 1983), appearing quite early in the infectious cycle (Adler *et al.*, 1978; Ogata and Shigeta, 1979). Their viral function is not established, but they are likely to be important because they bind aggregated IgG antibodies, which do not cap but act as blocking antibodies, preventing immune recognition of the infected cell. The infected cell thus enjoys considerable protection against antibody or cell-mediated immune lysis (Adler *et al.*, 1978). Fc receptors are also present on the surface of the virus particle itself (Bauke and Spear, 1979), and can bind normal IgG, thus conferring resistance against neutralising antibody (Dowler and Veltri, 1983). There are reports of C3 receptors appearing on the surface of cells early after infection with herpes simplex virus, but they have not been shown to be virus-coded (Cines *et al.*, 1982).

Finally, large quantities of viral antigen or non-infectious virus particles are sometimes liberated during infection and these tend to mop up antibodies which might otherwise usefully combine with virus particles or with infected cells. The immune complexes thus formed occur in certain persistent viral infections, for instance hepatitis B infection in man. It is not known whether the diversion of antibodies has significant effects on the course of the infection.

Reduced interferon induction or responsiveness

If a virus fails to induce significant amounts of interferon, or if it is relatively resistant to its action, host defences will be correspondingly weaker and persistence favoured. There is no firm evidence that this is a factor in persistent viral infections. Persistent viruses such as CMV have been reported to be relatively insensitive to interferon but there has been a failure to repeat these results, and other persistent viruses such

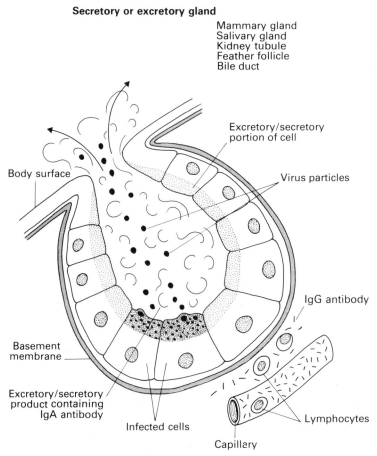

Fig. 6.4. Viral infection of cell surfaces facing the exterior.

as LCM are highly susceptible to interferon. A few persistent viruses have been found to induce little or no interferon and this could theoretically play a part in persistence. LDH virus, for instance, produces little or no interferon in cell cultures from mice, the persistently infected species, although it does so in chicken cells. Small amounts of gamma interferon are present in mice persistently infected with LCM virus (Saron *et al.*, 1982), but this is presumably produced by immunological rather than virological stimuli, and its function in persistence has not been elucidated. In mice infected with LDH virus interferon is present during the first few days, but is no longer detected during the chronic persistent stage of the infection (Evans and Riley, 1968). LDH virus is also relatively resistant to interferon (Stueckemann *et al.*, 1982). However, there is no evidence that this is important in virus persistence, and indeed for most persistent viral infections, the evidence for interferon insensitivity or defective interferon induction is either absent or conflicting. Scrapie (see pp. 229–32) is mentioned here to note that it neither induces interferon in infected mice, nor is sensitive to its action.

Quite separately interferon can restrict viral replication to a smouldering low-grade infection, as described for the 'carrier state' *in vitro* (see p. 205). Moreover, an otherwise cytopathogenic virus may then give rise to a persistent non-cytopathic infection. Interference with viral replication by defective interfering virus particles can have a similar effect. The importance of interferon acting in this way has been shown in L cell cultures persistently infected with vesicular stomatitis virus (Nishiyama, 1977). But there is no evidence that an interferon-mediated restriction of viral replication plays any part in persistent infection *in vivo*. In any case, the virus would then be persisting in spite of rather than because of the interferon response, and the more important question would be why the virus resists elimination by the immune system.

Virus persistence in bodily sites inaccessible to immune forces

Many viruses persist in the infected host and are shed to the exterior via the saliva (herpes simplex, cytomegalovirus, rabies in vampire bats), milk (cytomegalovirus in man, mammary tumour virus in mice) or urine (polyomavirus in mice). The surface of the infected cell can be said to face the external world as represented by the lumen of the salivary gland, mammary gland or kidney tubule (Fig. 6.4). As long as virus particles and viral antigens are presented only on the lumenal surface of the cell, and provided there is little or no cell destruction, sensitised lymphocytes or antibodies cannot reach the site and eliminate the infection. Secretory IgA antibodies could react with the viral antigens on the infected cell surface, but the complement sequence would be unlikely to be activated and the cell would not be destroyed (see Chapter

3). IgA antibodies could also react with the extracellular virus particles but would, at the most, render them non-infectious, again without acting on the source of the infection. The same considerations apply to epidermal infection with human wart virus, or to infection of the epidermis lining the chicken's feather follicle with Marek's disease virus. In the case of the wart, neither virus nor viral antigen is manufactured in significant quantities until the infected epidermal cell is keratinised and about to be released from the body, and is physically far removed from host immune forces. A similar type of inaccessibility is encouraged by the topography of budding of some viruses from epithelial cells. Viral multiplication often shows a striking polarity in epithelial cells, viral antigens and budding being confined to the lumenal surface of the cell (Boulan and Sabatini, 1978). On the other hand, this also applies to many non-persistent viruses, such as influenza, where it would not have this significance, and a number of retroviruses mature from the basolateral, rather than the lumenal aspect of epithelial cells (Roth et al., 1983).

Certain organs and tissues are less susceptible to immune attack ('immunologically privileged') because of restricted access of immune forces. The immunological privilege enjoyed by the brain, testes or placenta refers to the relative resistance to immune rejection of tissues in these sites. Is this a factor in persistent viral infections? Under normal circumstances the brain has a very low content of lymphocytes. Lymphocyte counts in the cerebrospinal fluid are low and nothing is known of lymphocyte recirculation in the brain, which is reputed to have no lymphatics. As far as antibodies go, IgG and IgA are present in cerebrospinal fluid at about 0.2–0.4% of plasma levels and IgM, being a larger molecule, is present in even smaller amounts. Many of the complement components also are absent from cerebrospinal fluid. As soon as inflammatory responses are initiated, of course, both cells and immunoglobulins have freer access to these tissues. Similar considerations apply to the testes and to joints. But the brain in particular is a common site of persistent viral infection, and when inflammatory responses are minimal or absent it is possible that the restricted access of immune forces plays some part (Mims, 1978).

Antigenic variation

Another way in which viruses avoid the consequences of immune responses is by periodically undergoing mutation and changing their surface antigens. Viral mutations commonly occur during longterm in vitro cultures (Holland et al., 1979), and indeed are the basis for attenuation of virulent viruses (see Chapter 7). These mutations would not especially affect the surface polypeptides that are important in immunological control of the infection, but the latter can be selected for if infected cells are cultivated in the presence of neutralising antibody (Webster *et al.*, 1982). RNA viruses evolve more rapidly than DNA viruses (Holland *et al.*, 1982) and this could influence the occurrence of antigenic variation *in vivo*, as well as *in vitro*.

Antigenic variation within the infected individual. Visna virus causes a persistent infection of sheep (see pp. 216–7) in which viral replication is restricted. In the infected host the association of viral DNA with host cell DNA provides one mechanism for persistence. The virus can remain in the cell without the display of the viral antigens that would call forth an antiviral host immune response. But it has also been shown that antigenic variants of the viral envelope glycoprotein appear in persistently infected animals, and these are neutralised poorly by antiserum to the original virus (Narayan *et al.*, 1978; Clements *et al.*, 1980). This gives an additional mechanism for persistence, but there is little evidence that it is important (see pp. 216–7).

Equine infectious anaemia is a retrovirus that causes persistent infection of horses (Crawford *et al.*, 1978). The disease is not progressive but occurs in cycles, between which the horse appears relatively normal. During an attack there is a burst of viral replication, probably confined to macrophages, to give blood titres of 10^4 ID$_{50}$ per ml as detected by viral antigen production in cultured horse leukocytes. Associated with this there is a vigorous immune response against antigens on the surface and in the core of the virion. Circulating antibodies react with viral components bound to erythrocytes, and this results in destruction of erythrocytes. The horse develops fever, sickness and depression for about a week, after which viral replication subsides. The number of cycles and their severity depends on host immune responses. Between attacks, immune complexes are present in the blood and are deposited in the kidney, generally without causing serious glomerulonephritis (see Chapter 4). Kono *et al.* (1973) showed that each cycle of clinical disease was initiated by a new antigenic variant of the virus, which was able to multiply for a few days until antibody and CMI responses to the new variant appeared and immunological control of the infection was re-established. Antigenic variation involves envelope glycoproteins of the virus, and more is known about the cycling of the disease than about its underlying persistence. In spite of the fact that the filtrable nature of the infectious agent has been known since 1904 (Henson and McGuire, 1974), much remains to be discovered about the virology and immunology of the infection. The virus assay system is difficult and horses are expensive, so work with this fascinating persistent infection proceeds slowly.

Antigenic variation within the species. Visna and equine infectious anaemia are persistent infections of relatively long-lived animals. The time-scale would allow antigenic variation within a given host to play a part in the maintenance of persistence. Other viruses show antigenic variation, which emerges by mutation during acute infection of a particular individual but becomes evident only following its spread to others. As discussed in Chapter 3, such antigenic drift occurs continuously with influenza and explains the emergence of novel epidemic strains every year of so, after mutations have accumulated in all the key antigenic sites (Webster *et al.*, 1982). With infections limited to body surfaces, acquired immunity to reinfection is often of limited efficacy and duration and there is strong selective advantage to virus strains with altered antigenic characters. Such variants may escape neutralisation by the low level of antibody remaining after a previous infection occurring years earlier with a different strain. Furthermore, the time between infection and shedding is only a few days, and an antigenically altered virus variant can infect, replicate and be shed from the body before a significant local secondary immune response is generated. In contrast to this, reinfection with re-shedding of viruses such as rubella, measles, mumps or smallpox (all of which cause systemic infection) is less likely. The incubation period is 2–3 times as long as in an infection confined to the body surfaces and the secondary immune response has time to come into action and prevent the spread of infection and shedding of virus from the body. This type of antigenic variation therefore is a feature of viral infections limited to the respiratory or alimentary tracts. It is more likely to be important in a long-lived animal such as the horse or man, where there is a need for multiple reinfection during an individual's lifetime if the virus is to remain in circulation, assuming the virus does not have the ability to become latent. In shorter-lived animals such as mice or rabbits on the other hand, populations renew themselves rapidly and fresh sets of uninfected individuals appear fast enough to maintain the infectious cycle.

While influenza is the best known example of antigenic drift it is by no means the only one. Human rhinoviruses and foot-and-mouth disease virus are also evolving rapidly and show a similar antigenic drift. Antigenic variation would also be expected for rotaviruses and the various picornaviruses that are normally restricted to the intestinal tract. It is possible that the papillomaviruses infecting the skin and mucosa (of which there are 24 distinct types in man and five in cows) have diversified antigenically in response to immune pressure in the host species (Lancaster and Olson, 1982).

Variants of a different sort arise when a virus infects geographically separated populations of the host species. In each isolated population there is the opportunity for antigenic or other variants of the virus to appear. These have not been selected out primarily by the pressure of immune responses, and therefore the changes need not involve surface antigens and the viruses are not merely those that cause infections confined to the body surfaces. For instance, geographical differences in the different herpesviruses will doubtless be revealed by 'fingerprinting' of viral DNA.

SUMMARY

A great deal has been learnt about persistent infections of cultured cells, including the nature of the virus–cell interaction in steady-state infections and transformation to the malignant state, but these studies have failed to answer many problems about persistent infection *in vivo*.

Thirteen persistent viral infections of man and animals are described in detail, including the human herpesviruses (herpes simplex, varicella-zoster, CMV and EB viruses) and three persistent infections in mice (LCM, LDH and polyoma viruses).

Persistent viruses are important because they can be reactivated, because they are associated with immune complex disease, neoplasms or other chronic diseases, and because they enable the virus to persist in the community. Persistent viral infections also pose problems for vaccination (see Chapter 7).

Virus persistence can be regarded as a failure of host defences in the face of viral adaptations to bypass or evade these defences. Mechanisms of persistent infection are discussed. Firstly, persistence can result from ineffective immune responses or immune responses that are interfered with by the infecting virus. For example, the host may be at least partially tolerant to the virus as a result of exposure during pre- or perinatal life, antigenic mimicry, Ir gene defects, helper T cell paralysis, or induction of suppressor T cells. Immunosuppression of a generalised nature can result from abortive or productive replication of virus in macrophages or lymphocytes; antigen-specific suppression may also occur. Antibodies may be ineffective for any of a number of reasons. They may not address the relevant viral protein or the critical antigenic site(s) on the relevant viral protein; in the latter instance these non-neutralising antibodies may actually block access of neutralising antibodies to virions or to infected cells, or may even enhance infection of macrophages by binding to Fc receptors. Immune cytolysis may fail to occur because viral antigens are not expressed on an accessible surface or because antibody caps and strips antigen from the plasma membrane. Conceivably, herpesvirus-infected cells may be protected in part by their Fc-binding capacity.

Reduced interferon induction or responsiveness has not been shown to be central to persistence. Viruses often persist in 'immunologically privileged' sites that are less accessible to immune forces, especially in epithelial cells of glands and other body surfaces facing the external world, or in the central nervous system. From the former site viruses can be shed to the exterior during persistent productive infection or following reactivation. The polarity of glycoprotein synthesis and viral budding from infected cells may be relevant.

The second major group of possible explanations of persistence relate not so much to the host response as to the virus itself. Some agents such as the scrapie group or viroids seem to be non-immunogenic. In the case of the oncogenic retroviruses and herpesviruses, the viral genome (or its cDNA equivalent) is integrated into the cell's genome and, unless virus-coded proteins are expressed on the cell surface, the virus is safe from immune elimination. A further factor in persistence is antigenic variation by the virus, either in the persistently infected individual (e.g. visna virus) or in the community (influenza and other viruses).

SELECTED READING

Buchmeier, M. J., Welsh, R. M., Dukto, F. J., and Oldstone, M. B. A. (1980). The virology and immunobiology of lymphocytic choriomeningitis virus infection. *Adv. Immunol.* **30**, 275.

dal Canto, M. C. and Rabinowitz, S. G. (1982). Experimental models of virus-induced demyelination of the central nervous system. *Ann. Neurol.* **11**, 109.

Deinhardt, F. and Gust, I. D. (1982). Viral hepatitis. *Bull. WHO* **60**, 661.

Denham, A. M., Bacon, T. H., and Pelton, B. K. (1983). Viruses: Immunosuppressive effects. *Phil. Trans. R. Soc. Lond. B* **303**, 137.

Epstein, M. A. and Achong, B. G. (eds.) (1979). *The Epstein-Barr Virus.* Springer-Verlag, Berlin.

Gajdusek, D. C. (1977). Unconventional viruses and the origin and disappearance of kuru. *Science* **197**, 943.

Ganem, D. (1982). Persistent infection of humans with hepatitis B virus: mechanisms and consequences. *Rev. Infect. Dis.* **4**, 1026.

Hamilton, J. D. (1982). *Cytomegalovirus and immunity*. Monographs in virology, (ed. J. L. Melnick), vol. 12.

Henle, W. and Henle, G. (1982). Immunology of Epstein-Barr virus. In *The Herpesviruses*, (ed. B. Roizman), vol. 1 p. 209. Plenum Press, New York.

Hill, T. J. (1983). Herpes simplex virus latency. In *The Herpesviruses*, vol. 2. (ed. B. Roizman). Plenum Press, New York.

Ho, M. (1982). *Cytomegalovirus: Biology and Infection*. Plenum Press, New York.

Hudson, J. B. (1979). The murine cytomegalovirus as a model for the study of viral pathogenesis and persistent infections. *Arch. Virol.* **62**, 1.

Kieff, E., Darnbaugh, T., Heller, M., King, W., *et al*. (1982). The biology and chemistry of Epstein-Barr virus. *J. Infect. Dis.* **146**, 506.

Klein, R. J. (1982). The pathogenesis of acute, latent and recurrent herpes simplex infections. *Arch. Virol.* **72**, 143.

Lehmann-Grube, F., Peralta, L. M., Bruns, M., and Lohler, J. (1982). Persistent infection of mice with the lymphocytic choriomeningitis virus. In *Compre-*

hensive Virology, vol. 18 (eds. H. Fraenkel-Conrat and R. R. Wagner). Plenum Press, New York.

ter Meulen, V. and Carter, M. J. (1982). Morbillivirus persistent infections in man and animals. In *Virus Persistence*, 33rd Symposium Soc. Gen. Microbiol., (eds. B. W. J. Mahy, A. C. Minson and G. K. Darby). Cambridge University Press, Cambridge.

Mims, C. A. (1978). General features of persistent virus infections. *Postgrad. Med. J.* **54**, 581.

Norkin, L. C. (1982). Papovaviral persistent infections. *Microbiol. Rev.* **46**, 384.

Porter D. D. and Cho, H. J. (1980). Aleutian disease of mink: a model for persistent infection. In *Comprehensive Virology*, vol. 16, (eds. H. Fraenkel-Conrat and R. R. Wagner). Plenum Press, New York.

Riley, V. (1974). Persistence and other characteristics of the lactate dehydrogenase-elevating virus (LDH-virus). *Progr. Med. Virol.* **18**, 198.

Robinson, H. L. (1982). Retroviruses and cancer. *Rev. Infect. Dis.* **4**, 1015.

Roizman, B. (1982). The family herpesviridae—General Description, Taxonomy and Classification. In *The Herpesviruses*, vol. 1, (ed. B. Roizman). Plenum Press, New York.

Stroop, W. G. and Baringer, J. R. (1982). Persistent, slow and latent viral infections. *Progr. Med. Virol.* **28**, 1.

Chapter Seven
Immunisation Against Viral Diseases

TYPES OF VIRAL VACCINE

Viral vaccines may be classified into two broad categories: 'live' and 'killed' (Fig. 7.1). Most live vaccines are attenuated mutants, selected for their relative avirulence. They must nevertheless be capable of multiplying in the host and eliciting a natural type of immune response, for that is the rationale of their use. 'Killed' vaccines, in contrast, are produced by chemically inactivating the infectivity of the virulent wild virus, while retaining its immunogenicity. A refinement is to purify or synthesise the particular protein known to elicit neutralising antibody.

Live vaccines

Most successful viral vaccines are live avirulent mutants. Some are delivered via the natural route, e.g. by mouth or nose, but most are injected. The live virus multiplies in the recipient, eliciting a lasting immune response, but causes little or no disease. In effect, a live vaccine produces a subclinical infection, which is 'Nature's way' of immunising. Because of the requirement that the mutant must not be so attenuated

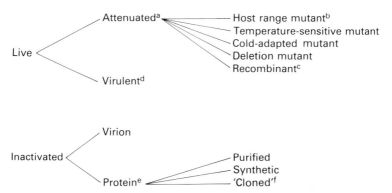

Fig. 7.1. Types of viral vaccine. a Including genetic reassortants incorporating mutant genes. b Occurring naturally in a different animal species, or selected by passage in cultured cells. c Incorporating gene from another virus. d Delivered via an unnatural route or at a safe age (in veterinary medicine). e May be incorporated in liposome or adjuvant. f In prokaryotic or eukaryotic cells by recombinant DNA technology.

that it fails to replicate satisfactorily, it is sometimes necessary to compromise with a vaccine that does in fact induce mild symptoms in a few recipients.

The avirulence of attenuated vaccines has generally not been characterised in terms of their pathogenesis in the vaccinee. In the case of many live respiratory viral vaccines, multiplication of the attenuated virus in the respiratory tract is severely restricted, i.e. the total yield of virus is greatly diminished. In other instances, however (e.g. live poliovaccine) the more fundamental defect appears to be loss of the capacity to infect the vulnerable target organ.

Most of today's live attenuated vaccines have been derived quite empirically by serial passage in cultured cells until the virus is found to have lost virulence ('genetic roulette'; Chanock *et al.*, 1975). Avirulence is demonstrated initially in a convenient laboratory model, e.g. a primate, before being confirmed by clinical trial in human volunteers. Such 'host range' (*hr*) mutants have accumulated a large number of sequential mutations, e.g. the poliovirus type 1 strain used in the 'Sabin' oral vaccine contains 57 separate base substitutions (Nomoto *et al.*, 1982), yet it is unknown which of these is/are responsible for the loss of virulence, though it is clear that many of the changes are clustered in the region of the genome coding for the NH_2-terminal half of the viral capsid protein VP1. Indeed, for the great majority of viruses, we have no idea which gene(s) confers virulence—in general, this vital property cannot be ascribed to any single gene (Palese and Roizman, 1980). Some attempts have been made to identify other phenotypic characters that are 'genetically linked' to virulence, but these have proved to be unreliable markers for the selection or identification of potential vaccine strains. For instance, the *rct/40* marker, i.e. capacity to grow at 40°C, though a useful indicator of virulence in poliovirus, is not an invariable correlate (Nakano *et al.*, 1978). Temperature sensitivity, i.e. reduced capacity to grow at a nominated 'non-permissive' temperature, say 38–40°C, does appear to denote reduced virulence in the case of influenza virus; in fact the property can be conferred by a *ts* lesion in any gene (Richman and Murphy, 1979).

Whether or not virulence in any virus can be associated with a particular gene(s), it has been forecast that licensing authorities may demand that future vaccines be fully defined genetically, i.e. that the nucleotide sequence of the nucleic acid be known, and perhaps even stipulated (Chanock, 1981). Utilising recombinant DNA technology, defined sequences or particular genes can now be excised or inserted at will (Lai *et al.*, 1980; Sveda *et al.*, 1982). Genetically engineered deletion mutants would presumably be less likely to revert (Chanock, 1981) than do host range mutants (Kew *et al.*, 1981), *ts* mutants (Murphy *et al.*, 1980) or cold-adapted (*ca*) mutants (Murphy and Chanock, 1981), even when the latter contain multiple mutations distributed throughout several different genes (Maassab *et al.*, 1981).

In the case of viruses with segmented genomes, genetic reassortment (Kilbourne, 1969) can be exploited to introduce *ts*, *ca* or *hr* genes from laboratory 'master strains' into a recent isolate of wild virus to produce an avirulent vaccine strain relatively quickly (Chanock and Murphy, 1980; Murphy and Chanock, 1981). As this ingenious technique has now become standard practice in the manufacture of influenza vaccines, it will be discussed more fully under that heading.

Host range mutants. Classically, live vaccines have been derived by several dozen passages of the wild virus through one or more types of cell culture, sometimes after prior 'adaptation' to laboratory animals or eggs. Emergence of mutants is of course favoured by transferring progeny at high concentration. Accumulation of a large number of sequential mutations generally leads not only to more vigorous growth in that particular type of cultured cell, but also, quite fortuitously, to progressive loss of virulence for the original host.

Temperature-sensitive mutants. The observation that *ts* mutants generally display reduced virulence suggested that they might constitute very satisfactory live vaccines (Fenner, 1969; 1972). Chanock and his colleagues vigorously pursued this possibility for the best part of a decade, producing *ts* vaccines against a number of respiratory viruses (reviews: Chanock and Murphy, 1980; Chanock, 1981; Murphy and Chanock, 1981). The rationale was that *ts* mutants incapable of replication at the temperature of the lungs (37°C) would nevertheless multiply safely if instilled into the nose, where the temperature is consistently lower. Such proved to be the case but, unfortunately, even vaccines containing more than one *ts* mutation displayed a disturbing tendency to revert towards virulence during replication in man. Reversion was not attributable solely to simple back-mutation; the wild-type phenotype could be restored by a suppressor mutation in a gene quite distinct from that containing the *ts* lesion (Murphy *et al.*, 1980).

It transpires that several of the empirically-derived host-range mutants that have been used for years as live vaccines are in fact also *ts* (see Richman and Murphy, 1979). These include the Sabin poliovirus strains, the Schwartz measles vaccine, and a number of live attenuated veterinary vaccines such as that against infectious bovine rhinotracheitis. The 'ceiling' ('shutoff', 'non-permissive') temperature for several of these *ts* mutants must be higher than 37°C, because the list includes vaccines that are administered systemically and are capable of multiplication at body temperature.

Concern has been expressed about the possibility that *ts* vaccines might be capable of setting up persistent infections in the brain or elsewhere. Such infections have been established experimentally in animal models using *ts* mutants of measles, vesicular stomatitis or reovirus, and the measles virus recoverable from some cases of SSPE (see Chapter 6) is *ts*. Yet the *ts* Schwartz mutant, which has been employed as the standard measles vaccine for two decades, has led, not to an increase, but to a marked decline in the incidence of SSPE (see Hinman *et al.*, 1980). Furthermore, many naturally occurring wild viruses with no known capacity to persist are *ts* (see Richman and Murphy, 1979); as might be expected, these are mainly viruses that infect superficial epithelial surfaces such as the eye (enterovirus 70), or upper respiratory tract (certain rhinoviruses, coronaviruses and influenza viruses). Nevertheless, prudence suggests we should be more than usually cautious and thorough in evaluating *ts* mutants for use as human vaccines.

Cold-adapted mutants. Somewhat different from classical *ts* mutants are cold-adapted (*ca*) mutants, derived by adaptation of virus to grow at suboptimal temperature (25°C). Maassab and colleagues (1981) have produced a strain of influenza virus with mutations in every gene, which grows as well at 25°C as at 33°C; it happens also to be *ts* in that it fails to grow at 38°C. This virus is used as a master strain for genetic reassortment with the prevalent wild strain to produce an attenuated vaccine containing wild-type HA and NA genes plus six *ca* mutant genes (Murphy and Chanock, 1981; Kendal *et al.*, 1982). So far, this *ca* vaccine has revealed less tendency to revert than the earlier *ts* vaccines.

Deletion mutants. Chanock (1981) has outlined a strategy for producing to order mutants with deletions of designated nucleic acid sequences. In the case of DNA viruses, the construction of deletion mutants would be relatively simple. Possibilities foreshadowed by Chanock include deletion of the 'oncogene' from live adenovirus vaccines, and deletion of the thymidine kinase gene (thought to be required for latency) from live herpes simplex vaccines. For single-stranded polycistronic RNA viruses of positive polarity, such as the togaviruses and picornaviruses, cloning of a DNA copy in mammalian cells should be itself sufficient to allow production of infectious virions, as has been demonstrated for poliovirus by Racaniello and Baltimore (1981), because the mRNA transcribed from DNA corresponds to infectious viral RNA. Indeed, systematic analysis of deletion mutants as well as of recombinants between virulent and attenuated strains recovered by transfection with cloned recombinant cDNAs (Nomoto *et al.*, 1982) might reveal a particular sequence to be responsible for virulence.

Construction of deletion mutants of negative-stranded RNA viruses with segmented genomes poses greater problems. Even so, Lai *et al.* (1980) have put forward a plausible protocol. Briefly, (1) a double-stranded DNA copy of each gene of a segmented RNA of negative polarity, such as that of influenza virus, is cloned in an *E. coli* plasmid system; (2) the influenza DNA from such plasmids is subjected to 'enzyme surgery' using appropriate restriction endonucleases and ligases; (3) this viral DNA from which the designated sequence has been deleted is then inserted into an appropriate viral or plasmid DNA vector and propagated in eukaryotic cells; (4) influenza viral ($-$) RNA transcribed from the hybrid DNA replicating in these mammalian cells is 'rescued' by coinfection of the cells with influenza virus; (5) viable reassortant virions containing the RNA with the required deletion are then selected and tested for immunogenicity, avirulence and genetic stability.

Recombinants incorporating cloned genes from other viruses. Moss and his colleagues have recently opened up a novel approach to vaccination which may prove to be of widespread applicability (see Smith *et al.*, 1983). The concept is to insert the gene for any given viral protein into the genome of an avirulent virus that can then be administered as a live vaccine. Cells in which the virus multiplies will produce the foreign viral protein, against which an immune response will then be mounted.

The prototype developed by Smith *et al.* (1983) is a 'live' vaccine in which the gene for hepatitis B surface antigen (HB$_s$Ag) is inserted into the genome of vaccinia virus. In brief, the recombinant was constructed as follows. The gene for HB$_s$Ag was inserted, within a non-essential vaccinia viral gene (e.g. that for thymidine kinase, TK), into a bacterial plasmid. A vaccinia early promoter was placed in the appropriate position adjacent to the 'foreign' (HB$_s$Ag) gene. Mammalian cells were then infected with wild-type vaccinia virus, and shortly thereafter transfected with the chimaeric plasmid. Recombination occurred between the vaccinia DNA and the plasmid DNA. Appropriate selection procedure enabled recombinant vaccinia virions containing the HB$_s$Ag gene to be recovered. Following inoculation of such recombinants into cultured cells or rabbits, the virus multiplied and substantial quantities of HB$_s$Ag were secreted from infected cells. The animals produced an excellent antibody response to HB$_s$Ag. More recently this vaccine has been shown to protect chimpanzees against challenge with hepatitis B, while analogous vaccinia-influenza (HA) and vaccinia-herpes simplex (gD) recombinants protected animals against influenza and herpes simplex respectively (see Smith *et al.*; Paoletti and Panicali; in Lerner and Chanock, 1984; also Panicali *et al.*, 1983).

This dramatic demonstration of the power of recombinant DNA technology is a real *tour de force*. In theory at least, it should now be possible to insert the gene for any, or indeed several, foreign proteins into the DNA of an avirulent live virus, such as vaccinia. Thereby one could hope to vaccinate simultaneously against a whole range of infectious diseases, including not only those of viral aetiology but also perhaps malaria and other scourges of mankind. The potential benefits, particularly to the Third World, are self-evident.

Of course, vaccinia virus is not likely to be the ideal vector. True, it does have the advantage of a large genome potentially capable of accommodating a number of foreign inserts and still being packaged within the virion. Furthermore, it has been used successfully as a live vaccine throughout the world for many years. However, this means that vaccinia will now fail to 'take' satisfactorily in the vaccinated population, especially in the developing nations. Also, the vaccine is not absolutely safe—indeed, the incidence of encephalitis and other complications following vaccination with existing strains of the virus (approximately 1:10 000) was judged to be unacceptable in Western countries in the final years before smallpox was eradicated. Another potential hazard would be the spread of infection from animals to man if vaccinia virus were used as a vector for immunizing livestock; however, there are a number of relatively species-specific poxviruses which could be used as vectors in particular animal species, e.g. fowlpox in poultry. Perhaps the vaccinia genome can be manipulated further to attenuate it further and lower the incidence of serious side effects. Alternatively, other DNA viruses, albeit with small genomes, could be harnessed as vectors. Adenoviruses and papovaviruses have been demonstrated to be very satisfactory eukaryotic cloning and expression vectors. While it would not be prudent to employ a virus with known oncogenic potential for animals, a non-oncogenic adenovirus might make a safer vector.

It may become necessary to develop several alternative vectors because, once a particular virus has been used, it cannot be reused as a live vaccine to immunize against another agent in the future. Alternatively, careful thought may need to be given to the construction of a single one-off, all-purpose vaccine incorporating genes for the key immunogenic proteins of most or all of the important human infectious diseases before substantial numbers of people are vaccinated with that vector in the first place.

Live virulent viruses as vaccines. The first known 'vaccine' consisted of virulent smallpox (variola) virus, taken from a relatively mild case and inoculated into the skin. This practice, known as 'variolation', was highly dangerous, but less so than 'natural' smallpox, and was pursued energetically in England and the U.S.A. for some 80 years prior to the development of the first avirulent live virus vaccine by Jenner (1798). A few vaccines still used in veterinary practice today consist of fully virulent live virus administered via an unnatural route, resulting in replication of the virus without producing disease, e.g. contagious pustular dermatitis virus of sheep inoculated on the inside of the thigh, or avian infectious laryngotracheitis virus scarified into the cloaca of chickens. Such an approach is generally considered to be far too dangerous to contemplate in man, but one interesting example, namely delivery of the respiratory pathogen, adenovirus, by mouth, enclosed in an 'enteric' capsule, is discussed later.

Another strategy occasionally pursued by veterinarians is to administer virulent live virus at a time of life when it will inflict little or no damage, e.g. avian encephalomyelitis virus can be given safely to adult hens (in which it produces no disease) in order to protect their chicks, by maternal antibody, during the vulnerable first few weeks of life. If this approach is ever applied to humans in the future, whether using virulent or avirulent live virus, (e.g. to prevent respiratory syncytial viral infections in the newborn infant) it may be prudent to immunise the mother before, rather than during, pregnancy unless it can be clearly shown that the vaccine does not cause congenital abnormalities or persistent infection in the foetus. Whereas the colostrum is of critical importance in passive transfer of maternal antibody in certain animals, it is not so vital in humans; nevertheless, breast-feeding could augment the protection of the baby against some of the viruses to which the mother is immune (see p. 187, Chapter 5).

A rather different approach pioneered by Jenner in his use of live cowpox virus to 'vaccinate' against smallpox, involves the use of a naturally occurring virus of low virulence or a virus indigenous to another species of animal. It is sometimes possible to find a virus that is, on the one hand, non-virulent for the host species one wishes to immunise, yet so closely related antigenically to the serotype(s) against which one wishes to protect that cross-immunity will result. One of many examples from veterinary medicine is the use of virulent herpesvirus of turkeys to protect fowls against Marek's disease (Purchase *et al.*, 1972). Similarly, bovine rotavirus, administered by the natural (oral) route, protects calves and piglets against bovine, porcine or human rotaviruses (Kapikian *et al.*, 1980). It is not inconceivable that such an approach could be successfully exploited in man.

Inactivated vaccines

Inactivated ('killed') vaccines are made from virulent virus by destroying its infectivity whilst retaining its immunogenicity. Being non-infectious, such vaccines are generally safe, but need to be injected in very large amounts to elicit an antibody response commensurate with that attainable by a much smaller dose of live attenuated vaccine. Normally, even the primary course comprises two or three injections, and further ('booster') doses may be required at intervals over the succeeding years to revive flagging immunity.

Traditionally the inactivating agent has been formaldehyde (e.g. see Gard, 1960), which is still used to produce two human vaccines, influenza and 'Salk' poliovaccine, even though the whole process is somewhat empirical. It is not clear to what extent the loss of viral infectivity is attributable to inactivation of nucleic acid (by reaction with the amino groups of nucleotides) and to what extent it is due to denaturation of protein (by cross-linking) (Bachrach, 1966); the latter, known as 'tanning', does produce some problems, including clumping and loss of immunogenicity. In recent years therefore, formaldehyde has increasingly been replaced by other agents, notably β-propiolactone and the ethylenimines. One of the advantages of β-propiolactone (LoGrippo, 1960; Goldstein and Tauraso, 1970) is that it is completely hydrolysed within hours *in vitro* to a non-toxic degradation product found normally in the body. Ethylenimine, binary ethylenimine, propylenimine and N-acetylethylenimine have been widely used for veterinary vaccines, e.g. foot-and-mouth disease vaccines (Morgan *et al.*, 1980). Psoralen derivatives, such as 4'-hydroxymethyltrioxsalen and 4'-aminomethyltrioxsalen, are polycyclic planar molecules which bind covalently to the bases of nucleic acids in a photochemical reaction requiring irradiation with ultraviolet light of long wavelength (Isaacs *et al.*, 1977). Psoralens are now being used for the preparation of safe, non-infectious antigens for serology in diagnostic laboratories (Redfield *et al.*, 1981); their potential as agents for the production of inactivated vaccines merits exploration. Ultraviolet light is no longer used for vaccine production because the infectivity of 'killed' virions can be regained as a result of multiplicity reactivation, i.e. the production of infective virus by a cell co-infected with two or more virions with lethal mutations in different genes (see Fenner *et al.*, 1974).

Inactivated vaccines tend to be expensive because of the large numbers of virions that need to be injected. Recent efforts have been directed therefore towards scaling up the commercial production of virus, e.g. by using continuous cell lines (Montagnon *et al.*, 1981) capable of growing in suspension, or as monolayers coating 'micro-carrier' beads (van Wezel *et al.*, 1978) in fermentation tanks. Secondly, much higher standards are being applied to the purification and concentration of viruses, whether by zonal ultracentrifugation, gel filtration, ion exchange chromatography, affinity chromatography using mono-clonal antibodies, or a combination of such procedures (van Wezel, 1981). It is particularly important to remove aggregated virus prior to chemical inactivation (Gard, 1960); failure to do so led to a notorious tragedy with an early batch of Salk vaccine which retained infectivity and was responsible for a number of cases of paralytic poliomyelitis in 1955. A similar occurrence may be the explanation of the mysterious 1981 outbreak of foot-and-mouth disease in cattle on the Isle of Wight from which 'vaccine-like' virus was recovered. An unusual precaution against such events is to prepare a formalin-inactivated vaccine from an avirulent mutant, as has been done for Venezuelan equine encephalitis (Edelman *et al.*, 1979).

Purified, synthetic and 'cloned' proteins

Large doses of inactivated virions often produce a febrile response as well as a local reaction at the infection site, especially in young children. It was found quite empirically that the reactogenicity of inactivated influenza vaccines could be reduced by 'splitting' the envelope of the virus with a lipid solvent such as deoxycholate, ether or n-butyl-phosphate (see Perkins and Regamy, 1977; Tyrrell and Smith, 1979). The logical extension of this compromise is of course to remove all non-essential components of the virion and inoculate only the relevant immunogen, namely the particular surface (envelope or outer capsid) protein against which neutralising antibodies are directed. Such 'subunit' vaccines are in use against influenza (see Tyrrell and Smith, 1979) and hepatitis B (see Vyas *et al.*, 1978) and have been shown to be feasible against a wide range of other viruses, including foot-and-mouth disease, rabies, herpes simplex and adenoviruses (see Ginsberg, 1975; Bachrach *et al.*, 1976).

Synthetic peptides. The techniques of nucleic acid sequencing are now such that we already know the complete structure of the genome of a number of viruses (Kitamura *et al.*, 1981; Laver and Air, 1980). The amino acid sequence of each viral protein can of course be read off the nucleotide sequence of the viral nucleic acid, and/or can be determined directly. The protein or any sequence thereof can then be synthesised chemically. Sela and Arnon (1980) have been advocating for several years that such synthetic polypeptides would constitute ideal vaccines, having themselves clearly demonstrated the feasibility of the idea by showing that a synthetic icosapeptide elicited antibodies capable of 'neutralising' the infectivity of the bacteriophage, MS2 (Langbeheim et al., 1976).

Now that techniques are available for locating the antigenic sites on the surface of viral proteins (Wiley et al., 1981) it is possible to synthesise shorter peptides corresponding to the critical determinants to which neutralising antibodies bind. Of particular interest is the possibility, for which Lerner (1982) has produced evidence, that relatively invariate ('conserved'), even buried, sequences, not normally immunogenic when presented in situ in the virion, may be capable in isolation of eliciting neutralising antibodies which may then have the added advantage of cross-protection against heterologous serotypes. There is evidence that such cross-reactive conserved regions may be especially immunogenic for T lymphocytes (Anders et al., 1981a, b; Lamb et al., 1982; Hackett et al., 1983).

Synthetic viral peptides displaying significant antigenic and/or immunogenic activity at the time of writing are listed in Table 7.1. This is an exciting new approach which merits further research, although it must be emphasised that, because short synthetic peptides lack the tertiary conformation they assume in the intact virion, most

Table 7.1. Synthetic peptides as potential vaccines.

Virus	Reference
Hepatitis B	Lerner et al. (1981)
	Dreesman et al. (1982)
	Hollinger et al. (1982)
	Prince et al. (1982)
	Gerin et al. (1983)
	Ionescu-Matiu et al. (1983)
Influenza	Jackson et al. (1981, 1982)
	Green, N. et al. (1982)
	Müller et al. (1982)
	Lamb et al. (1982)
	Hackett et al. (1983)
Foot-and-mouth disease	Bittle et al. (1982)
Poliovirus	Emini et al. (1983)
Herpes simplex	Dietzschold et al. (1984)

antibodies raised against them are incapable of binding to virus, hence the neutralising titre may be orders of magnitude lower than that induced by inactivated vaccine, or even by the purified intact protein (Jackson *et al.*, 1981; 1982). Furthermore, some conformational determinants are 'non-sequential', i.e. are composed of amino acids that are separated in the primary sequence but find themselves close together in the intact molecule. Nevertheless, there are already some striking examples of synthetic viral peptides that have been shown to elicit neutralising antibodies (e.g. hepatitis B, Lerner *et al.*, 1981), and even to protect animals against challenge with a lethal dose of virus (FMDV, Bittle *et al.*, 1982). Moreover, peptides incapable of inducing protective levels of antibody may nevertheless successfully prime an animal to respond anamnestically when subsequently boosted with a sub-immunising dose of virus (Emini *et al.*, 1983). Synthetic peptides might conceivably make more satisfactory antiviral vaccines if their original tertiary structure is at least partially restored by the introduction of appropriately located cross-linking bonds (Ionescu-Matiu *et al.*, 1983). Moreover, the immunogenicity of such weakly immunogenic molecules may need to be considerably augmented by conjugation to suitable carriers, and/or emulsification with powerful adjuvants (Bittle *et al.*, 1982) or incorporation into liposomes (see below).

'Cloning'. Recombinant DNA technology is beginning to make its mark in the area of vaccines, as it has so conspicuously elsewhere. The complete genomes or selected genes of several mammalian viruses have now been 'cloned' in both prokaryotic and eukaryotic cells.

The desired gene, or a cDNA copy of an RNA gene, is recombined with a suitable vector, such as a plasmid, cosmid or phage. Commonly, the viral gene is inserted into the vector adjacent to all or part of the gene for a bacterial protein that is made in large amounts, hence the product is a 'fused polypeptide' containing, say, the N-terminal end of β-galactosidase or β-lactamase followed by the viral protein in question. The yield of functional protein may be enhanced by a number of technical tricks such as the use of multicopy vectors and high efficiency promoters (review: Murray, 1980; Maniatis *et al.*, 1982). Yet, in too high a concentration the product may be toxic for the cell. This difficulty can be circumvented by ensuring that the protein cannot be made during the growth phase of the bacteria. Furthermore, the polypeptide, whether in its nascent state on the ribosome, free inside the bacterial cytoplasm, or extracellular, is often found to be rapidly denatured; glycoproteins, which cannot be glycosylated by prokaryotic cells, may be especially vulnerable to proteases.

More recently, cloning has been accomplished in eukaryotic cells. Commonly, the viral gene is first incorporated into a bacterial plasmid, then into a 'divalent' vector able to replicate autonomously in

Table 7.2. Some viral genes cloned by recombinant DNA technology.

Virus	Gene	Vector	Host cell	Expression	Secretion	Reference
Hepatitis B	HBsAg	plasmid	E. coli	+	−	Edman et al. (1981)
	HBsAg	plasmid	E. coli	+	−	Mackay et al. (1981)
	HBsAg	phage λ	E. coli	+	−	Charnay et al. (1980)
	HBsAg	plasmid	S. cerevisiae	+	−	Valenzuela et al. (1982)
	HBsAg	plasmid	Mouse Ltk⁻	+	+	Pourcel et al. (1982)
	HBsAg	plasmid[a]	CV-1	+	+	Smith et al. (1983)
Herpes simplex 1	gD	plasmid	E. coli	+	−	Weis et al. (1983)
Influenza	HA	plasmid	E. coli	+	−	Emtage et al. (1980)
	HA	plasmid	E. coli	+	−	Davis et al. (1983)
	HA	SV40	MK	+	+	Gething & Sambrook (1981)
	HA	SV40	MK	+	+	Sveda et al. (1982)
Foot-and-mouth disease	VP1	plasmid	E. coli	+	−	Küpper et al. (1981)
	VP3	plasmid	E. coli	+	−	Kleid et al. (1981)
Poliomyelitis	Complete genome	plasmid	CV-1, HeLa	+	+	Racaniello & Baltimore (1981)
Rabies	G	plasmid	E. coli	+	−	Yelverton et al. (1983)

[a]Chimeric plasmid incorporating foreign gene flanked by non-essential vaccinia gene (e.g. TK) used to transfect mammalian cells co-infected with vaccinia virus; recombinant vaccinia virions containing gene for HBsAg selected for use as 'live' vaccine.

Analogous vaccinia-influenza (HA) and vaccinia-herpes simplex (gD) recombinants protect animals against influenza and herpes simplex (Panicali et al., 1983; Smith et al., and Paoletti and Panicali, in Lerner and Chanock, 1984).

eukaryotes. The small circular viral DNA molecules of bovine papilloma and SV40 are now widely used as cloning vectors in mammalian cells. A particularly ingenious artifice for augmenting the expression of a cloned gene is cotransformation of an enzyme-deficient mutant cell line with the gene for the missing enzyme, e.g. thymidine kinase. For instance, if a viral gene is recombined into a suitable vector alongside the gene for dihydrofolate reductase, then a DHFR⁻ Chinese hamster ovary cell line transfected with this vector will, in the presence of methatrexate, produce a yield of the corresponding viral protein amounting to some 1% of the cells' total output. Antigenic surface proteins of a number of viruses have been produced (Table 7.2).

Immunopotentiation by adjuvants, liposomes and carriers. If isolated viral proteins—whether purified from virions, chemically synthesised or made by recombinant DNA technology—are to be employed as vaccines, their immunogenicity will need to be enhanced by several orders of magnitude. Such immunopotentiation could be achieved by coupling the protein to a suitable carrier, and/or incorporation in a liposome, or emulsification with an adjuvant.

Adjuvants have been defined as '. . . materials that are added to vaccines with the intent of potentiating the immune response so that a greater amount of antibody is produced, a lesser quantity of antigen is required, and fewer doses need to be given' (World Health Organization, 1976). They also potentiate cell-mediated immune responses. The most widely used adjuvants in man to date are aluminium phosphate and aluminium hydroxide gel, to which the immunogen is adsorbed, but the resulting immune response is not particularly prolonged, hence booster injections are required. The classical oily adjuvants of Freund are still widely employed to enhance the antibody response to antigens inoculated into laboratory animals, but are unacceptable for human use, mainly because the oil occasionally produces sterile abscesses at the injection site (even following the recommended deep intramuscular injection) and, being non-biodegradable, persists indefinitely in the body, raising the possibility of inducing various unexpected auto-immune or allergic responses. A metabolisable adjuvant based on peanut oil ('Adjuvant 65') has been used experimentally in man for two decades (Hilleman, 1966) but has still not been generally accepted because of doubts about possible carcinogenicity of one of the ingredients. Attention has therefore been directed towards simple, chemically defined, preferably synthetic substances of known mode of action. One of the most interesting of these is the active component of the Mycobacterium of Freund's complete adjuvant, namely the muramyl dipeptide (MDP), N-acetyl-muramyl-L-alanyl-D-isoglutamine. MDP or various derivatives, in aqueous medium, may be administered by injection or mouth, mixed with or actually conjugated to the immunogen, or incorporated into liposomes (Chedid, 1979). This synthetic adjuvant is effective even when coupled to a synthetic antigen (Sela and Arnon, 1980). Chedid et al. (1982) recently described a derivative of MDP which has the advantage of being non-pyrogenic.

Our knowledge of the mode of action of adjuvants is still vestigial. Evidence gleaned mainly from studies of Freund's 'complete' and 'incomplete' adjuvants suggests that their manifold actions may include: (1) prolonged retention of antigen; (2) activation of macrophages (leading to secretion of lymphokines and attraction of lymphocytes); and (3) mitogenicity for lymphocytes (World Health Organization, 1976; Chedid, 1979; Edelman, 1980; Edelman et al., 1980). Latterly, appreciation of the complexity of the immune system has alerted us to the importance of determining the effects of potential adjuvants on each class of lymphocyte. For instance, an adjuvant that preferentially turned on T_s cells, T_d cells, IgE or the complement system could be a disaster. The adjuvants of the future might well be simple synthetic chemicals with selective mitogenicity for, say, T_h and/or B cells. Moreover, such adjuvants might be covalently conjugated to the immunogen in such a way that only the relevant clones of lymphocytes will be activated. Purified endogenous lymphokines might eventually be harnessed for this purpose (Edelman et al., 1980).

Liposomes are micelles consisting of artificial lipid membranes into which proteins can be incorporated (Allison and Gregoriadis, 1974; Gregoriadis, 1976). When purified viral envelope proteins are used, the resulting 'virosomes' (or 'immunosomes') somewhat resemble the original enveloped virion (Simons et al., 1978). This ingenious trick enables one not only to reconstitute virus-like structures lacking all nucleic acid and other extraneous material, but also to select non-pyrogenic lipids and to incoporate substances with adjuvant activity, such as saponin (becoming widely used in veterinary vaccines) or lipid A (Naylor et al., 1982), thus regaining much of the immunogenicity lost when the viral protein was removed from its original milieu.

A *carrier* is a protein to which a smaller molecule (a 'hapten') may be chemically coupled in order to render the latter more immunogenic. The potentiation of the immune response to the hapten is due to the helper T (T_h) cell response to the carrier. For example, the immunogenicity of synthetic peptides representing key antigenic regions of the VP1 protein of the foot-and-mouth disease virus is considerably augmented by conjugation to the carrier, keyhole limpet haemocyanin (KLH) (Bittle et al., 1982). Indeed, if a particular viral peptide is expensive to produce, it may prove feasible to prime with carrier alone, then boost with carrier–hapten conjugate. If such carrier proteins were to be employed for human vaccines, it would be important to ascertain that clinically significant hypersensitivity to that protein will not develop.

'LIVE' OR 'DEAD'?

The question of 'live' versus 'dead' vaccines predates the famous debates of the mid-fifties over the merits and demerits of 'Sabin' versus 'Salk' poliovaccines (Sabin, 1957; Salk, 1958), and remains an issue today (Sabin, 1981b; Salk, 1980). The major considerations are summarised in Table 7.3 and then discussed.

Immunological considerations

The object of immunisation is to protect against disease, not necessarily to prevent infection. If, as immunity wanes over the years following active immunisation, or the weeks following passive immunisation, infection with wild virus does occur, the infection is likely to be subclinical. Such an occurrence may have the beneficial effect of boosting immunity.

Table 7.3. Advantages and disadvantages of live versus dead vaccines.

	Live	Inactivated
Route of administration	Natural[a] or injection	Injection
Dose of virus; cost	Low	High
Number of doses	Single[b]	Multiple
Need for adjuvant	No	Yes[c]
Duration of immunity	Many years	Generally less[d]
Antibody response	IgG; IgA[e]	IgG
Cell-mediated response	Good	Poor
Heat lability in tropics	Yes[f]	No
Interference	Occasional; OPV only[g]	No
Side effects	Occasional mild symptoms[h]	Occasional sore arm
Reversion to virulence	Rarely; OPV only[i]	No

[a]Oral or respiratory, in certain cases.
[b]Except OPV (to preempt possibility of interference). For some other live vaccines a single booster may be required by law (yellow fever) or desirable (rubella?) after a decade or so.
[c]But few satisfactory adjuvants yet licensed for human use.
[d]But satisfactory with some inactivated vaccines.
[e]IgA if delivered via oral or respiratory route. OPV can thereby prevent wild poliovirus from multiplying in the gut hence facilitate near eradication of the virus from the community.
[f]$MgCl_2$ and other stabilisers, plus maintenance of 'cold chain' assist preservation.
[g]Especially in Third World.
[h]Especially rubella and measles.
[i]10^{-6} vaccinees.

Acquired immunity to many respiratory viruses is so poor even following natural infection that it is perhaps unrealistic to expect any vaccine to be effective. In such cases, however, a reasonable objective may be to prevent serious (low respiratory) disease. For instance, Prince *et al.* (in preparation) have shown that immunisation with an experimental respiratory syncytial virus vaccine gives durable protection of hamsters and cottonrats against pneumonitis but not against rhinitis. They postulate a qualitative, not simply quantitative, distinction between 'pulmonary immunity' and 'nasal immunity'.

It has been argued here that subclinical infection is 'Nature's way' of immunising, that by and large this is extremely effective, inducing lifelong immunity following systemic infection (see Chapter 3), and that live vaccines, preferably delivered via the natural route, are obviously the nearest approach to this ideal. One of the great advantages of live oral poliovaccine (OPV) is that, by virtue of its replication in the alimentary tract, it leads to prolonged synthesis of local antibody of the IgA class. This prevents the subsequent multiplication of wild poliovirus in the gut, thereby depriving it of hosts in which to circulate subclinically, hence rendering feasible the prospect of total eradication of the virus, as well as the disease, from the community (Sabin, 1981b). In general, IgA is considered to be the most important (some would say the only) class of immunoglobulin relevant to prevention of viral infection of mucosal surfaces, such as the alimentary, respiratory, genitourinary and ocular epithelia (Ogra, 1971; Chanock *et al.*, 1975; Strober *et al.*, 1982). This, it could be said, is more an argument for topical delivery of vaccines than for live vaccines as such.

A second, perhaps even more crucial, reason for favouring live vaccines is that they are evidently more effective in eliciting 'cell-mediated' immunity (Ada *et al.*, 1981; Askonas *et al.*, 1982). While it is clear that neutralising antibody is the key to prevention of establishment of infection, there is good evidence that T lymphocytes play a crucial role in recovery from infection, once it has been established (see Chapter 3). In particular, cytotoxic T (T_c) cells, which destroy virus-infected cells, can be shown to protect infected animals following adoptive transfer (Ada *et al.*, 1981). All the available evidence indicates that both resting and memory T_c cells are activated not by soluble antigen, but by viral antigen presented on the surface of infected cells in association with MHC antigens (K, D or L), i.e. the same composite antigen that they later recognise as a target (Doherty *et al.*, 1976; Zinkernagel and Doherty, 1979). T_d cells are also turned on more effectively by live virus, presumably due to more effective display of viral antigens in association with Ia antigens on macrophages (Ada *et al.*, 1981), though their antiviral role is less clear. They secrete a variety of lymphokines including interferons and interleukins that attract and activate macrophages and lymphocytes (Tada and Okamura, 1979; Möller, 1982), but they can also cause extensive and sometimes lethal immunopathology (Ada *et al.*, 1981). Various subclasses of T_h cells are probably involved in the induction of T_d as well as T_c cells. Those T_h cells which provide antigen-specific and non-specific help for B cells following activation by viral antigen presented in association with Ia antigen on the surface of macrophages (Möller, 1981) are evidently induced in sufficient numbers by live or inactivated vaccines, as comparable antibody levels are achievable by either. Suppressor T (T_s) cells, however, may be preferentially turned on by 'soluble' viral antigen (Tada and Okamura, 1979); Germain and Benacerraf, 1981) so it is quite possible that inactivated vaccines, and particularly purified, synthetic or cloned soluble proteins, might actually suppress the very immune response they aim to elicit. The differential response of T_s, T_h, T_d and T_c cells, as well as the recently described 'contrasuppressor cells' (D. R. Green *et al.*, 1982), to viral antigens presented in the form of live virus, inactivated virions or soluble protein respectively, merits urgent and detailed investigation.

A further major reason for favouring vaccines that elicit a T lymphocyte response is that T cells display broader cross-recognition of related viral strains than do B cells (Anders *et al.*, 1981b; Askonas *et al.*, 1982). Such cross-immunity presents evident advantages where several viral strains or serotypes circulate simultaneously or sequentially (antigenic drift), although it may also facilitate 'original antigenic sin' (see Chapter 3)—a mixed blessing. Having said all this it must be added that, following natural infection there is at best only limited cross-protection against different serotypes.

In contrast with the lasting immunity that follows systemic infections, immunity following localised infections of epithelial surfaces is relatively short-lived (Ogra, 1971; Rossen *et al.*, 1971; Chanock *et al.*, 1975; Strober *et al.*, 1982). Perhaps for this very reason, large numbers of respiratory and enteric viruses have evolved, presumably by antigenic drift. Really satisfactory vaccines against rhinoviruses, for example, will therefore need, not only to contain all the important serotypes, but also to elicit a better immune response than follows natural infection. It has been submitted that only inactivated vaccines present any hope of achieving either of these two requirements. Very highly concentrated, purified vaccines, delivered repeatedly, in a suitable adjuvant, might conceivably elicit higher antibody responses than ever occur naturally. Antigenic competition between the dozens of serotypes involved may or may not be a problem, but an inactivated vaccine would circumvent the greater impediment which would undoubtedly occur with a live vaccine, namely mutual interference between the numerous viruses attempting to multiply simultaneously in the same vicinity. Conceivably, high doses of purified antigen administered topically to the upper respiratory tract might elicit greater numbers of IgA memory cells in the locality, but allergic reactions following subsequent exposure to vaccine or natural challenge constitute a risk. Indeed, serious complications of an immunological nature have followed even systemic administration of inactivated vaccines against measles and respiratory syncytial virus (RSV), leading to the view that killed vaccines should not be employed against respiratory agents.

Several years ago, experimental vaccines against measles and RSV were injected into children; following subsequent natural exposure to wild virus these children developed significantly more serious disease than did unimmunised controls (Chanock et al., 1968; Isacson and Stone, 1971; Rossen et al., 1971). Chanock et al. (1968), drawing an analogy with the clinical observation that young infants with high levels of maternal IgG against RSV develop serious disease (bronchiolitis/pneumonitis) more frequently than do older infants with lower levels, postulated an immunological basis for the phenomenon, perhaps akin to the Arthus reaction. Norrby et al. (1975) then showed that formalin-inactivated measles (or mumps) vaccine in man failed to induce antibody against the fusion (F) protein. The importance of this became clear when Merz et al. (1980) demonstrated that anti-F antibody is necessary to prevent direct cell-to-cell spread of virus by fusion. They postulated, therefore, that the anti-haemagglutinin (H) antibody, which is formed satisfactorily following killed vaccine, merely serves to form damaging immune complexes with virions released into the lung, and/or with viral syncytia, and activates the complement system, so producing an Arthus reaction and precipitating the destruction of syncytia by antibody/complement and/or antibody-mediated K cell cytolysis. Merz et al. went on to recommend the use of purified F protein (or F plus H) as a vaccine, to be delivered perhaps by aerosol, in the hope of eliciting antibodies of only the IgA class, which are protective but neither activate the complement series nor participate in ADCC.

Safety

Inactivated vaccines should certainly be preferred in immunocompromised individuals, in whom live attenuated vaccines not uncommonly produce disease (Melnick, 1980). Some virologists are also concerned about the wisdom of using live vaccines against herpesviruses because of the known propensity of members of this family to establish persistent infections and their association with cancer. Licensing authorities have become extremely vigilant and have insisted on rigorous tests for residual live virulent virus since a number of tragedies occurred in the pioneering days. Precautions now routinely instituted to prevent accidents such as that encountered with an early batch of Salk vaccine are discussed in a later section. Purified, synthetic or 'cloned' proteins are of course absolutely safe, and have been advocated as potential vaccines against not only herpesviruses and perhaps paramyxoviruses, but also oncogenic viruses. When vaccines are derived from viruses grown in cancer cell lines licensing authorities would insist on total absence of nucleic acid.

There are four distinct types of problem relating to safety which are unique to live vaccines and must be overcome for every product before it can be licensed for human use.

Under-attenuation. Some live vaccines are not as avirulent as one would wish for in an ideal world. Several veterinary vaccines, e.g. rinderpest and rabies, consist of attenuated mutants which, though quite safe in most animals, may be too virulent for certain highly susceptible breeds or species. A number of the human viral vaccines in routine use (e.g. rubella and measles) produce some symptoms—in effect a mild case of the disease—in a minority of vaccinees. However, attempts to attenuate virulence further by additional passages in cultured cells have led to an accompanying decline in capacity of the virus to multiply in man, hence a corresponding loss of immunogenicity. Such trivial side effects as do occur with current human viral vaccines are of no real consequence and do not prove to be a significant disincentive to immunisation, provided that parents are adequately informed in advance and that the benefits of immunisation are perceived as substantially greater than the risks.

Genetic instability. A quite different problem occurs in the case of vaccine strains with an inherent tendency to revert towards virulence during multiplication in the recipient or in contacts to whom the vaccine virus has spread. Most vaccine viruses are incapable of such spread, but in the case of those that do, such as oral poliovaccine, there are obviously greater opportunities for the occurrence of rare back-mutations and for the accumulation of successive mutations leading to a gradual increase in virulence (Kew *et al.*, 1981; Nakano *et al.*, 1978). 'Vaccine-associated' poliomyelitis does occur, particularly in unvaccinated parents, but is exceedingly rare ($<10^{-6}$) (Nightingale, 1977). No other human viral vaccine in use today displays any sign of genetic instability, although livestock losses have occurred with particular veterinary vaccines. As discussed, experimental temperature-sensitive vaccines against some human respiratory viruses have proved to be unstable; indeed, the revertants were found to contain suppressor mutations as well as putative back-mutations (Murphy and Chanock, 1981).

Persistent infection with ts mutants. The theoretical risk that *ts* mutants used as live vaccines might establish persistent infections in the brain or elsewhere has been discussed. All that can be said further is that careful epidemiological follow-up of recipients of human vaccines now known to be *ts* has not exposed any clinical evidence for persistence or reactivation.

Contaminating viruses. Cultured cells employed as a substrate for the growth of viruses for vaccine production may carry endogenous viruses. These may be overt or covert. Primary cell cultures, such as monkey kidney, are particularly liable to contain adventitious agents; over 75 simian viruses have been identified in this way (Kalter *et al.*, 1980), and some, such as *Herpesvirus simiae* ('B virus') are lethal for man. Clearly, such contaminants are more of a worry in live vaccines, but even inactivated vaccines are not free from this risk, for the contaminant may be more resistant to the inactivating agent than the vaccine strain. For example, early batches of formaldehyde-inactivated, as well as live attenuated, poliovaccine were contaminated by live SV40 virus, which is oncogenic for baby rodents but not, fortunately, for humans!

The discovery of SV40-adenovirus 'hybrids' in adenovirus vaccines grown in monkey kidney cells (Rapp *et al.*, 1964; Rowe and Baum, 1964) added a new dimension to the problem of contaminating viruses. Such recombinants, some of which are highly oncogenic, are indistinguishable serologically from the parent adenovirus since they have identical capsids. So far this represents a unique instance of hybridisation between viruses of different families, but intrafamilial recombination or phenotypic mixing is quite common; the latter would be a significant hazard in a retrovirus vaccine, for example.

The danger of contamination of live vaccines with adventitious viruses has triggered a great deal of debate about which types of cultured cell should be licensed for use as substrates for the growth of viruses for human vaccine production (Petricciani *et al.*, 1979). If primary cell cultures are to remain legally acceptable for this purpose, the minimum requirement should be that the animals are bred in captivity, preferably under specific-pathogen-free conditions (e.g. closed colonies of monkeys, or eggs from leukosis-free chickens) and that the cultured cells are rigorously scrutinised for all possible endogenous viruses. In general, however, primary cell cultures were replaced during the 1970s by diploid strains of human embryonic fibroblasts (Plotkin, 1980). Such strains can be subjected to comprehensive virological and karyological screening, certified as safe, then frozen for storage and distribution to vaccine manufacturers on request.

Recently, there has been a revival of discussion about the acceptability of heteroploid cell lines (Montagnon *et al.*, 1981; Hennessen and van Wezel, 1982). Continuous cell lines present great advantages to the vaccine manufacturers because of their infinite growth potential and ease of cultivation *in vitro* including suspension culture. Several veterinary vaccine viruses are grown commercially in suspension culture in large fermentation tanks, e.g. foot-and-mouth disease virus in BHK-21 cells. In 1982, heteroploid cell lines were, for the first time, licensed for the production of human vaccines, provided that adequate techniques are used to demonstrate that the cells are indeed nonmalignant and to exclude the presence of putative cancer viruses or DNA 'oncogenes' in the final product.

Interference

Live vaccines delivered by mouth or nose depend for their efficacy on multiplication in the alimentary or respiratory tract respectively. Interference can occur between different live viruses contained in the vaccine, or between the vaccine virus and itinerant enteric or respiratory viruses that happen to be growing in the vaccinee at the time. Oral poliovaccine (OPV), for example, fails to 'take' in substantial numbers of children in tropical countries where subclinical infection with any one of the numerous enteroviruses is the rule rather than the exception at any particular time (Sabin, 1980). The same phenomenon occurs with lower frequency in developed countries, but, even here, the three strains of poliovirus in the vaccine may interfere with one another. Therefore, OPV is routinely administered on three occasions, separated by at least two months.

Interference would probably negate the effectiveness of a live intra-nasal vaccine against the multitude of rhinoviruses that cause the common cold, should that ever become possible. However, it is not a problem with systemically administered polyvalent vaccines, live or inactivated. The measles-rubella-mumps live vaccine given subcutaneously to infants in the U.S.A. evidently elicits as good an antibody response against each of the three viruses as do the individual vaccines given separately (Weibel *et al.*, 1979).

Heat lability

Live vaccines are vulnerable to inactivation by the high ambient temperatures encountered in the tropics. Since these countries are also, in the main, those with underdeveloped health services, formidable problems are encountered in maintaining refrigeration ('the cold chain') from manufacturer to the point of delivery, i.e. the child in some inaccessible rural village (Sabin, 1980). To some extent the problem has been alleviated by the addition of stabilising agents to the vaccines (Melnick, 1978; McAleer *et al.*, 1980), and by packaging them lyophilised (freeze-dried) for reconstitution immediately before administration.

VACCINATION POLICY

This leads us into a discussion of the medical, political, economic and sociological considerations which determine vaccination policy.

The aim of immunisation is generally thought of as the protection of the vaccinee. This is usually so, but in the case of certain vaccines (e.g. rubella in women; rotavirus and transmissible gastroenteritis in swine; bursal disease, infectious bronchitis, Newcastle disease and avian encephalomyelitis in fowls) the objective is to protect the vaccinee's offspring, by dint of maternal antibody. Under other circumstances an important auxiliary objective may be to protect unvaccinated members of the community (e.g. against poliomyelitis), either by natural spread of live vaccine virus, or by reducing the circulation of wild virus.

Universal vaccination may conceivably lead to the eradication of certain human viruses, such as measles, in much the same way as has been accomplished with smallpox (Fenner, 1982). The difficulties, however, are immeasurably greater, not only because these viruses are more widespread, but also because the diseases they cause do not engender the same degree of fear. Fear is the principal factor motivating people to seek or accept immunisation for themselves and their children. Even in the case of a feared disease such as polio, it is difficult to maintain enthusiasm for a programme of universal immunisation after the disease has been reduced to a rarity. Complacency has led to a limited resurgence of polio and measles in a number of countries with strong immunisation programmes. Continuation of routine immunisation after the threat of disease has almost vanished but the virus has not been totally eradicated is doubly essential because reduction in circulation of wild virus in the community has left unimmunised people uniquely susceptible, by removing the protective effect of repeated subclinical infections. Highly organised and resolute health services are called for. Particular attention must be given to unimmunised pockets, e.g. urban ghettos, immigrants, and certain religious minorities (Melnick, 1980). Legislation for compulsory immunisation against particular diseases prior to crossing national borders or entering school is perhaps the most effective single measure (Robbins et al., 1981).

Acceptability of a vaccine by the community is governed by a complex equation, balancing efficacy against safety, gain against risk, fear of the disease against fear of needles and side effects (Hennessen and Huygelen, 1979). If the disease is lethal or debilitating, e.g. poliomyelitis, the need for immunisation should be clear to all; both the people and the vaccine-licensing authorities will accept a small risk of even quite serious consequences of vaccination gone wrong (Centers for Disease Control, 1982a). If, on the other hand, the disease is perceived as trivial, no side effects will be countenanced. This is a major consideration with respiratory viral vaccines. It has already severely limited the acceptance of influenza vaccine and has led to calls for a government insurance scheme (such as obtains in Japan) to compensate victims of vaccination complications and protect vaccine manufacturers against legal liability for vaccines that have been licensed for use by the approved government authority (Melnick, 1977). Where equally satisfactory vaccines are available against a single disease, considerations such as cost and ease of administration tip the balance, e.g. towards oral poliovaccine (Melnick, 1978; 1980; Centers for Disease Control, 1982a).

A significant impediment to comprehensive vaccine coverage of the community is the unnecessarily complicated immunisation schedules officially recommended by some government health authorities. Most of the currently available vaccines, bacterial and viral, are aimed at preventing diseases the risks of which are greatest in early infancy. Optimally therefore, these vaccines should be given as soon as convenient, e.g. during the first six months of life for oral poliovaccine, or after maternal antibody has completely disappeared (12–15 months) in the case of systemically administered live vaccines for measles, mumps, and rubella (Table 7.4). Polyvalent vaccines, such as that available against measles/mumps/rubella confer a major practical advantage in

Table 7.4. Schedules for immunisation against human viral diseases[a].

Vaccine	Primary course	Subsequent doses
Live vaccines		
Poliomyelitis	2–6 months of age, then 1 or 2 further doses at 2–3 month intervals[b]	School entry
Measles	12 months[c] (single dose)	—
Rubella	12 months[d] (single dose)	High school entry[d] (girls only)
Mumps	12 months (single dose)	—
Yellow fever	Before travel to endemic area	10 years
Inactivated vaccines		
Influenza	Autumn[e]	Annual booster
Rabies	After bite, then at 3, 7, 14 and 28 days	—
Hepatitis B	When at risk[f], then 1 and 6 months later	?

[a]Schedules vary from country to country. This table is to be taken only as a guide.
[b]Two or three doses spaced two months apart during first year of life, commencing between 2 and 6 months of age. A further dose at 15–18 months is not essential but should be given if there is any doubt about whether the first three doses were received.
[c]Given on or shortly after first birthday in most developed countries, but as early as 6–9 months in some tropical developing countries where measles death rate is high in the second six months of life.
[d]Current U.S. policy is to immunise males and females shortly after first birthday. Current U.K. policy is to immunise females only, on entry into high school. Recommended here is a combination of both.
[e]Vulnerable groups only, e.g. old respiratory invalids.
[f]Vulnerable groups only, e.g. family contacts and babies of carriers, staff of hemodialysis units, blood banks, laboratories, hospitals, institutions for mentally retarded, etc., immunosuppressed, drug addicts, male homosexuals.

minimising the number of visits the mother must make to the clinic. Live vaccines are also much the most convenient in that repeated boosters are not normally required.

Developing countries of the tropics struggle with problems of a quite different order, compounded by poverty and pathetically inadequate health care infrastructure—maintenance of the cold chain in delivering live vaccines to remote rural villages is just one well known example (Assaad, 1979; Sabin, 1980). If the WHO Expanded Programme of Immunization (EPI), which calls for vaccination of all children against diphtheria, tetanus, pertussis, tuberculosis, poliomyelitis and measles by the year 1990, is to be fulfilled, much more will need to be done to assist the Third World in money and in kind.

PASSIVE IMMUNISATION

Instead of actively immunising with viral vaccines it is possible to confer short-term protection by the intramuscular administration of antibody, either as immune serum or immunoglobulin (Ig) purified therefrom (usually designated 'immune globulin', IG). Human Ig is preferred in human medicine, because heterologous protein provokes an immune response which can manifest itself as serum sickness or even anaphylaxis. Pooled normal human Ig can be relied upon to contain reasonably high concentrations of antibody against all the common viruses that cause systemic disease in man. Higher titres of course occur in 'convalescent' Ig from donors who have recovered from infection with the virus in question, and such specific immune globulin is the preferred product if commercially available, e.g. for rabies, varicella-zoster, or hepatitis B.

Although passive immunisation should be regarded only as an emergency procedure for the immediate protection of unimmunised individuals exposed to special risk, it is an important prophylactic measure in several human infections (World Health Organization, 1966). Normal human Ig has proved most effective in short-term post-exposure protection against hepatitis A of contacts of cases in families, schools, hospitals and other institutions, and (pre-exposure) in military personnel or travellers to developing countries (Centers for Disease Control, 1977). Hepatitis B immune globulin (HBIG), obtained ideally by plasmapheresis of multiply transfused patients with high titres of anti-HB$_s$, is effective in prompt post-exposure prophylaxis of hepatitis B, e.g. in staff of haemodialysis units, blood banks and serology laboratories, in newborn infants of HB$_e$Ag-positive mothers, and, some would argue, in family and homosexual contacts of carriers. Post-exposure prophylaxis against rabies includes rabies immune globulin (RIG) as well as active immunisation with inactivated vaccine (Centres for Disease

Control, 1980b). Varicella-zoster immune globulin (VZIG) is used to protect newborn babies of mothers with chickenpox at the time of delivery, as well as leukaemic or otherwise immunocompromised children following exposure to varicella or zoster (Centers for Disease Control, 1981b). Immunodeficient children, or babies too young to have been actively immunised, may be similarly protected against measles. However, passive immunisation is not effective against rubella and is not recommended as prophylaxis for pregnant women exposed to the virus.

Specific antibody can occasionally be used as therapy for an established viral disease. For instance, immune plasma dramatically reduced the mortality from Argentine haemorrhagic fever in a double-bind trial (Maiztegui *et al.*, 1979). Now that monoclonal antibodies of high specificity and high titre are readily obtainable, it is appropriate to re-examine the role of antibody in the treatment of established disease (Doherty *et al.*, 1982). It does not necessarily follow that a single monospecific monoclonal antibody will constitute the ultimate weapon. Indeed, there is good evidence that each viral protein bears a number of distinct antigenic domains, that more than one of these may be a binding site of neutralising antibody, and that monoclonal antibodies directed against any individual site can select mutants with substitutions in that site (Wiley *et al.*, 1981; Webster *et al.*, 1982). Hence, a reconstituted mixture of appropriate monoclonal antibodies might represent the optimal passive immunotherapy of the future.

HUMAN VIRAL VACCINES

The principles of vaccine production and usage outlined here are best illustrated by actual examples. Accordingly, the characteristics of the major human viral vaccines (Table 7.5; reviews: Melnick, 1977; Horstmann, 1979; Hilleman, 1980; Meyer *et al.*, 1980; Chanock, 1981; Sabin, 1981a), plus others in the process of development or clinical trial, will be discussed.

Smallpox

Long before the formulation of the germ theory of infectious disease, a practice known as 'variolation' was widely employed in China and the Middle East to protect infants against smallpox. This procedure consisted of inoculation with material taken from the pustules of smallpox patients, and, as might be expected, conferred a significant mortality of its own! Jenner's subsequent use of cowpox virus for intradermal 'vaccination', following his famous observation that milkmaids were

Table 7.5. Viral vaccines recommended for use in man[a].

Disease	Vaccine strain	Cell substrate	Attenuation	Inactivation	Route
Rabies	Pasteur	HEF	−	BPL or TBP	i.m. or i.d.
Yellow Fever	17D	Chick embryo	+	—	s.c.
Poliomyelitis	Sabin 1, 2, 3 (OPV)	HEF	+	—	Oral
Measles	Schwarz	CEF	+	—	s.c.
Rubella	RA27/3 or Cendehill	HEF or RK	+	—	s.c.
Mumps	Jeryl Lynn	CEF	+	—	s.c.
Influenza	A/H3N2, B, (A/H1N1)	Chick embryo	−	BPL or formalin or HANA subunits	i.m.
Hepatitis B	—[c]	—	−	HB_sAg[c]	i.m.

[a]A wide variety of different viral strains and cell substrates are used in different countries; the selection listed is not comprehensive.
[b]Abbreviations: BPL = β-propiolactone; CEF = chick embryo fibroblast cultures; HEF = diploid strain of human embryonic fibroblasts; i.d. = intradermally; i.m. = intramuscular; RK = rabbit kidney cultures; s.c. = subcutaneous; TBP = tri-(n)-butylphosphate.
[c]Hepatitis B surface antigen purified from serum of human donors, then formalin-treated.

immune to smallpox was, and remains, one of the milestones in the history of medical science (Jenner, 1798). The precise origin of vaccinia virus, used so successfully for vaccination during the past century or more is, remarkably, quite unknown. But all this is now irrelevant, for smallpox, the most feared of all the great plagues of mankind, was declared in 1980 to have been eradicated from the earth, so rendering vaccination redundant. Accordingly, the vaccine will not be discussed further here; readers interested in the history of smallpox and the triumphant success story of its eradication by vaccination may consult Fenner (1982), or Fenner *et al.* (in press).

Rabies

We shall shortly celebrate the centenary of the first successful clinical trial of a vaccine against rabies (Pasteur, 1885). Since then, a succession of vaccines based on Louis Pasteur's 'fixed' rabies virus have been used to protect those unfortunate enough to have been bitten by a rabid animal. Though virtually 100% lethal, this greatly feared disease can be prevented by active immunisation after infection, because of its un-usually long incubation period.

A human diploid cell vaccine (HDCV) developed at the Wistar Institute (Wiktor *et al.*, 1978; Plotkin, 1980) has now supplanted all previous vaccines. Grown in WI-38 or MRC-5 cell strains, the virus is concentrated by ultrafiltration or rate zonal centrifugation, then inactivated with β-propiolactone or tri-(n) butylphosphate. The latter is a solvent which 'splits' the virion into 'subunits'. Rabies subunit vaccines are reviewed by Wunner *et al.* (1983).

A typical post-exposure immunisation course consists of five intra-muscular injections of HDCV on days 0, 3, 7, 14 and 28, accompanied by a single dose of human rabies hyperimmune globulin on day 0 (Centers for Disease Control, 1980b). None of some hundreds of people vaccinated following the bite of proven rabid animals in Iran, Germany and the U.S.A. up till 1980 developed rabies (Plotkin, 1980; Anderson *et al.*, 1980). Moreover, the vaccine is clearly much safer than earlier preparations which were notorious for their high incidence of anaphyl-axis and neurological sequelae. Local reactions (pain, erythema, itching) and mild systemic reactions are common (approx. 20%). Recent data suggest that multiple intradermal injections on day 0 only may achieve a rapid response with considerable cost savings.

The vaccine may of course also be used to provide pre-exposure prophylaxis for people whose professions bring them into contact with animals, e.g. veterinarians, trappers, animal handlers, laboratory workers and long-term visitors to endemic areas. Domestic animals, particularly dogs and cats, can be immunised by injection of live attenu-ated vaccine. A unique approach to the immunisation of wild animals, such as the foxes currently responsible for the dissemination of rabies across Europe, is the campaign launched on an experimental basis in the Swiss Alps in 1982 to drop from the air, bait containing live attenuated rabies vaccine virus.

Despite the success of HDCV, research proceeds on a number of fronts. The demonstration that interferon is effective in protecting animals after challenge with rabies virus (see Baer, 1978; Plotkin, 1980) suggests that a combination of interferon with vaccine may be the most certain way of preventing rabies post-exposure. Vero cells on microcarriers in suspension culture are being used in lieu of human diploid cells at the Merieux Institute to reduce the cost of the vaccine. Wiktor and Koprowski (1982) have postulated that strain variation which they have detected among wild rabies viruses prevalent in different parts of the world may explain some recent apparent vaccine failures and justify the incorporation of additional or more broadly reactive variants in future vaccines. Coulon et al. (1982) have been able to select avirulent rabies mutants by growing virus in the presence of particular monoclonal antibodies; this could be developed as a useful general approach to the attenuation of viruses for possible use as live vaccines. Finally, following the cloning of the gene representing the membrane glycoprotein of rabies virus (Yelverton et al., 1983), a genetically engineered vaccine looks to be a real possibility, although protection of experimental animals has yet to be demonstrated (Wunner et al., 1983). Reagan et al. (1983) elicited virus-neutralising antibodies by immunisation of mice with anti-idiotypic antibody (directed against the idiotypic determinants on monoclonal antibodies to rabies glycoprotein).

Yellow fever and other arboviruses

Years ago Theiler and Smith (1937) developed on a purely empirical basis a first-rate vaccine against yellow fever. Virus isolated in a monkey was passaged through mice, cell cultures and finally embryonated eggs to give the 17D strain that comprises the present-day living avirulent vaccine (Monath et al., 1983). The vaccine is administered subcutaneously, after reconstitution from the lyophilised state. Side-effects are minimal (5–10% mild headache, fever or myalgia); encephalitis in children is an exceedingly rare complication (10^{-7}). Protection is long-lasting, but boosters every ten years are required (WHO, 1971). There is a case for updating the manufacturing procedures, e.g. to insist on SPF and leukosis-free chickens and to move towards exclusively cell culture (CEF) grown vaccine (WHO, 1983b).

A formalin-inactivated, mouse brain-derived Japanese encephalitis vaccine is routinely administered to Japanese children and has dramatically reduced the incidence of that disease in Japan (Hammon et al., 1971). A more potent formalin-killed vaccine derived from virus grown in cultured hamster kidney cells has proved to be at least as efficacious as its predecessor (>80%) in field trials, and no encephalitis or other serious side-effects have so far been reported in vaccinees (WHO, 1983b). However, like the mouse brain vaccine, it induces only short-lived immunity, hence regular boosters will be necessary. A live vaccine is used in horses and in the principal domestic animal host, the pig. Another formalin-inactivated vaccine, against tick-borne encephalitis, is produced in chick embryonic fibroblast cultures, and administered to vulnerable populations in Eastern Europe as a primary course of injections followed by annual boosters. Improved, more concentrated versions of this vaccine, recently developed in the USSR and Austria, are reported to give 85–100% seroconversion following a single subcutaneous inoculation, to prevent paralysis and to reduce the incidence of meningoencephalitis (WHO, 1983b). For some years a live vaccine (TC-83) has been used successfully for the protection of laboratory workers as well as horses against Venezuelan equine encephalitis; more recently, a formalin-inactivated vaccine (C-84) prepared from the attenuated TC-83 strain has been shown to be protective and safe (Edelman et al., 1979). Inactivated vaccines are also available against Rift Valley fever.

The desirability of a vaccine against the most widespread of all the arboviral diseases, dengue fever, must be considered in the light of the current debate about the pathogenesis of dengue haemorrhagic fever/shock syndrome (see Chapter 4). If indeed the syndrome is the result of enhanced viral replication in the presence of antibody to a heterologous serotype ('immune infection enhancement'; Halstead, 1981), then widespread active immunisation against dengue could turn out to be a disaster unless protective levels of antibodies against all four types could be guaranteed for life.

The haemorrhagic fevers and the encephalitides are among the most lethal of all viral diseases. Effective vaccines, selectively employed in particular regions of the tropics, could be very valuable. However, pharmaceutical companies generally do not feel in a position to undertake the costly development and testing required, and safety considerations impose great restraints on laboratory work with these highly dangerous arenaviruses, rhabdoviruses, filoviruses, bunyaviruses and togaviruses, hence vaccines may be some distance away. Recombinant DNA technology may prove to be the shortest cut to a totally safe product.

Poliomyelitis

Throughout most of Europe, North America, Japan and Australasia, poliomyelitis, once the most feared of all viral diseases in the 'developed' countries of the world, has all but passed into history as a result of immunisation. The credit for this remarkable achievement goes firstly to

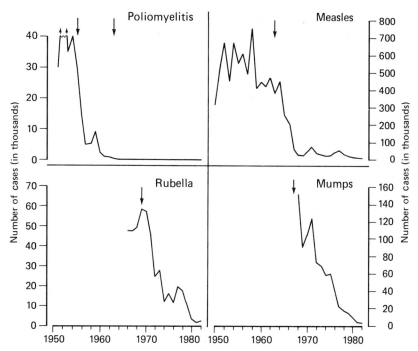

Fig. 7.2. Annual incidence of various viral diseases in the USA: date of introduction of vaccine indicated by arrow. Compiled from data kindly supplied by the Centers for Disease Control.

Enders, Weller and Robbins (1949) for their Nobel Prize winning discovery that poliovirus could be grown in monolayer cultures of nonneural cells, then to Salk for the production in 1954 of his inactivated polio vaccine (IPV; see Salk, 1958), and finally to Sabin (1957) and Koprowski (1957) for the development a couple of years later of live attenuated oral vaccines (OPV). Though both 'Salk' and 'Sabin' vaccines proved to be dramatically effective in reducing the incidence of disease by over 1000-fold in the Western world (Fig. 7.2), the greater convenience and lower cost of OPV ensured that it soon replaced IPV everywhere except in Sweden, Finland, Iceland and Holland (Melnick, 1978; 1980; Horstmann, 1979).

OPV is a 'trivalent' vaccine, consisting of attenuated strains of all three types. Traditionally the viruses have been grown in primary cultures of monkey kidney, carefully monitored to exclude contaminating simian viruses, some of which (herpes B and Marburg) are lethal to man and others (SV40) oncogenic for laboratory rodents. More recently, strains of diploid human embryonic fibroblasts such as WI-38, MRC-5, HEL-299 or IMR-90 have been preferred. Attenuation is confirmed by absence of neurovirulence for monkeys (Nakano *et al.*, 1978).

The three types are then pooled in carefully adjusted proportions (10^5–10^6 $TCID_{50}$ of each) to balance numbers against growth rate, hence minimise the probability of mutual interference. In the presence of molar $MgCl_2$ buffered at pH 6.5–6.9 to protect the virus against heat inactivation (Melnick, 1978), the vaccine is stable for about a year under proper conditions of refrigeration (but for only a few days at 37°C). It can be administered simply, by unqualified personnel. OPV is usually given in the first six months of life, in three doses, spaced two months apart, to maximise the chances of a successful 'take' even if concurrent infection with another enterovirus should happen to interfere with the replication of one or more of them on one or more occasion, as commonly occurs in the developing countries of the tropics (Sabin, 1980). Earlier concern that breast-feeding may represent a contraindication has not been substantiated—though colostrum contains moderate titres of maternal IgA, milk itself does not contain enough antibody to neutralise the vaccine virus (Sabin, 1980).

Two further significant advantages of OPV over IPV follow from the fact that it multiplies in the alimentary tract. Firstly, this subclinical infection elicits the prolonged synthesis not only of IgG antibodies which protect the individual against paralytic poliomyelitis (as does IPV) by intercepting wild polioviruses during their viraemic phase, but also of 'copro-antibodies' of the IgA class (Ogra, 1971) which prevent primary implantation of wild virus in the gut, and hence diminish very considerably the circulation of virulent viruses in the community (Sabin, 1957). Indeed, wild polioviruses have now virtually disappeared from countries such as the U.S.A.; the only strains that can be isolated from sewage, for example, are 'vaccine-like'. This striking replacement of wild virus by vaccine strains is facilitated by the fact that the latter are excreted in the faeces and spread to non-immune contacts (see Fox and Hall, 1980).

A consequence of the spread of vaccine virus to contacts is that it provides greater opportunity for the selection of mutants displaying varying degrees of reversion towards virulence (Kew et al., 1981; Nakano et al., 1978). Very rarely, a family contact of a vaccinee, or even more rarely the vaccinee himself, develops poliomyelitis, usually type 3 (or type 2, especially in contacts). The incidence is hard to ascertain as some of the so-called 'vaccine-associated' poliomyelitis (defined as occurring within a month of OPV) may not in fact be polio (Sabin, 1981b), but the upper limit would appear to be about one case per million vaccinees (Nightingale, 1977; Nathanson and Martin, 1979; WHO Consultative Group, 1982). By any standards therefore, this is a very safe vaccine; the fact that around half of the cases of paralytic poliomyelitis in the U.S.A. today are 'vaccine-associated' is testimony to the extraordinary success of OPV rather than a reason for returning to IPV, as is currently being seriously proposed in some quarters (Salk and Salk, 1977; Salk, 1980; Hennessen and van Wezel, 1981). Despite the outstanding success of IPV in Scandinavia, where over 95% of the population have been immunised, doubts about the permanence of the immunity following a childhood course of IPV, plus its cost and the general unpopularity of needles argue against its widespread reintroduction in other parts of the world.

Nevertheless, certain refinements of the present OPV policy are called for and have recently been recommended for general implementation in the U.S.A. (Nightingale, 1977; Centers for Disease Control, 1982a). Because OPV-associated polio is 10 000 times more common in those who are immunocompromised in some way (Melnick, 1980) only IPV should be used in such cases. Secondly, because there are still significant numbers of parents who have never received polio vaccine, there are good arguments for immunising such non-immune family contacts prior to or simultaneously with their infants (Melnick, 1978; 1980), as well as for routine boosters for every child at one year, then on entering school, and again on entering high school (Nightingale, 1977). Thirdly, it has been recommended that non-immunised adults travelling to developing countries where polio is still endemic should receive IPV rather than OPV because of the slightly higher risk of OPV-associated polio in adults; however the data on this latter point are marginal and the established dogma that non-immune adults are more prone to paralysis by wild poliovirus than are young children has been cogently challenged (Nathanson and Martin, 1979).

IPV of greater potency is now being introduced as a result of a number of technological improvements (Hennessen and van Wezel, 1981). Since many species of monkeys are declared to be endangered and cannot lawfully be exported from their countries of origin, they are now bred in captivity and can be more effectively screened for adventitious herpes B and 'foamy' viruses. Cynomolgus monkey kidney cells are subcultured for a few generations and grown on the surface of myriads of DEAE-Sephadex beads known as 'microcarriers' suspended in large fermentation tanks (van Wezel et al., 1978). Unfortunately, human diploid cell strains do not grow sufficiently well to make them a commercial proposition for production of the very large amounts of virus required for IPV, but nonmalignant, aneuploid monkey kidney cell lines such as Vero, LLC-MK$_2$ or CV-1 (Montagnon et al., 1981) have recently been approved for this purpose. Following clarification, virus is purified from the supernatant by gel filtration and ion exchange chromatography, e.g. on DEAE-Sepharose 6B, or affinity chromatography on Sepharose 4B-immobilised antibodies, and/or zonal ultracentrifugation (van Wezel, 1981). The importance of ultracentrifugation before inactivation with formaldehyde was established many years ago following the 1955 disaster in which clumped virus escaped inactivation and paralysed numerous children in the U.S.A. (Gard, 1960). Two doses of the newer preparations of IPV appear to confer protection equivalent to the four previously required; this has encouraged the proposal that IPV replace OPV, particularly in the Third World, where unsatisfactory seroconversion rates are frequently reported even after the full course of three doses of OPV (Salk, 1980; Hennessen and van Wezel, 1981; Beale, 1982). Since two injections of 'triple vaccine' (against diphtheria, pertussis and tetanus) is already the standard regime in most countries, it would not be too difficult to add IPV to the cocktail to make a 'quadruple' vaccine.

In stark contrast to the dramatic success of the polio vaccination programmes of the wealthy temperate countries, relatively little impact has been made on the disease throughout most of the Third World (Sabin, 1981b). The reasons for this are complex but are mainly due to the lack of adequate health service infrastructure. OPV is simply not delivered satisfactorily to the children, particularly in inaccessible rural villages. In most developing countries it is still true to say that most children never receive a full course of OPV and that, even when they do, there are doubts whether the viability of the virus has been retained by adequate refrigeration during storage and transport in hot tropical climates. Maintenance of the cold chain is typical of the type of problem to which much greater attention is now being paid (Assaad, 1979; Sabin, 1980). It is also suggested that much more extensive coverage can be obtained by annual mass immunisation campaigns aimed at all children under the age of say 3–5 years, on two nominated days two months apart (Borgono et al., 1980; Sabin, 1980; 1981b). There is a case for using only type 1 for the first dose (and also in the face of a known type 1 epidemic) as at least 85% of paralytic cases are attributable to this sero-type (Sabin, 1980). Such a policy would pick up those children who happened to miss out in a previous year, whether by reason of viral interference, cold chain breakdown or whatever. That polio can indeed be, to all intents, eradicated by comprehensive coverage with OPV in developing countries has been amply demonstrated by the superb record of Chile, Brazil and Cuba, to name three particularly impressive examples (Borgono et al., 1980; Sabin, 1980).

Eradication of poliomyelitis from the Third World is a major objective of WHO's Expanded Programme of Immunization (EPI) (Assaad, 1979; Sabin, 1980, 1981b). In the more advanced nations the disease has been effectively conquered but it remains imperative that very high levels of immunisation are maintained in spite of the lack of perceived threat. Pockets of immunised people, e.g. immigrants concentrated in urban ghettos, are particularly vulnerable to imported viruses; similarly, out-breaks occurred among the Arab population of Gaza and the West Bank of the Jordan during the 1970s (Melnick, 1980). Another recent salutory instance was the outbreak of poliomyelitis in 1978 in Holland which was confined entirely to members of a particular religious minority who had refused immunisation. The epidemic spread to Canada and then to the U.S.A. where it affected only unimmunised members of the Amish community, causing many cases of paralysis (Melnick, 1980).

Measles

Though a relatively harmless disease in the average child, measles is complicated by serious sequelae (see Chapter 5) sufficiently often to make it a common cause of death in unimmunised communities.

The live attenuated vaccine (Katz *et al.*, 1983) was developed by Enders and colleagues by serial passage successively through human kidney and human amnion cell cultures, then the amnion of the developing chick embryo, and finally chick embryo cell cultures (see Enders and Katz, 1967) then further attenuated by Schwartz (1964). In most of the developed countries the vaccine is injected subcutaneously at or shortly after twelve months of age, when maternal antibody has disappeared. However, in tropical countries where measles is still a major killer of malnourished infants in the first year of life (Morley, 1967), some advocate immunisation as early as nine (or even six) months. Seroconversion occurs in over 95% of 15-month-old recipients, but in only 50–75% at six months, depending on the particular country in which the study is undertaken (Black, 1982). Antibody titres are lower than following natural infection but persist for many years at protective levels Krugman, 1977; Weibel *et al.*, 1979). Trivial side effects are not uncommon, particularly mild fever (5–15%) and transient rashes (5%); encephalopathy has been reported but is very rare (Centers for Disease Control, 1982b). Immunocompromised patients, though vulnerable to measles, should not be vaccinated.

Today, indigenous measles has almost disappeared from the U.S.A. (Hinman *et al.*, 1980; see also Fig. 7.2), where immunisation of children prior to (otherwise after) school entry is now required by law (Robbins *et al.*, 1981). Many of the cases that still occur follow importations from abroad. As expected, the age distribution has shifted upwards and eradication of the disease will require more comprehensive immunisation of older children and young adults as well as infants, at least for a 'catch-up' period of a decade or so.

In the developing countries of the tropics, where measles ranks with gastroenteritis and pneumonia as the major causes of death in childhood (Morley, 1980; Walsh and Warren, 1979) immunisation is a top priority. The optimum age of immunisation is the subject of debate and may differ from country to country depending upon the extent of protein malnutrition and age/mortality statistics (Black, 1982). Maintenance of the cold chain is particularly important; the freeze-dried vaccine stores well at 4°C but, after reconstitution, is particularly vulnerable to inactivation by heat and light (McAleer *et al.*, 1980). More stable vaccines are now becoming available (Hilleman *et al.*, 1983). Sabin *et al.* (1983) have recently reported immunisation of children, including 4–6 month olds possessing substantial levels of maternal antibody, by a live attenuated measles vaccine delivered as an aerosol from a nebulizer via a face mask.

Rubella

Vaccination against rubella is aimed not so much at protection of the recipient against this trivial disease as at protection of her offspring against the devastating teratogenic effects of infection occurring during the first trimester of pregnancy (Gregg, 1941; see Chapter 2).

The first rubella vaccine, HPV-77, developed in the mid-60s by Parkman and Meyer (1969) has now been replaced by two other attenuated vaccines. These are the Cendehill-51 strain developed in Belgium by Huygelen *et al.* (1969) by 53 passages, 51 of which were in primary rabbit kidney cells at 34°C, and RA27/3, derived by Plotkin *et al.* (1969) by 25–27 passages in the human diploid cell strain WI-38. Though the latter has been successfully given intranasally, both of these vaccines are routinely administered subcutaneously. A single injection protects over 95% of recipients. Antibody titres are significantly lower than following natural infection, particularly with Cendehill; RA27/3 induces a wider range of antibodies which remain at higher levels and protect against challenge for a longer period (reviews: Krugman, 1977; Horstmann, 1979; Preblud *et al.*, 1980). Nevertheless, reinfection, generally subclinical, occurs quite frequently during the years following immunisation with any of the vaccines, thereby providing a natural boost to immunity.

Though substantially attenuated, rubella vaccines commonly induce one significant side effect, namely arthralgia. This is seen mainly in adult females, is usually confined to the small peripheral joints and only rarely progresses to frank arthritis (Preblud *et al.*, 1980). Rarely such arthritis may persist for years with recurrent exacerbations during which the virus may be isolated from lymphocytes (Chantler *et al.*, 1981). Lymphadenopathy, a fleeting rash, or low grade fever are not uncommon, while unusual peripheral neuritic symptoms have been reported to occur quite rarely (Preblud *et al.*, 1980).

The vaccine virus, which of course multiplies in the body, is shed in small amounts from the respiratory tract of the vaccinee, but seems to be incapable of spreading to contacts (see Preblud *et al.*, 1980).

There is no evidence that the vaccine virus is teratogenic (Preblud *et al.*, 1981). Hence, accidental immunisation during pregnancy is not considered to be an indication for termination (Centers for Disease Control, 1981a). Nevertheless, since the vaccine virus is known to cross the placenta and infect the foetus, prudence suggests that women not be deliberately immunised during the first trimester and that non-pregnant vaccinees should be advised to avoid conception for the next 2–3 months and/or immunised immediately post-partum (Preblud *et al.*, 1980).

From the outset in 1969, two opposing schools of thought dictated the strategies of rubella vaccine programmes in different parts of the world. In the U.K. and Australia for example, the primary target population has been teenage females; the policy has been to immunise all girls on entry into high school (i.e. usually 12–13 years of age). By contrast, the U.S.A. has aimed to immunise all children, male and female, early in the second year of life. An ancillary feature of both policies has been to immunise seronegative females of childbearing age.

The rationale of the U.K. approach is that, because naturally acquired immunity is demonstrably more effective and more lasting than that induced by any vaccine, it is desirable not to interfere with the circulation of wild virus in the community but to allow it to infect the majority of children. Immunisation of pubescent girls is therefore intended to protect that 50% or less who have not acquired immunity naturally by the time they enter high shcool. This cohort will be protected during the crucial childbearing years more efficiently than had they been vaccinated as infants, because immunity is known to decay within the years following immunisation. Furthermore, the immunity of these women will be boosted further by subclinical infections they may receive as a result of the fact that a vaccination programme confined to post-primary school children will not significantly diminish the circulation of wild virus in the community.

The logic of the U.S. policy, on the other hand, is that universal immunisation of all children in the second year of life could theoretically eradicate the virus entirely from the community, as has been achieved with smallpox, and very nearly with poliomyelitis and measles, following similar strategies.

Neither strategy can be deemed an unqualified success. As would be expected from the fact that rubella circulates mainly among children of preschool and primary school age, the U.K. programme has had no demonstrable effect on the overall incidence of rubella; more disturbingly however, it has not yet apparently led to a major decline in the incidence of the congenital rubella syndrome, 'CRS', probably because the coverage of teenage girls has been inadequate and most women in the 25–45 age group have been missed entirely (Dudgeon, 1979; Preblud *et al.*, 1980). The U.S. programme, on the other hand, has led to a substantial decline in the incidence of rubella in children, but not in adolescents or adults, and has had only a modest impact on the occurrence of CRS (Krugman, 1977; Preblud *et al.*, 1980). This too is not unexpected as the cohort at which the vaccine was targeted during the 1970s is only now moving into the childbearing years.

Knox (1980) designed a computer simulation model which demonstrates why neither strategy can be expected to succeed unless a higher vaccine coverage can be attained. Perhaps the most disturbing conclusion from his graphs is that half-hearted pursuit of the U.S. policy may be expected to lead to an actual increase in the incidence of CRS. The currently inadequate vaccine coverage may, by diminishing but not abolishing the circulation of virus, greatly increase the chance that the first encounter the unvaccinated minority have with wild virus will be delayed until the childbearing years. Moreover, if vaccination in infancy does not induce a level of immunity that, in the absence of sufficient circulating wild virus to boost the response, will protect for at least 40 years, there is an additional grave risk of a 'rebound' in the occurrence of CRS in women who will reach their 20s and 30s several years hence.

These calculations indicate firstly, that careful studies must be undertaken to determine the level and duration of immunity up to 40 years after RA27/3 and Cendehill vaccines, in the absence as well as in the presence of natural subclinical booster infections; secondly, that the vaccine uptake rate must be increased to at least 80–90%, whichever vaccination schedule is employed; and thirdly, that the ideal strategy is universal (>90%) coverage of one-year-olds, male and female, coupled with a policy, for the next several years at least, of vigorous pursuit and immunisation of non-immune 15–40-year-old women. The latter can most conveniently be vaccinated on entry into educational establishments or workplaces, family planning clinics, or post-partum; laboratory determination of antibody status is not essential, particularly if the cost of the vaccine is lower than that of an HI test. The foregoing has now been adopted as the revised rubella vaccination policy for the U.S.A. (Centers for Disease Control, 1981a).

Mumps

Mumps do not pose an important threat to life but can give rise to unpleasant complications, notably orchitis in up to 20% of males infected after puberty, but also pancreatitis, meningitis and more rarely encephalitis. A highly satifactory live attenuated vaccine derived by passage of the Jeryl Lynn strain in chick fibroblasts is now widely used in the U.S.A. in combination with live attenuated measles and rubella (Stokes *et al.*, 1971), at 12–15 months of age, or alone, particularly to adolescent males (Centers for Disease Control, 1980a). Protective levels of antibody in at least 95% of recipients are conferred by a single subcutaneous injection and persist for at least a decade (Weibel *et al.*, 1979). A marked decline in the incidence of mumps has occurred in the U.S.A. since the introduction of the vaccine (Fig. 7.2; Hayden *et al.*, 1978). Occasional allergic reactions to the vaccine and rarely, parotitis or CNS disturbances have been reported.

Influenza

No disease illustrates better than influenza the difficulties of control by immunisation and the ingenuity required to overcome them. Notorious for its propensity for antigenic shift and drift (see Chapter 6), the virus is constantly changing, so rendering the current vaccine obsolete. Hence WHO's extensive network of laboratories around the globe must remain continuously alert to the emergence of novel strains which are then made available to update existing vaccines.

The conventional product is an egg-grown, formalin- or β-propio-lactone-inactivated vaccine incorporating the equivalent of 15–25 μg of haemagglutinin (HA) of each of the latest prevalent strains of influenza types A and B (reviews: Perkins and Regamy, 1977; Tyrrell and Smith, 1979; Dowdle, 1981; Tyrrell et al., 1981; Potter, 1982). This polyvalent vaccine is injected (i.m.) annually in late autumn into those most vulnerable to the 'excess mortality' observed during winter epidemics, namely old people and persons with chronic respiratory, cardiac or renal disease, diabetes, anaemia or immunodeficiency; some also advocate inclusion of medical personnel and those providing vital community services, while others point out that the principal disseminators of virus during an epidemic are school children. Side effects of redness and induration at the injection site, fever, malaise and occasionally myalgia are not uncommon, particularly in children, but are reduced with 'disrupted' ('split-virus') vaccines, in which the envelope of the formalin-inactivated virion has been disrupted with cetyltrimethyl-ammonium bromide, n-butylphosphate, ether or deoxycholate. Allergy to eggs is a contraindication. A particularly serious problem, the Guillain-Barré syndrome, was encountered in one of every 10^5 Americans vaccinated against 'swine flu', i.e. A/New Jersey/76 (H1N1), during a mass campaign in 1976–7 (Schonberger et al., 1979), but no such association has been reported with any subsequent influenza vaccine.

Protection is at best of the order of 70% for 1–2 years following immunisation with the latest strain of influenza, but is often much lower in the most important target group, the elderly (Dowdle, 1981; Tyrrell and Smith, 1979). Our best efforts can be sabotaged by 'original antigenic sin', the phenomenon in which the immune response to vaccination (or to natural infection) is characterised by an anamnestic recall of antibody directed against an earlier strain with which the vaccinee was previously vaccinated (or infected) (see Chapter 3). The problem is well illustrated by the finding of Hoskins et al. (1979) that immunisation of schoolchildren with a vaccine against the current influenza strain provided no protection in those immunised annually for a number of years with the most up-to-date vaccine.

One approach to improving the response, in 'virgin' populations at least, would be to increase the dose quite substantially (Dowdle, 1981), but this involves a marked increase in both cost and side effects. Production costs are reduced somewhat by a clever technique, first introduced by Kilbourne and Murphy (1960), namely genetic reassortment between the new strain and an established laboratory 'master strain' known for its high yield in eggs (Kilbourne, 1969). Side effects can be reduced by the use of purified HA, or HA plus neuraminidase (NA), together with a suitable adjuvant, e.g. the 'HANA' vaccine currently in use in the U.K. (see Tyrrell and Smith, 1979).

There are a number of more recent developments which could be exploited for vaccine production. Firstly, liposomes ('virosomes' or 'immunosomes'), as mentioned earlier in this chapter, can be constituted from influenzal HA and NA, lipids such as cholesterol selected for their lack of pyrogenicity, and saponin as an adjuvant, and induce good immune responses experimentally (Gregoriadis, 1976; Brand et al., personal communication). (The relative importance of NA in inducing immunity is a controversial question; Kilbourne (1969) has advocated the use of vaccines that will elicit only an anti-NA response, in the expectation that this will permit infection to occur but limit its spread.) Secondly, a DNA copy of the (RNA) gene for HA has been cloned, not only in E. coli using a plasmid as vector (Emtage et al., 1980) but more recently also in mammalian (simian) cells using SV40 DNA as vector (Gething and Sambrook, 1981; Sveda and Lai, 1981). In monkey kidney cells the HA is glycosylated and, furthermore, is secreted into the supernatant if the DNA sequence coding for the hydrophobic C-terminus of the HA molecule (the membrane attachment site) is excised (Sveda et al., 1982). Thirdly, the HA gene has been incorporated by recombination into the genome of vaccinia virus; vaccinated animals develop neutralising antibodies and resist intranasal challenge with influenza (Panicali et al. (1983); Paoletti and Panicali; Smith et al., in Lerner and Chanock, 1984). Fourthly, since the complete sequence of the HA of any strain of influenza can now be rapidly determined and the location of the critical antigenic sites on the surface of the molecule is also known (Laver and Air, 1980; Wiley et al., 1981; Webster et al., 1982), it is possible to synthesise de novo any particular antigenic site (N. Green et al., 1982; Jackson et al., 1982; Müller et al., 1982). Conceivably, a conserved portion of the HA molecule which, being relatively non-immunogenic under natural conditions and hence not subject to antigenic drift, may nevertheless, if injected in the form of a synthetic peptide, be capable of eliciting cross-reactive antibodies protecting against many or all potential strains of influenza A (Lerner, 1982). Such a peptide would probably need to be coupled to a suitable carrier and/or emulsified with a potent but safe adjuvant in order to elicit a satifactory antibody response.

There are, however, good reasons for supposing that live vaccines may represent a superior alternative to all the options discussed so far. Firstly, there is evidence that T cells play an important role in recovery from influenza infection (see Askonas *et al.*, 1982), that these lymphocytes display marked cross-recognition of differerent strains and even different subtypes (Anders *et al.*, 1981a, b; Askonas *et al.*, 1982) and that their clonal expansion may be elicited only by live virus (Ada *et al.*, 1981). Secondly, live vaccines, administered intranasally, elicit a 'natural' IgA response (Chanock *et al.*, 1975), although it must be added that Couch *et al.* (1981) believe serum IgG to be more important.

Live influenza vaccines have been in use for decades in the U.S.S.R. since exploitation of mutants obtained by serial passage in eggs was first suggested for this purpose by Burnet (1943), but the efficacy, safety and stability of these host-range mutants has never been fully documented. Following up the Russian observation that mutants resistant to an inhibitor of haemagglutination found in horse serum were attenuated in virulence for man, Beare (1975) developed live influenza vaccines which were widely tested in Britain during the 70s. However, it has still not been demonstrated that any particular gene is responsible for virulence; the evidence indicates that any or all may be involved (Palese and Roizman, 1980). It has been suggested that attenuation might be quite regularly accomplished by reassorting the three P (polymerase) genes. Recently, Murphy *et al.* (1982), reasoning that a reassortant containing six genes derived from an avian influenza strain might be avirulent but immunogenic in man, have demonstrated that such a reassortant delivered transtracheally to monkeys is in fact protective; preliminary human trials (Murphy *et al.*, personal communication) indicate that the reassortant multiples satisfactorily in the upper respiratory tract without symptoms.

During the last decade or so, painstaking efforts have been made to develop vaccines from two other types of mutant: temperature-sensitive (*ts*) mutants and 'cold-adapted' (*ca*) mutants. Following the demonstration that *ts* mutants of influenza virus are attenuated in virulence (Mackenzie, 1969), Chanock and colleagues at the U.S. National Institutes of Health developed the notion that *ts* mutants might be safely employed as live vaccines in man. These workers exploited genetic reassortment to derive potential vaccine strains containing the HA and NA genes from the influenza strain against which they wished to immunise, together with *ts* genes for the non-surface proteins from an established laboratory strain (Chanock and Murphy, 1980; Murphy and Chanock, 1981). Chemical mutagenesis with 5-fluorouracil was employed to introduce *ts* mutations into the master strain A/Udorn/72 (H3N2). Reassortants containing *ts* lesions in two separate genes (P1 and P3) were *ts*, with a shutoff temperature of 37°C, yet multiplied satisfactorily in the upper respiratory tract of the hamster or man, inducing an immune response capable of protecting against subsequent challenge with virulent wild-type virus. However, to everyone's bitter disappointment, the vaccine virus displayed a tendency to lose its temperature sensitivity during replication in man. The cause of this genetic instability was investigated very thoroughly and discovered to be surprisingly complex. At least three new mutations had emerged in the revertant, at least one of which did not display the characteristics of a simple reversion but was a suppressor mutation in the P2 gene that corrected the *ts* phenotype of the P3 gene product (Murphy *et al.*, 1980).

Mention has been made of Maassab's cold-adapted (*ca*) mutants of influenza A/Ann Arbor/60 (H2N2) which are avirulent for ferrets, grow as well at 25°C as at 33°C, and are also *ts*, with a ceiling temperature of 37°C. While the mutations have yet to be characterised biochemically and genetically, there is some evidence that the changes in the P1, P2, P3 and M genes may be principally responsible for the *ca* phenotype. Reassortants containing 6 *ca* genes from the master (donor) strain and only the HA and NA genes from the recipient wild-type strain, are *ca*, *ts* and highly attenuated for man when administered intranasally. Clinical trials currently underway indicate that these *ca* recombinants revert only rarely and partially, hence seem to be promising candidates for more general introduction as live attenuated intranasal vaccines (Maassab *et al.*, 1981; Murphy and Chanock, 1981; Kendal *et al.*, 1982; Wright *et al.*, 1982).

Chanock (1981) has discussed the possibility of constructing deletion mutants of influenza virus using the protocol of Lai *et al.* (1980), set out earlier in this chapter.

Respiratory syncytial virus

RSV is the most important cause of serious lower respiratory tract infection (bronchiolitis and pneumonitis) in infants, and there is an evident need for a vaccine, particularly to protect premature and sickly infants in hospitals and 'homes for foundlings'. Chanock and his colleagues at NIH have devoted many years of painstaking effort to a succession of unsuccessful attempts to develop a satisfactory vaccine. The history of their frustrations provides an instructive illustration of the problems besetting this type of research (Chanock and Murphy, 1980).

Their original vaccine, developed in the mid 1960s was a formalin-inactivated, alum-precipitated preparation, given parenterally. Immunised children developed good neutralising antibody responses but, on encountering RSV during a subsequent epidemic, actually suffered more severe disease than did unimmunised controls; the possible explanations of this episode have been discussed (Chanock *et al.*, 1968; Merz *et al.*, 1980). Efforts were then redirected towards the development of an intranasal live vaccine. A number of *ts* mutants were isolated which were unable to grow in the lungs of hamsters but multiplied asymptomatically in the upper respiratory tract. A trial in children, however, indicated an undesirable incidence of rhinitis and even otitis media. Moreover, ts^+ virus was secreted by some of the children, indicating that reversion, or perhaps suppression, had occurred. Further mutagenesis with nitrosoguanidine produced mutants which appeared to be more attenuated for chimpanzees, but were still not completely stable genetically *in vivo*. And there the matter rests.

Even if a safe vaccine is eventually developed, there is no assurance that it will provide significant protection. Despite the fact that only a single serotype of RSV has been described, reinfections in children as well as adults are common following natural infection in infancy. Furthermore, the target population for immunisation would need to be very young babies, as most of the mortality and morbidity from RSV bronchiolitis and pneumonitis occurs during the first year, particularly the first six months of life, and the immune response to immunisation in the presence of the maternal antibody usually present at this stage is known to be significantly diminished (Chanock and Murphy, 1980; Hall, 1980; Tyeryar *et al.*, 1978). Nevertheless, it may be possible to improve on Nature by repeated immunisation of the baby with a potent preparation incorporating a suitable adjuvant to augment recall of IgA memory, or perhaps to confer short-term protection during the vital first six months of life by immunising the mother before or after she becomes pregnant.

Parainfluenza

Parainfluenza viruses, particularly types 1–3, are the major aetiological agents of croup. Early efforts to protect children with inactivated vaccine proved negative (Jackson and Muldoon, 1975). Attempts to develop *ts* mutants as potential vaccines have so far not met with much success (Tyeryar *et al.*, 1978). However, 'rosettes' of the two surface glyco-proteins, F and HN, have been incorporated into liposomes to produce experimental vaccines that show some promise in animals (Choppin, unpublished data; Compans, unpublished data).

Adenovirus

Adenoviruses, notably types 3, 4, and 7, regularly cause outbreaks of 'acute respiratory disease' in situations where young people are brought together, such as army camps. Many years ago Couch *et al.* (1963) demonstrated the validity of a rather novel approach to immunisation. By enclosing live unattenuated adenovirus in enteric-coated capsules, they ensured that the virus, taken by mouth, would bypass the throat (in which it would normally cause disease) and be released in the intestine, in which it would grow and induce solid immunity against both respiratory and alimentary challenge (Edmonson *et al.*, 1966). Top *et al.* (1971) confirmed and extended this work, showing that HEF-grown adenoviruses types 4 and 7 so administered, grow with little or no mutual interference, producing highly effective immunity to challenge; vaccine virus is excreted in the faeces but spreads only rarely to contacts.

Hepatitis B

It is estimated that as many as 200 million people, 5% of the world's population, are chronically infected with hepatitis B virus. The carriage rate is particularly high in Oceania, Asia and Africa where transmission seems to occur principally by non-parenteral routes, often perinatally from mother to baby. In North America, Europe and Australasia it tends to be associated with certain high-risk groups, such as heroin addicts, male homosexuals, recipients of frequent blood transfusions, and staff and patients in renal dialysis units. Clearly then, there is a great need for a vaccine. Also, hepatitis B is of major importance in the development of liver cancer (see Chapter 6) and vaccines are to be used in large-scale trials to see if this type of cancer can be prevented (WHO,

Table 7.6. Steps in the preparation of a human hepatitis B vaccine[a].

---

1. Collect plasma by regular plasmapheresis of known high titre HB_sAg human carriers negative for infectious virions (Dane particles), DNA polymerase and HB_eAg.

2. Defibrinate with calcium.

3. Concentrate HB_sAg by precipitation with ammonium sulphate.

4. Band by isopycnic (equilibrium) ultracentrifugation in sodium bromide.

5. Reband by rate zonal centrifugation in sucrose gradient.

6. Treat with pepsin, pH2 to digest adsorbed plasma and liver proteins.

7. Denature with 8M urea, then renature (also to remove extraneous proteins).

8. Purify by gel (molecular sieve) filtration.

9. Treat with formalin, 1:4000, 3 days to inactivate any residual infectious virus.

10. Adsorb onto aluminium hydroxide as adjuvant (0.5 mg alum per 20 μg HB_sAg) and add thimerosal 1:20 000 as preservative.

11. Ampoule in 1 ml doses (20 μg HB_sAg) and store at 4°C.

---

[a]Reproduced in modified form from Hilleman *et al.* (1982).

1983a). Paradoxically, an effective vaccine against this disease has recently been developed even though the virus has yet to be cultured *in vitro*.

Hepatitis B surface antigen (HB_sAg) occurs in the blood of carriers as 22 nm particles lacking DNA, hence devoid of infectivity. Because such particles are often present in enormous numbers (up to 10^{13} per ml), it is feasible to extract HB_sAg from serum and, after precautionary inactivation of possible contaminating virus, use it as a vaccine (Maupas *et al.*, 1976; Purcell and Gerin, 1978; Skelly *et al.*, 1981; reviews: Vyas *et al.*, 1978; Maupas and Guesry, 1981; Szmuness *et al.*, 1982).

The protocol for the preparation of the first vaccine licenced for general human use, that is, in 1981 (Hilleman *et al.*, 1982) is set out in Table 7.6. In a well controlled trial in male homosexuals by Szmuness *et al.* (1980), this vaccine, administered intramuscularly as three 40 μg doses, at 0, 1 and 6 months, was demonstrated to produce no untoward side effects (other than an occasional sore arm) and no hepatitis, but to induce antibodies and to reduce the incidence of subsequent disease by over 95% in this high-risk population. Anti-HB_s titres were slow to develop (except in those already anti-HB_s positive) and the third dose was essential, boosting the titre substantially. As antibody titres dropped significantly after a year or two it can be anticipated that further boosters will be necessary to maintain adequate levels of immunity over a much longer period. Subsequent to this trial it has become clear that the dose may be reduced to 20 μg without significant reduction in protection and this is now standard (Szmuness *et al.*, 1981a). The vaccine fails to eliminate the virus from carriers, indeed fails to elicit an antibody response (Dienstag *et al.*, 1982). However, since it also does the carrier no harm, immunisation programmes can be mounted without the need to screen potential recipients for serological markers of infection.

As might be expected, the vaccine is very expensive to produce and will always be in short supply. High-risk target populations that should be given priority (Centers for Disease Control, 1982c) include:

Family contacts of known chronic HB_sAg carriers

Babies born of HB_eAg-positive mothers

Patients with diseases requiring frequent transfusions

Patients and staff of haemodialysis units

Medical and ancillary personnel in other high risk situations, e.g. blood banks, serology laboratories, dental surgery, pathology

Inmates and staff of homes for the mentally retarded and other custodial institutions

Immunosuppressed or cancer patients

Drug addicts

Male homosexuals

In an emergency, immediate protection can be conferred by giving immune human globulin at the same time as the first dose of vaccine (Szmuness *et al.*, 1981b). Such combined active–passive immunisation could be advisable in the case of accidental exposure to contaminated blood, and in acutely infected or carrier pregnant women and their newborn babies.

In the longer term it will be necessary to replace this vaccine with something much more widely available if we are to contemplate routine immunisation of all infants in those areas of Africa, Asia and Oceania where the infection is so prevalent. A conventional live attenuated or inactivated vaccine is likely to be highly satisfactory and should follow within a few years of the cultivation of the virus in cell culture. The cross-protection between subtypes reported with the existing HB_sAg vaccines and with cross-challenge experiments in chimpanzees seems to be of sufficient magnitude to obviate the necessity to include more than one virus in such a vaccine.

Meanwhile, some workers are interested in the possibility that HB_sAg could be obtained safely in commercial quantities from a human hepatoma cell line (Alexander et al., 1978). Furthermore hepatitis B DNA has been cloned in E. coli (Burrell et al., 1979) and sufficient expression of HB_sAg obtained (Charnay et al., 1980; Edman et al., 1981; Mackay et al., 1981) to engender some optimism that this may be the way to go. Yields of immunogenic HB_sAg are substantially greater from transfected mammalian cells (Pourcel et al., 1982), or from yeast, which produce typical HB_sAg particles (Valenzuela et al., 1982; Miyanohara et al., 1983) that protect chimpanzees against challenge (McAleer et al., 1984). Moreover, following the demonstration that individual polypeptides derived from HB_sAg are immunogenic (Sanchez et al., 1980; Hollinger et al., 1982), Lerner et al. (1981), Dreesman et al. (1982), Prince et al. (1982) and Gerin et al. (1983) have synthesised shorter peptides which are themselves immunogenic, though much less so than the HB_sAg particles produced by yeast or mammalian cells. Incorporation of synthetic polypeptides into micelles might restore immunogenicity to something like its original level (Skelly et al., 1981), as might cross-linking to restore conformation (Ionescu-Matiu et al., 1983). The exciting new approach recently introduced by Moss and colleagues in which recombinant vaccinia virus incorporating the gene for HB_sAg is used as a 'live' vaccine to immunise against hepatitis B (Smith et al., 1983) was discussed earlier in this chapter.

Hepatitis A and nonA-nonB

Now that hepatitis A virus has finally been cultured unequivocally *in vitro* (Daemer et al., 1981; Provost et al., 1981) the way is open to develop a vaccine against this common and widespread disease also. The feasibility of a hepatitis A vaccine has already been established in marmosets (Provost and Hilleman, 1978). Virus isolated in foetal rhesus monkey kidney cell cultures has been adapted to human embryonic lung fibroblasts but the yields are low (Hilleman *et al.*, 1981a). Nevertheless, attenuated virus derived by serial passage in these cells has been shown to protect marmosets against challenge with virulent hepatitis A (Provost *et al.*, 1982). Furthermore, serially passaged virus of the HM/175 strain of Daemer *et al.* (1981) appears to be avirulent yet immunogenic in chimpanzees (Purcell *et al.*, personal communication), hence could constitute satisfactory seed for preparation of an experimental vaccine to be tested in man. Meanwhile, a DNA copy of part of the RNA genome of this picornavirus has been cloned in *E. coli* and detectable quantities of viral antigens are made (von der Helm *et al.*, 1981), therefore recombinant DNA technology offers an alternative approach.

NonA-nonB hepatitis appears to be increasing in occurrence, particularly in drug addicts, in recipients of blood (that has been demonstrated free of hepatitis B virus by routine RIA screening), and in water-borne epidemics. At least two distinct viruses currently seem to be involved but neither has yet been isolated. Outbreaks of hepatitis attributable to the defective 'delta' agent in hepatitis B carriers have also been reported recently (Hadler *et al.*, 1983). Vaccines against all these viruses are needed.

Rotavirus

Gastroenteritis is the biggest killer of children in the developing countries of the world and rotavirus is the single most important viral cause (Holmes. 1979; Kapikian *et al.*, 1980). The need for a vaccine to protect infants in the first two years of life therefore needs no further justification. In order to stimulate the synthesis of protective antibodies of the IgA class, live virus would need to be administered by the oral route. All the common serotypes may have to be included since little is yet known about cross-protection, although laboratory studies show a degree of serological cross-reaction.

Human rotavirus has now been propagated in rolled cultures of the monkey kidney cell line MA104 in the presence of trypsin (Sato *et al.*, 1981; Urasawa *et al.*, 1981). This breakthrough might be expected to pave the way for the development of a satisfactory vaccine.

Whereas live attenuated mutants of human rotaviruses, administered orally to infants, would appear to be the most logical first approach to immunisation, Kapikian *et al.* (1980) have considered a variety of alternative strategies. For example, waning immunity following oral live vaccine might be boosted by inactivated vaccine systemically. Pregnant women might be immunised to protect the newborn. The protective type-specific viral protein could be produced by recombinant DNA technology. Or finally, live unattenuated bovine rotavirus given orally might protect children, as it does calves and piglets, against human rotavirus.

Herpesviruses

All the human herpesviruses are common pathogens responsible for significant morbidity and mortality. Quite apart from the diseases attributable to primary infections, the misery of herpes zoster and recurrent exacerbations of herpes simplex justify attempts to produce vaccines against them. The purpose of such vaccines would be to prevent primary infections and thereby recurrences; it would be unrealistic to hope to prevent recurrences after latent infection has already been established, as even naturally acquired immunity fails to do so.

Two major difficulties stand in the way of the development of herpesvirus vaccines (Parks and Rapp, 1975). The first is that all the human herpesviruses, except HSV, release only very small numbers of virions into the supernatant of infected cell cultures; most of the virus remains cell-associated, hence there are severe logistical problems militating against production of virus on the scale required for the manufacture of a vaccine, particularly of the inactivated type. Our current belief in the centrality of cell-mediated immunity in herpesvirus infections suggests that live vaccines may be superior, or even essential. Many virologists, however, are nervous about the possibility that live attenuated vaccines might share the capacity of the wild virus to establish life long latent infection; or at worst, lead to some sinister pathology, perhaps not manifesting itself until years after apparently satisfactory clinical trials have led to the licensing of the vaccine. Nevertheless, others, spurred on by such notable successes as the prevention, by vaccination, of Marek's disease of chickens (Purchase, 1976) and of lymphomas caused by *H. saimiri* in monkeys (Laufs and Steinke, 1975) have developed experimental live attenuated vaccines against varicella (reviews: Takahashi *et al.*, 1981; Gershon, 1980) and human cytomegalovirus (reviews: Lang, 1980; Osborn, 1981).

Takahashi and his colleagues in Japan produced a live attenuated varicella vaccine, the OKA strain, by serial passage in human guinea pig cells. The vaccine was tested not only in normal individuals but also in immunocompromised children suffering from such debilitating conditions as leukaemia and nephrotic syndrome, who are seen as the principal target group for vaccination if it can be shown to be safe in them. Seroconversion occurred in 98% of normal recipients, and side effects (mild fever and papular rash) were observed only very occasionally. In the immunocompromised group however, a significant minority developed mild varicella, particularly if their immunosuppressive drugs were not suspended for vaccination. In both populations, immunisation conferred substantial protection against natural varicella (Asano and Takahashi, 1977). More recently, Neff *et al.* (1981) have reported similarly encouraging results with their KMcC strain of varicella virus attenuated by 50 passages in WI-38 cells.

Cytomegalovirus, though not a major cause of morbidity in healthy people, is highly dangerous in two particular circumstances: it is the commonest infectious cause of mental retardation (cytomegalic inclusion disease) and the commonest infectious cause of death in bone marrow transplant recipients and other profoundly immunosuppressed patients (see Lang, 1980; Osborn, 1981). Elek and Stern (1974) were the first to develop an experimental vaccine against human CMV. Their strain Ad-169, attenuated by 54 passages in HEF, produced antibody following subcutaneous injection; the only side effect seemed to be a rather regular tendency to a delayed local reaction at the injection site. These findings were subsequently confirmed and extended by Neff *et al.* (1979). Meanwhile, Plotkin and colleagues produced their Towne-125 strain by 125 passages in WI-38 and demonstrated both humoral and cellular immune responses in normal recipients; responses in patients being prepared for renal transplants were often much reduced or delayed (Starr *et al.*, 1981). A majority of the latter group were found to be excreting CMV in their urine following subsequent renal transplantation, thus raising doubts about the vaccine's efficacy or safety or both (Osborn, 1981).

EB virus is the aetiological agent not only of the ubiquitous disease infectious mononucleosis but also, in all probability, of two highly malignant tumours, Burkitt lymphoma and nasopharyngeal carcinoma (Epstein and Achong, 1979). Epstein has advocated the development of a vaccine, even though the virus cannot yet be grown in conventional cell culture. The 340 000 dalton glycoprotein component of the EB virus-induced membrane antigen complex has been extracted from a marmoset lymphoblastoid cell line, then incorporated into liposomes and demonstrated to induce EBV-neutralising antibodies in mice (North *et al.*, 1982) and marmosets (Epstein *et al.*, 1983; Epstein and Morgan, 1983).

Oddly enough, the only human herpesvirus that grows rapidly to high titre in culture and the one responsible for by far the greatest morbidity, namely herpes simplex, has not attracted as much attention until recently. Recurrent HSV infections of the genitalia, face and eye, not to mention the rarer but lethal encephalitis and perinatal herpes, are certainly worth preventing. An experimental 'subunit' HSV type 2 vaccine, consisting of formaldehyde-treated viral glycoprotein adsorbed to alum adjuvant (Hilleman *et al.*, 1981b) is currently under trial, and there are promising reports of a similar vaccine from Skinner *et al.* (1982). Meanwhile, Naylor *et al.* (1982) have shown that antibody responses of mice to HSV-1 glycoproteins are greatly enhanced by incorporation of the immunogen into liposomes containing lipid A. Very recently, Watson *et al.* (1982) have cloned the gene for the HSV-1 glycoprotein gD in *E. coli*, and the same group (Weis *et al.*, 1983) have obtained greatly enhanced expression by constructing a hybrid gene encoding a chimaeric protein containing HSV-1 gD, bacteriophage λ Cro and *E. coli* β-galactosidase; the chimaeric protein elicits antibodies which neutralise the infectivity of both HSV-1 and HSV-2. Roizman *et al.* (1982) have constructed live attenuated HSV-1/HSV-2 recombinants and live deletion mutants lacking a non-essential early gene; neither safety nor protection against challenge by a natural route of infection has yet been demonstrated.

Virologists are naturally reluctant about the use of any live herpes-virus vaccine which may be capable of establishing a latent infection, or of reverting to a virus that may. Whether this degree of caution is excessive remains to be seen. For instance, a deletion mutant lacking the TK (thymidine kinase) gene, which seems to be required both for pathogenicity and for the establishment of latency, could perhaps form the basis of a satisfactory HSV vaccine. It may yet turn out that herpes simplex—the Cinderella in the Big League of viral vaccines—will come to occupy the center of the stage in the battle for supremacy between deletion mutants and cloned or synthetic polypeptides.

VETERINARY VIRAL VACCINES

Space does not permit detailed consideration of 'veterinary' vaccines, but a few points are worth making.

The consumption of vaccines for the prevention of viral diseases in animals is at least two orders of magnitude greater than that of human vaccines, reflecting not only the greater world population of farm and companion animals but, more significantly, their rapid turnover. Currently, the majority of these vaccines are consumed by the poultry industry.

Somewhat less absolute standards of safety have been accepted for some veterinary vaccines where the loss of an occasional animal is not considered a disaster. Examples of fully virulent viruses delivered as vaccines to a heterologous species of animal, or by an unnatural route, or at a 'safe' age, were given earlier in this chapter. Most veterinary vaccines are, however, live attenuated, or less commonly, inactivated vaccines, quite comparable with their human counterparts. The principles of their derivation are much the same, though certain differences in their usage should be noted.

The certainty of successful delivery by injection (e.g. jet gun) makes this the preferred route of administration. A convenient method of oral delivery is to add the virus to drinking water (e.g. for chickens). Immunisation of the mother in order to confer short-term protection on the offspring is quite a practicable way of preventing a number of diseases prevalent in the very young (e.g. in chickens)—examples of which were given earlier. As in the human situation, sudden unexpected local outbreaks of disease can be controlled by mass vaccination and quarantine, but slaughter is an additional option hardly appropriate in man. Even quite widespread animal diseases, such as rinderpest and foot-and-mouth disease have been eradicated from whole continents, though not yet on the world scale achieved with human smallpox. Ironically however, some recent outbreaks of foot-and-mouth disease in previously free areas have been attributed to vaccine virus, and the recent 'pandemic' of canine parvovirus is widely ascribed to a contaminant of another vaccine.

A selection of the more important viral vaccines for domestic animals and birds is given in Table 7.7. For further information the reader is referred to standard veterinary texts.

Table 7.7. Veterinary viral vaccines.

Virus family	Disease	Host	Vaccine		
Papovaviridae	Papilloma	Cattle			I
Adenoviridae	Canine hepatitis	Dog		LA,	I
Herpesviridae	Marek's disease	Chicken	LV[a],	LA	
	Infectious laryngo-tracheitis	Chicken	(LV[b]),	LA	
	Duck hepatitis	Duck		LA	
	Infectious bovine rhinotracheitis	Cattle		LA	
	Equine rhino-pneumonitis	Horse		LA,	I
	Feline rhino-tracheitis	Cat		LA,	I
	Aujeszky's disease (pseudorabies)	Pig		LA,	I
Iridoviridae	African swine fever	Pig		LA	
Poxviridae	Fowlpox	Chicken		LA	
	Sheeppox	Sheep	LV[c],	LA,	I
	Orf (scabby mouth)	Sheep	LV[c]		
	Lumpy skin disease	Cattle		LA	
	Myxomatosis	Rabbit	LV[d]		
Parvoviridae	Panleukopaenia, enteritis	Cat, dog, mink		LA,	I
Picornaviridae	Foot-and-mouth disease	Pig, cattle		LA,	I, (P)
	Teschen disease	Pig		LA,	I
	Encephalomyelitis	Chicken		LA,	I
Togaviridae	Swine fever (hog cholera)	Pig		LA,	I

Table 7.7. *continued*

Virus family	Disease	Host	Vaccine	
Togaviridae (*cont.*)	Bovine virus diarrhoea	Cattle	LA	
	Louping ill	Sheep		I
	Wesselsbron disease	Sheep, goat, cattle	LA,	I
	Eastern equine encephalitis	Horse	LA,	I
	Western equine encephalitis	Horse	LA,	I
	Venezuelan equine encephalitis	Horse	LA,	I
	Japanese encephalitis	Pig, horse	(LA),	I
	Equine arteritis	Horse	LA,	I
Orthomyxoviridae	Influenza	Horse		I
	Fowl plague	Chicken		I
Paramyxoviridae	Distemper	Dog	LA	
	Newcastle disease	Chicken	LA,	I
	Rinderpest	Cattle	LA	
	Parainfluenza 3 (shipping fever)	Cattle, dog	LA,	I
Coronaviridae	Infectious bronchitis	Chicken	LA	
	Transmissible gastroenteritis	Pig	LA,	I
	Diarrhoea	Cattle	LA	
Bunyaviridae	Rift Valley fever	Sheep, goat, cattle	LA	
Rhabdoviridae	Rabies	Dog, cat, cattle	LA,	I
	Vesicular stomatitis	Cattle	LA	
	Ephemeral fever	Cattle	LA	
Reoviridae	Bluetongue	Sheep	LA	
	African horse sickness	Horse	LA	
	Rotavirus enteritis	Cattle, pig	LA	
Birnaviridae	Bursal disease	Chicken	LA,	I

LV = Live virulent ([a]turkey herpesvirus; [b]cloaca; [c]thigh; [d]rabbit fibroma virus).
LA = Live attenuated; ( ) = experimental.
I = Inactivated.
P = Purified protein cloned.

SUMMARY

Most of the highly successful viral vaccines in use today are living host range mutants derived empirically by serial passage in cultured cells until sufficiently attenuated in virulence. They multiply in the recipient, as in a natural subclinical infection, and, if delivered via the natural route as in the case of oral poliovaccine, they generate local immunity. With some live vaccines trivial symptoms occur in a minority of recipients; very rarely, frank disease is seen in immunologically compromised individuals.

For global eradication of a viral disease, as accomplished with smallpox, the disease in question must be caused by a single or very few serotypes which establish no persistent infections and have no other host but man. A dramatic reduction in incidence in a particular country can be more easily achieved, as for example with poliomyelitis and measles in the U.S.A.

In recent years attempts have been made to devise more reliable ways of deriving attenuated mutants. It would be convenient if the gene(s) determining virulence could be deleted, replaced or modified, but such genes have generally not been identified. There does appear to be a correlation between avirulence and temperature-sensitivity. Live respiratory viral vaccines containing *ts* lesions in one or more genes are usually attenuated, but unfortunately tend to revert towards virulence *in vivo* as a result of suppressor mutations. Cold-adapted vaccines derived by genetic reassortment between the prevalent wild-type and a *ca* master strain containing mutations in most genes currently look more promising. Mutants containing a deletion in a non-essential gene, preferably a 'virulence gene', may be expected to display a lesser tendency to revert.

Killed vaccines, e.g. those against influenza, have not in general been as satisfactory, although the β-propiolactone-inactivated rabies vaccine has proven very successful, as was the earlier IPV ('Salk' vaccine) against poliomyelitis. Since inactivated vaccines must be inoculated in multiple large doses they are expensive. The cost may be reduced by cultivation on new substrates, e.g. continuous cell lines capable of growing in suspension or on microcarrier beads.

Attention has recently turned to the use of viral proteins or peptides as vaccines. The relevant surface antigen may be extracted from the virion or, in the special case of HB_sAg, from the serum of hepatitis B carriers.

Now that the amino acid sequence and the location of the antigenic sites on viral proteins can so readily be determined, it has become feasible to synthesise chemically the whole polypeptide, or shorter peptides corresponding to the critical antigenic site(s). Since these synthetic peptides lack the tertiary structure of the original antigenic determinant they elicit relatively little antibody capable of neutralising the parent virus. Nevertheless, a foot-and-mouth-disease peptide vaccine is protective and hepatitis B peptides look promising.

Recombinant DNA technology is also leaving its mark. The genes (or cDNA copies of RNA genes) coding for the key immunogenic proteins of several viruses have now been cloned in bacteria, yeasts or mammalian cells. In some cases where the protein is produced in reasonable amounts, it has been shown to confer protection (e.g. FMDV; hepatitis B). In an exciting new approach the gene for HB_sAg, influenza HA or herpes simplex gD has been inserted into the genome of vaccinia virus, which is then used as a live vaccine. When the virus multiplies *in vivo*, the foreign gene is also expressed, substantial amounts of HB_sAg, HA or gD are made, and the vaccinee mounts a good immune response.

If purified proteins are to be exploited as vaccines in man, new methods of immunopotentiation will be needed. These include the use of synthetic adjuvants such as MDP, coupling viral peptides to a carrier protein, or incorporating viral proteins into liposomes.

The derivation and usage of the established and experimental human viral vaccines is discussed in some detail. Veterinary vaccines are listed.

SELECTED READING

Bittle, J. L., Houghten, R. A., Alexander, H., Shinnick, T. M., Sutcliffe, J. G., Lerner, R. A., Rowlands, D. J., and Brown, F. (1982). Protection against foot-and-mouth disease with a chemically synthesized peptide predicted from the viral nucleotide sequence. *Nature* **298**, 30.

Chanock, R. M. (1981). Strategy for development of respiratory and gastrointestinal tract viral vaccines in the 1980s. *J. Infect. Dis.* **143**, 364.

Edelman, R. (1980). Vaccine adjuvants. *Rev. Infect. Dis.* **2**, 370.

Epstein, M. A. and Morgan, A. J. (1983). Clinical consequences of Epstein-Barr virus infection and possible control by an antiviral vaccine. *Clin. Exp. Immunol.* **53**, 257.

Gregoriadis, G. (1976). The carrier potential of liposomes in biology and medicine. *New Engl. J. Med.* **295**, 704–10 and 756–70.

Hilleman, M. R., Buynak, E. B., McAleer, W. J., McLean, A. A., Provost, P. J., and Tytell, A. A. (1982). Hepatitis A and hepatitis B vaccines, In *Viral Hepatitis*, (ed. W. Szmuness, H. J. Alter, and J. M. Maynard), pp. 385–97. Franklin Institute Press, Philadelphia.

Hinman, A. R., Brandling-Bennett, A. D., Bernier, R. H., Kirby, C. D., and Eddins, D. L. (1980). Current features of measles in the United States: feasibility of measles elimination. *Epidemiol. Rev.* **2**, 153.

Kapikian, A. Z., Wyatt, R. G., Greenberg, H. B., Kalica, A. R., Kim, H. W., Brandt, C. D., Rodriguez, W. J., Parrott, R. H., and Chanock, R. M. (1980). Approaches to immunization of infants and young children against gastroenteritis due to rotaviruses. *Rev. Infect. Dis.* **2**, 459.

Kleid, D. G., Yansura, D., Small, B., Dowbenko, D., Moore, D. M., Grubman, M. J., McKercher, P. D., Morgan, D. O., Robertson, B. H., and Bachrach, H. L. (1981). Cloned viral protein vaccine for foot-and-mouth disease: responses in cattle and swine. *Science* **214**, 1125.

Lerner, R. A. (1982). Tapping the immunological repertoire to produce antibodies of predetermined specificity. *Nature* **299**, 592.

Lerner, R. A. and Chanock, R. M. (eds) (1984). *Modern Approaches to Vaccines*. Cold Spring Harbor Laboratory, New York.

Melnick, J. L. (1977). Viral vaccines. *Progr. Med. Virol.* **23**, 158.

Melnick, J. L. (1978). Advantages and disadvantages of killed and live poliomyelitis vaccines. *Bull. WHO* **56**, 21.

Murphy, B. R., Tolpin, M. D., Massicot, J., Kim, H. W., Parrott, R. H., and Chanock, R. M. (1980). Escape of a highly defective influenza A virus mutant from its *ts* phenotype by extragenic suppression and other types of mutation. *Ann. N.Y. Acad. Sci.* **354**, 142.

Nomoto, A, Omata, T., Toyoda, H., Kuge, S., Horie, H., Kataoka, Y., Genba, Y., Nakano, Y., and Imura, N. (1982). Complete nucleotide sequence of the attenuated poliovirus Sabin 1 strain genome. *Proc. Nat. Acad. Sci. U.S.A.* **79**, 5793.

Pourcel, C., Sobzack, E., Dubois, M.-F., Gervais, M., Drouet, J., and Tiollais, P. (1982). Antigenicity and immunogenicity of hepatitis B virus particles produced by mouse cells transfected with cloned viral DNA. *Virology* **121**, 175.

Preblud, S. R., Serdula, M. K., Frank, J. A., Brandling-Bennett, A. D., and Hinman, A. R. (1980). Rubella vaccination in the United States: a ten-year review. *Epidemiol. Rev.* **2**, 171.

Sabin, A. B. (1980). Vaccination against poliomyelitis in economically underdeveloped countries. *Bull. WHO* **58**, 141.

Sabin, A. B. (1981a). Immunization: evaluation of some currently available and prospective vaccines. *J. Am. Med. Assoc.* **246**, 236.

Szmuness, W., Stevens, C. E., Harley, E. J., Zang, E. A., Oleszko, W. R., William, D. C., Sadovsky, R., Morrison, J. M., and Kellner, A. (1980). Hepatitis B vaccine: demonstration of efficacy in a controlled clinical trial in a high-risk population in the United States. *New Engl. J. Med.* **303**, 833.

Van Wezel, A. L. (1981). Present state and developments in the production of inactivated poliomyelitis vaccine. *Develop. Biol. Stand.* **47**, 7.

Wiktor, T. J., Plotkin, S. A., and Koprowski, H. (1978). Development and clinical trials of the new human rabies vaccine of tissue culture (human diploid cell) origin. *Dev. Biol. Stand.* **40**, 3.

WHO (1983b). *Viral Vaccines and Antiviral Drugs*. WHO, Geneva.

Wunner, W. H., Dietzschold, B., Curtis, P. J., and Wiktor, T. J. (1983). Rabies subunit vaccines. *J. Gen. Virol.* **64**, 1649.

References

Abildgaard, C., Harrison, J., Espana, C. *et al.* (1975). Simian haemorrhagic fever: studies of coagulation and pathology. *Am. J. Trop. Med. Hyg.* **24**, 537.

Abramson, J. S., Lewis, J. C., Lyles, D. S. *et al.* (1982a). Inhibition of neutrophil lysosome-phagosome fusion associated with influenza virus infection *in vitro*: role in depressed bactericidal activity. *J. Clin. Investig.* **69**, 1393.

Abramson, J. S., Giebink, G. S. and Quie, P. G. (1982b). Influenza A-induced polymorphonuclear leucocyte dysfunction in the pathogenesis of experimental pneumococcal otitis media. *Infect. Immunity* **36**, 289.

Ada, G. L. (1981). Controlling influenza epidemics. *Immunol. Today* **2**, 219.

Ada, G. L., Leung, K. N. and Ertl, H. (1981). An analysis of effector T cell generation and function in mice exposed to influenza A or Sendai viruses. *Immunol. Rev.* **58**, 5.

Adams, D. (1982). Molecules, membranes and macrophage activation. *Immunol. Today* **3**, 285.

Adler, R. M., Glorioso, J. C., Cossman, J. *et al.* (1978). Possible role of Fc receptors on cells infected and transformed by herpes virus: escape from immune lysis. *Infect. Immunity* **21**, 442.

Aguet, M. (1980). High affinity binding of ^{125}I-labelled mouse interferon to a specific cell surface receptor. *Nature* **284**, 459.

Air, G. M., Blok, J. and Hall, R. M. (1981). Sequence relationships in influenza viruses. In *Replication of Negative Strand Viruses* (D. H. L. Bishop and R. W. Compans, eds.), pp. 225–39. Elsevier, Amsterdam.

Alberto, B. P., Callahan, L. F. and Pincus, T. (1982). Evidence that retrovirus expression in mouse spleen cells results from B cell differentiation. *J. Immunol.* **129**, 2768.

Albrecht, P. (1978). Immune control in experimental subacute sclerosing panencephalitis. *Am. J. Clin. Pathol.* (Suppl) **70**, 175.

Alexander, J., Macnab, G. and Saunders, R. (1978). Studies on *in vitro* production of hepatitis B surface antigen by a human hepatoma cell line. *Perspect. Virol.* **10**, 103.

Allen, G. and Fantes, K. H. (1980). A family of structural genes for human lymphoblastoid (leukocyte-type) interferon. *Nature* **287**, 408.

Allison, A. C. (1967). Lysosomes in virus-infected cells. *Perspect. Virol.* **5**, 29.

Allison, A. C. (1972). Immunity against viruses. In *The Scientific Basis of Medicine*. Annual Review, Athlone Press, London.

Allison, A. C. (1978). Macrophage activation and non-specific immunity. *Int. Rev. Exp. Path.* **18**, 304.

Allison, A. C. and Gregoriadis, G. (1974). Liposomes as immunological adjuvants. *Nature* **252**, 252.

Almeida, J. D. and Waterson, A. P. (1969). The morphology of virus-antibody interactions. *Adv. Virus Res.* **15**, 307.

Almeida, J. D., Howatson, A. F. and Williams, M. G. (1962). Electron microscope study of human warts, sites of virus production and the nature of the inclusion bodies. *J. Investig. Derm.* **38**, 337.

Alter, H. J., Gerety, R. J., Smallwood, L. A. *et al*. (1982). Sporadic non-A, non-B hepatitis; frequency and epidemiology in an urban US population. *J. Infect. Dis.* **145**, 886.

Anders, E. M., Katz, J. M. Jackson, D. C. *et al*. (1981a). *In vitro* antibody response to influenza virus. II Specificity of helper T cell recognizing hemagglutinin. *J. Immunol.* **127**, 669.

Anders, E. M., Katz, J. M., Brown, L. E. *et al*. (1981b). The specificity of T cells for influenza virus hemagglutinin. In *Genetic Variation among Influenza Viruses* (ed. D. P. Nayak). ICN-UCLA Symposium, vol. 21, pp. 547–65. Academic Press, New York.

Anderson, L. J., Sikes, R. K., Langkop, C. W. *et al*. (1980). Postexposure trial of a human diploid cell strain rabies vaccine. *J. Infect. Dis.* **142**, 133.

Anderson, M. J. (1982). The emerging story of a human parvovirus-like agent. *J. Hyg. Camb.* **89**, 1.

Andersson, V., Bird, A. G., Britton, S. *et al*. (1981). Humoral and cellular immunity in humans studied at the cell level from birth to two years of age. *Immunol. Rev.* **57**, 5.

Andrewes, C., Pereira, H. G., and Wildy, P. (1978). *Viruses of Vertebrates*, 4th edn. Baillière Tindall, London.

Andries, K. and Pensaert, M. B. (1980). Immunofluorescence studies on the pathogenesis of haemagglutinating encephalomyelitis virus infection in pigs after oronasal inoculation. *Am. J. Vet. Res.* **41**, 1372.

Arnheiter, H., Baechi, T. and Haller, O. (1982). Adult mouse hepatocytes in primary monolayer culture express genetic resistance to mouse hepatitis virus type 3. *J. Immunol.* **129**, 1275.

Arvin, A. M., Pollard, R. B., Rasmussen, L. E. *et al*. (1978). Selective impairment of lymphocyte reactivity to varicella zoster virus antigens among untreated patients with lymphoma, *J. Infect. Dis.* **137**, 531.

Asano, Y. and Takahashi, M. (1977). Clinical and serologic testing of a live varicella vaccine and two-year follow-up for immunity of the vaccinated children. *Pediatrics* **60**, 810.

Ashman, R. B. (1982). Persistence of cell-mediated immunity to influenza A virus in mice. *Immunology* **47**, 165.

Ashman, R. B. and Müllbacher, A. (1979). A T helper cell for viral cytotoxic T cell responses. *J. Exp. Med.* **150**, 1277.

Askenase, P. W. and van Loveren, H. (1983). Delayed type hypersensitivity activation of mast cells by antigen-specific T cell factors initiates the cascade of cellular interactions. *Immunol. Today* **4**, 259.

Askonas, B. A., McMichael, A. J. and Webster, R. G. (1982). The immune response to influenza viruses and the problem of protection against infection. In *Basic and Applied Influenza Research* (ed. A. S. Beare). CRC Press, Florida.

Assaad, F. (1979). Poliomyelitis vaccination benefits versus risk. *Develop. Biol. Stand.* **43**, 141.

Atkins, E. (1983). Fever—new perspectives on an old phenomena. *New Engl. J. Med.* **308**, 958.

Aune, T. M. and Pierce, C. W. (1982). Activation of a suppressor T cell pathway by interferon. *Proc. Nat. Acad. Sci. USA* **79**, 3808.

Bachrach, H. L. (1966). Reactivity of viruses *in vitro*. *Progr. Med. Virol.* **8**, 214.

Bachrach, H. L., Moore, D. M., McKercher, P. D. *et al*. (1976). An experimental subunit vaccine for foot-and-mouth disease. *Dev. Biol. Stand.* **35**, 155.

Baer, G. M. (1975). The Natural History of Rabies, p. 181. Academic Press, New York.

Baer, G. M. (1978). Advances in post-exposure rabies vaccination. *Am. J. Clin. Pathol.* **70**, 185.

Baglioni, C. (1979). Interferon-induced enzymatic activities and their role in the antiviral state. *Cell* **17**, 255.

Baglioni, C. (1983). The molecular mediators of interferon action. In *Interferons and their Applications* (ed. P. E. Came and W. A. Carter). *Handbook Exp. Pharmacol.* Vol. 71. Springer-Verlag, Berlin.

Baker, D. A. and Plotkin, S. A. (1978). Enhancement of vaginal infection in mice by herpes simplex virus type II with progesterone. *Proc. Soc. Exp. Biol. Med.* **158**, 131.

Balachandran, N., Bacchetti, S. and Rawls, W. E. (1982). Protection against lethal challenge of BALB/c mice by passive transfer of monoclonal antibodies to five glycoproteins of herpes simplex virus type 2. *Infect. Immunity* **37**, 1132.

Bale, J. F., Kern, E. R., Overall, J. C. *et al*. (1982). Enhanced susceptibility of mice infected with murine cytomegalovirus to intranasal challenge with Escherichia coli: pathogenesis and altered inflammatory response. *J. Infect. Dis.* **145**, 525.

Balkwill, F. R. (1979). Interferons as cell-regulatory molecules. *Cancer Immunol. Immunother.* **7**, 7.

Balkwill, F. R., Griffin, D. B., Band, H. A. *et al*. (1983). Immune human lymphocytes produce an acid-labile α-interferon. *J. Exp. Med.* **157**, 1059.

Ball, L. A. (1982). 2′,5′-oligoadenylate synthetase. In *The Enzymes* (ed. P. D. Boyer), vol. 15, pp. 281–313. Academic Press. New York.

Baltimore, D. (1971). Expression of animal virus genomes. *Bacteriol. Rev.* **35**, 235.

Bancroft, G. J., Shellam, G. R. and Chalmer, J. E. (1981). Genetic influences on the augmentation of natural killer (NK) cells during murine cytomegalovirus infection: correlation with patterns of resistance. *J. Immunol.* **126**, 988.

Bang, F. B. (1978). Genetics of resistance of animals to viruses. I Introduction and studies in mice. *Adv. Virus. Res.* **23**, 269.

Bang, F. B. and Warwick, A. (1960). Mouse macrophages as host cells for the mouse hepatitis virus and the genetic basis of their susceptibility. *Proc. Nat. Acad. Sci. USA* **46**, 1065.

Baringer, J. R. and Swoveland, P. (1973). Recovery of herpes simplex virus from human trigeminal ganglions. *New Engl. J. Med.* **228**, 648.

Barker, L. F. and Murray, R. (1972). Relationship of virus dose to incubation time of clinical hepatitis and time of appearance of hepatitis-associated antigen. *Am. J. Med. Sci.* **263**, 27.

Baron, M. H. and Baltimore, D. (1982). Anti-VPg antibody inhibition of the poliovirus replicase reaction and the production of covalent complexes of VPg-related polypeptides and newly-made RNA. *Cell* **30**, 745.

Baron, S., Dianzani, F. and Stanton, G. J. (1982). *The Interferon System. Review to 1982*, parts 1 and 2. *Texas Repts. Biol. Med.* **41**, Univ. Texas, Medical Branch, Galveston.

Bartholomew, R. M., Esser, A. F. and Müller-Eberhard, H. J. (1978). Lysis of oncornaviruses by human serum: isolation of the viral complement (C1) receptor and identification as p15E. *J. Exp. Med.* **147**, 844.

Bastardo, J. W., McKimm-Breschkin, J. L., Sonza, S. *et al.* (1981). Preparation and characterization of antisera to electrophoretically purified SA11 Virus polypeptides. *Infect. Immunity* **34**, 641.

Bastian, F. O., Rabson, A. S., Yee, C. L. *et al.* (1974). Herpes-virus varicellae isolated from human dorsal root ganglion. *Arch. Pathol.* **97**, 311.

Baucke, R. B. and Spear, P. G. (1979). Membrane proteins specified by herpes simplex virus V. Identification of an Fc-binding glycoprotein. *J. Virology* **32**, 779.

Beale, J. (1982). Control of poliomyelitis: killed or living vaccine. In *Viral Diseases of S.E. Asia and the Western Pacific* (ed. J. S. Mackenzie) pp. 405–14. Academic Press, New York.

Beare, J. S. (1975). Live viruses for immunization against influenza. *Progr. Med. Virol.* **20**, 49.

Beasley, R. P., Hwang, L. Y., Lin, C. C. *et al.* (1981). Hepato-cellular carcinoma and hepatitis B virus. A prospective study of 22,707 men in Taiwan. *Lancet* ii, 1129.

Beasley, R. P., Hwang, L-Y, Lau, M. L. *et al.* (1982). Incidence of hepatitis B virus infection in preschool children in Taiwan. *J. Infect. Dis.* **146**, 698.

Becht, H. (1980). Infectious bursal disease virus. *Curr. Top. Microbiol. Immunol.* **90**, 107.

Beck, O. E. (1981). Distribution of virus antibody activity among human IgG subclasses. *Clin. Exp. Immunol.* **43**, 626.

Beckmann, A. M. and Shah, K. V. (1983). Propagation and primary isolation of JCV and BKV in urinary epithelial cell cultures. In *Polyomaviruses and Human Neurological Diseases*, pp. 3–14 (eds. J. L. Sever and D. L. Maddan). Alan R. Liss, New York.

Bedson, H. S. and Duckworth, M. J. (1963). Rabbitpox: An experimental study of the pathways of infection in rabbits. *J. Pathol. Bacteriol.* **85**, 1.

Beltz, G. A. and Flint, S. J. (1979). Inhibition of HeLa cell protein synthesis during adenovirus infection: restriction of cellular messenger RNA sequences to the nucleus. *J. Mol. Biol.* **131**, 353.

Benacerraf, B. and Germain, R. (1978). The immune response genes of the major histocompatibility complex. *Immunol. Rev.* **38**, 70.

Benacerraf, B. and Unanue, E. R. (1979). *Textbook of Immunology*. Williams and Wilkins, Baltimore.

Berge, T. O. (ed.) (1975). *International Catalogue of Arboviruses Including Certain Other Viruses of Vertebrates*, 2nd edn. U.S. Dept. Health, Education, Welfare. DHEW Publ. No. (CDC) 75-8301. U.S. Govt. Printing Office, Washington.

Berns, K. I. (ed.) (1983). *The Parvoviruses*. Plenum Press, New York.

Berzofsky, J. A. (1980). Immune response genes in the regulation of mammalian immunity. In *Biological Regulation and Development*, vol. II pp. 467–594 (ed. R. F. Goldberger). Plenum Press, New York.

Billiau, A. (1981). Interferon therapy: pharmacokinetic and pharmacological aspects. *Arch. Virol.* **67**, 121.

Biron, C. A. and Welsh, R. M. (1982). Blastogenesis of natural killer cells during viral infection *in vivo*. *J. Immunol.* **129**, 2788.

Bishop, D. H. L. (1977). Virion polymerases. *Comprehen. Virol.* **10**, 117.

Bishop, D. H. L. (1979). *Rhabdoviruses*, vols. 1–4. CRC Press, Florida.

Bishop, D. H. L. and Compans, R. W. (eds.) (1981). *The Replication of Negative-Strand Viruses*. Elsevier, Amsterdam.

Bishop, D. H. L. and Shope, R. E. (1979). Bunyaviridae. *Comprehen. Virol.* **14**, 1.

Bishop, J. M. (1978). Retroviruses. *Ann. Rev. Biochem.* **47**, 35.

Bishop, J. M. (1982). Oncogenes. *Sci. Am.* **246**, 68.

Bishop, J. M. (1983). Cellular oncogenes and retroviruses. *Ann. Rev. Biochem.* **52**, 301.

Bittle, J. L., Houghten, R. A., Alexander, H. *et al.* (1982). Protection against foot-and-mouth disease with a chemically synthesized peptide predicted from the viral nucleotide sequence. *Nature* **298**, 30.

Bixler, G. S. and Booss, J. (1981). Adherent spleen cells from mice acutely infected with cytomegalovirus suppress the primary antibody response in vitro. *J. Immunol.* **127**, 1293.

Black, F. L. (1966). Measles endemicity in insular populations: critical community size and its evolutionary implication. *J. Theoretical Biol.* **11**, 207.

Black, F. L. (1982). Problems encountered in measles immunization in developing countries. In *Viral Diseases of S.E. Asia and the Western Pacific* pp. 297–307 (ed. J. S. Mackenzie). Academic Press, New York.

Black, F. L., Hierholzer, W. J., Pinheiro, F. D. *et al.* (1974). Evidence for persistence of infectious agents in isolated human populations. *Am. J. Epidermiol.* **100**, 230.

Blacklow, N. R. and Cukor, G. (1981). Viral gastroenteritis. *New Engl. J. Med.* **304**, 397.

Blalock, J. E. and Smith, E. M. (1981). Structure and function relationship of interferon (IFN) and neuroendocrine hormones. In *The Biology of the Interferon System* pp. 93–9 (eds. E. de Mayer, G. Galasso, and H. Schellekens). Elsevier North-Holland, Amsterdam.

Blanden, R. V. (1970). Mechanisms of recovery from a generalized virus infection: mousepox I. The effects of antithymocyte serum. *J. Exp. Med.* **132**, 1035.

Blanden, R. V. (1971a). Mechanisms of recovery from a generalized virus infection: mousepox II. Passive transfer of recovery mechanisms with immune lymphoid cells. *J. Exp. Med.* **133**, 1074.

Blanden, R. V. (1971b). Mechanisms of recovery from a generalized virus infection: mousepox III. Regression of infectious foci. *J. Exp. Med.* **133**, 1090.

Blanden, R. V. (1974). T cell response to viral and bacterial infection. *Transplant. Rev.* **19**, 56.

Blanden, R. V. and Mims, C. A. (1972). Macrophage activation in mice infected with ectromelia or lymphocytic choriomeningitis viruses. *Aust. J. Exp. Biol. Med. Sci.* **51**, 393.

Blanden, R. V. and Gardner, I. D. (1976). The cell-mediated immune response to ectromelia virus infection. I. Kinetics and characteristics of primary effector T cell response *in vivo*. *Cell. Immunol.* **22**, 271.

Blanden, R. V., Hapel, A. J., Doherty, P. C. *et al.* (1976). In *Immunobiology of the Macrophage* pp. 367–400 (ed. D. S. Nelson). Academic Press, New York.

Blattner, R. J., Williamson, A. P. and Heys, F. M. (1973). Role of viruses in the etiology of congenital malformations. *Progr. Med. Virol.* **15**, 1.

Blinzinger, K. and Muller, W. (1971). The intercellular gaps of the neuropil as possible pathways for virus spread in viral encephalomyelitis. *Acta Neuropath.* **17**, 37.

Blinzinger, K., Simon, J., Magrath, D. *et al.* (1969). Poliovirus crystals within the endoplasmic reticulum of endothelial and mononuclear cells in the monkey spinal cord. *Science* **163**, 1336.

Bocci, V., Pacini, A. Muscettola, M. *et al.* (1982). The kidney is the main site of interferon catabolism. *J. Interferon Res.* **2**, 309.

Boulan, E. R. and Pendergast, M. (1980). Polarized distribution of viral envelope proteins in the plasma membrane of infected epithelial cells. *Cell* **20**, 45.

Boere, W. A. M., Benaissa-Trouw, B. J., Harmsen, M. *et al.* (1983). Neutralizing and non-neutralizing monoclonal antibodies to the E_2 glycoprotein of Semliki Forest virus can protect mice from lethal encephalitis. *J. Gen. Virol.* **64**, 1405.

Boulan, E. R. and Sabatini, D. D. (1978). Asymmetric budding of viruses in epithelial monolayers. Model system for epithelial polarity. *Proc. Nat. Acad. Sci. USA* **75**, 5071.

Boulter, E. A., Maber, H. B. and Bowen, E. T. W. (1961). Studies on the physiological disturbances occurring experimental rabbitpox: an approach to rational therapy. *Br. J. Exp. Pathol.* **42**, 433.

Bona, C. and Hiernaux, J. (1981). Immune response: idiotype anti-idiotype network. *CRC Critical Rev. Immunol.* **2**, 33.

Borgono, J. M., Vicent, P. and Toro, J. (1980). Efficacy of live poliovirus vaccine in Latin America. In *Potency and Efficacy of Vaccines* pp. 73–82 (ed. F. E. André). Smith Kline-RIT, U.S.A.

Bower, R. K., Gyles, N. R. and Brown, C. J. (1965). The number of genes controlling the response of chick embryo chorioallantoic membranes to tumor induction by Rous sarcoma virus. *Genetics* **51**, 739.

Brack, C., Nagata, S., Mantei, N. *et al.* (1981). Molecular analysis of the human interferon-α gene family. *Gene* **15**, 379.

Brahic, M., Stowring, L., Ventura, P. *et al.* (1981a). Gene expression in visna virus infection. *Nature* **292**, 240.

Brahic, M. B., Stroop, W. G. and Baringer, J. R. (1981b). Theiler's virus persists in glial cells during demyelinating disease. *Cell* **26**, 123.

Branca, A. A. and Baglioni, C. (1981). Evidence that types I and II interferons have different receptors. *Nature* **294**, 768.

Brandt, W. E., McCown, J. M., Gentry, M. K. *et al.* (1982). Infection enhancement of Dengue Type 2 virus in the U937 human monocyte cell line by antibodies to flavivirus cross-reactive determinants. *Infect. Immunity* **36**, 1036.

Brautigam, A. R., Dukto, F. J., Olding, L. B. *et al.* (1979). Pathogenesis of murine cytomegalovirus infection: macrophages as a permissive cell for cytomegalovirus infection, replication and latency. *J. Gen. Virol.* **44**, 349.

Brechot, C., Pourcel, C., Luoisa, A. *et al.* (1980). Presence of integrated hepatitis B virus DNA sequences in cellular DNA of human hepatocellular carcinoma. *Nature* **286**, 533.

Brenner, S. and Horne, R. W. (1959). A negative staining method for high resolution electron microscopy of viruses. *Biochim. Biophys. Acta* **34**, 103.

Breschkin, A. M., Ahern, J. and White, D. O. (1981). Antigenic determinants of influenza virus hemagglutinin. VIII. Topography of the antigenic regions of influenza virus hemagglutinin determined by competitive radioimmunoassay with monoclonal antibodies. *Virology* **113**, 130.

Brier, A. M., Synderman, R., Mergenhagen, S. E. *et al.* (1970). Inflammation and herpes simplex. Release of a chemotaxis-generating factor from infected cells. *Science* **170**, 1104.

Brinton, M. A. and Nathanson, N. (1981). Genetic determinants of virus susceptibility: epidemiological implications of murine models. *Epidem. Rev.* **3**, 115.

Brinton, M. A., Arnheiter, H. and Haller, O. (1982). Interferon independence of genetically controlled resistance to flaviviruses. *Infect. Immunity* **36**, 284.

Britt, W. J. and Cheseboro, B. (1983). H_2-D control of recovery from Friend virus leukemia: H-$_2$D region influences the kinetics of the T lymphocyte response to Friend virus. *J. Exp. Med.* **157**, 1736.

Bromberg, J. S., Lake, P. and Brunswick, M. (1982). Viral antigens act as helper determinants for antibody responses to cell surface antigens. *J. Immunol.* **129**, 683.

Brooksby, J. B. (1982). Portraits of Viruses: Foot-and-Mouth Disease. *Intervirology* **18**, 1.

Brown, P. (1980). An epidemiologic critique of Kreutzfeldt-Jakob disease. *Epidemiol. Rev.* **2**, 113.

Brown, S. M., Subak-Sharpe, J. H., Warren, K. G. *et al*. (1979). Detection by complementation of defective or uninducible (herpes simplex type 1) virus genomes latent in human ganglia. *Proc. Nat. Acad. Sci. USA* **76**, 2364.

Brownson, J. M., Mahy, B. W. J. and Hazleman, B. L. (1979). Interaction of influenza A virus with human peripheral blood lymphocytes. *Infect. Immunity* **25**, 749.

Bruns, M., Cihak, J., Muller, G. *et al*. (1983). Lymphocytic choriomeningitis virus VI. Isolation of a glycoprotein mediating neutralization. *Virology* **130**, 247.

Bruns, M. and Lehmann-Grube, F. (1983). Lymphocytic choriomeningitis virus V. Proposed structural arrangement of proteins in the virion. *J. Gen. Virol.* **64**, 2157.

Buchmeier, M. J., Welsh, R. M., Dukto, F. J. *et al*. (1980). The virology and immunobiology of lymphocytic choriomeningitis virus infection. *Adv. Immunol.* **30**, 275.

Buchmeier, N. A., Gee, S. R., Murphy, F. A. *et al*. (1979). Abortive replication of vaccinia virus in activated rabbit macrophages. *Infect. Immunity* **26**, 328.

Buckland, F. E., Bynoe, M. L. and Tyrrell, D. A. J. (1965). Experiments on the spread of colds. II. Studies with volunteers with coxsackievirus A21. *J. Hyg. Camb.* **63**, 327.

Buckley, S. M. and Casals, J. (1978). Pathobiology of Lassa fever. *Int. Rev. Exp. Pathol.* **18**, 97.

Bukowski, J. F., Woda, B. A., Habu, S. *et al*. (1983). Natural killer cell depletion enhances virus synthesis and virus-induced hepatitis *in vivo*. *J. Immunol.* **131**, 1531.

Burke, D. C. (1980). The type I human interferon gene system: chromosomal location and control of expression. In *Interferon* 2 pp. 47–64 (ed. I. Gresser). Academic Press, New York.

Burke, D. C. (1983). The control of interferon formation. In *Interferons* (D. C. Burke and A. G. Morris, eds.), Symposium of the Society of General Microbiology vol. 35, pp. 67–88. Cambridge University Press, Cambridge.

Burke, D. C. and Meager, A. (1980). Genetic control of interferon formation. *Annals N. Y. Acad. Sci.* **350**, 179.

Burke, D. C. and Morris, A. G. (eds.) (1983). *Interferons: from Molecular Biology to Clinical Application.* Symposium of the Society of General Microbiology vol. 35. Cambridge University Press, Cambridge.

Burke, D. C. and Russell, W. C. (eds.) (1975). *Control Processes in Virus Multiplication.* Society for General Microbiology Symposium, no. 25. Cambridge University Press, Cambridge.

Burnet, F. M. (1943). Immunization against epidemic influenza with living attenuated virus. *Med. J. Aust.* **1**, 385.

Burnet, F. M. (1952). The pattern of disease in childhood. *Austral. Ann. Med.* **1**, 93.

Burnet, F. M. (1955). *Principles of Animal Virology.* Academic Press, New York.

Burnet, F. M. (1968). Measles as an index of immunological functions. *Lancet* ii, 610.

Burnet, F. M. and Williams, S. W. (1939). Herpes simplex: a new point of view. *Med. J. Aust.* **1**, 637.

Burns, W. H. and Allison, A. C. (1975). Virus infections and the immune responses they elicit. In *The Antigens*, vol. 3, pp. 480–574, (ed. M. Sela). Academic Press, New York.

Burns, W. H., Billups, L. C. and Notkins, A. L. (1975). Thymic dependence of viral antigens. *Nature* **256**, 654.

Burrell, C. J., MacKay, P., Greenway, P. J. *et al.* (1979). Expression in *Escherichia coli* of hepatitis B virus DNA sequences cloned in plasmid pBR322. *Nature* **279**, 43.

Burrows, R. (1966). Studies on the carrier state of cattle exposed to foot and mouth disease virus. *J. Hyg.* (Camb) **64**, 81.

Burstin, S. J., Brandriss, M. W. and Schlesinger, J. J. (1983). Infection of a macrophage-like cell line. P388D1 with reovirus; effects of immune ascitic fluids and monoclonal antibodies on neutralization and enhancement of viral growth. *J. Immunol.* **130**, 2915.

Cabrera, C. V., Wohlenberg, C., Openshaw, H. *et al.* (1980). Herpes simplex virus DNA sequences in the CNS of latently infected mice. *Nature* **288**, 288.

Cafruny, W. A. and Plagemann, P. G. W. (1982). Immune response to lactate dehydrogenase-elevating virus: serologically specific rabbit neutralizing antibody to the virus. *Infect. Immunity* **37**, 1007.

Cahill, K. M. (ed.) (1983). *The AIDS Epidemic.* St. Martin's Press, New York.

Cairns, J. (1960). The initiation of vaccinia infection. *Virology* **11**, 603.

Calafat, J., Hilger, J., von Blitterswijk, W. J. *et al.* (1976). Antibody-induced modulation and shedding of mammary tumor virus antigens on the surfaces of GR ascites leukaemia cells as compared with normal antigens. *J. Nat. Cancer Inst.* **56**, 1019.

Calnek, B. W. and Hitchner, S. B. (1969). Localization of viral antigen in chickens infected with the Marek's disease herpes virus. *J. Nat. Cancer Inst.* **43**, 935.

Came, P. E. and Carter, W. A. (eds.) (1983). *Interferons and Their Applications.* Handbook Exp. Pharmacol. Vol. 71. Springer-Verlag, Berlin.

Campbell, A. E., Loria, R. M., Madge, G. E. *et al.* (1982). Dietary hepatic cholesterol elevation: effects on coxsackievirus B5 infection and inflammation. *Infect. Immunity* **37**, 307.

Canning, W. M. and Fields, B. N. (1983). Ammonium chloride prevents lytic growth of reovirus and helps to establish persistent infection in mouse L cells. *Science* **219**, 987.

Cantell, K., Hirvonen, S., Kauppinen, H.-L. *et al.* (1981). Production of interferon in human leucocytes from normal donors with the use of Sendai virus. *Meth. Enzymol.* **78**, 29.

dal Canto, M. C. and Rabinowitz, S. G. (1982). Experimental models of virus-induced demyelination of the central nervous system. *Ann. Neurol.* **11**, 109.

Cantor, H. and Gershon, G. K. (1979). Immunological circuits: cellular composition. *Fed. Proc.* **38**, 2058.

Cardosa, M. J., Porterfield, J. S. and Gordon, S. (1983). Complement receptor mediates enhanced flavivirus replication in macrophages. *J. Exp. Med.* **158**, 258.

Carney, W. P. and Hirsch, M. S. (1981). Mechanisms of immunosuppression in cytomegalovirus mononucleosis. II Virus-monocyte interaction. *J. Infect. Dis.* **144**, 47.

Carter, M. J., Willcocks, M. M. and ter Meulen, V. (1983). Defective translation of measles virus matrix protein in a subacute sclerosing panencephalitis cell line. *Nature* **305**, 153.

Carton, C. A. (1953). Effect of previous sensory loss on the appearance of herpes simplex. *J. Neurosurg.* **10**, 463.

Casali, P., Sissons, J. G. P., Buchmeier, M. J. *et al.* (1981). *In vitro* generation of human cytotoxic lymphocytes by virus. Viral glycoproteins induce non-specific cell-mediated cytotoxicity without release of interferon. *J. Exp. Med.* **154**, 840.

Caspar, D. L. D. (1965). Design principles in virus particle construction. In *Viral and Rickettsial Infections of Man*, 4th edn, p. 51 (eds. F. L. Horsfall, Jr. and I. Tamm). Lippincott, Philadelphia.

Caspar, D. L. D. and Klug, A. (1962). Physical principles in the construction of regular viruses. *Cold Spring Harbor Symp. Quant. Biol.* **27**, 490.

Cayley, P. J., Silverman, R. H., Wreschner, D. H. *et al.* (1981). The 2-5A system in interferon-treated and control cells. In *Cellular Responses to Molecular Modulators* pp. 347–360 (eds. L. W. Mozes *et al.*). Academic Press, New York.

Centifanto, Y. M., Fitzgerald, T., Yamagudii, T. *et al.* (1982). Ocular disease pattern induced by herpes simplex virus is genetically determined by a specific region of viral DNA. *J. Exp. Med.* **155**, 475.

Centers for Disease Control (1977). Immune globulins for protection against viral hepatitis. *Morbid. Mortal. Weekly Report* **26**, 425–8, 441–2.

Centers for Disease Control (1980a). Mumps vaccine. *Morbid. Mortal. Weekly Report* **29**, 87–94.

Centers for Disease Control (1980b). Rabies prevention. *Morbid. Mortal. Weekly Report* **29**, 265–80.

Centers for Disease Control (1981a). Rubella prevention. *Morbid. Mortal. Weekly Report* **30**, 37–47.

Centers for Disease Control (1981b). Varicella-zoster immune globulin—United States. *Morbid. Mortal. Weekly Report* **30**, No. 2.

Centers for Disease Control (1982a). Poliomyelitis prevention. *Morbid. Mortal. Weekly Report* **31**, 22.

Centers for Disease Control (1982b). Measles prevention. *Morbid. Mortal. Weekly Report* **31**, 217–31.

Centers for Disease Control (1982c). Inactivated hepatitis B virus vaccine. *Morbid. Mortal. Weekly Report* **31**, 317–28.

Challberg, M. D. and Kelly, T. J. (1982). Eukaryotic DNA replication: viral and plasmid model systems. *Ann. Rev. Biochem.* **51**, 901.

Chandler, R. L. (1961). Encephalopathy in mice produced with scrapie brain material. *Lancet* i, 1378.

Chandra, R. K. (1979). Nutritional deficiency and susceptibility to infection. *Bull WHO* **57**, 167.

Chandra, R. K. (1983). Nutrition, immunity and infection: present knowledge and future directions. *Lancet* i, 688.

Chanock, R. M. (1981). Strategy for development of respiratory and gastro-intestinal tract viral vaccines in the 1980s. *J. Infect. Dis.* **143**, 364.

Chanock, R. M. and Murphy, B. R. (1980). Use of temperature-sensitive and cold-adapted mutant viruses in immunoprophylaxis of acute respiratory tract diseases. *Rev. Infect. Dis.* **2**, 421.

Chanock, R. M., Parrott, R. H., Kapikian, A. Z. *et al.* (1968). Possible role of immunological factors in pathogenesis of RS virus lower respiratory tract disease. *Perspect. Virol.* **6**, 125.

Chanock, R. M., Richman, D. D., Murphy, B. R. *et al.* (1975). Current approaches to viral immunoprophylaxis. In *Viral Immunology and Immuno-pathology* pp. 291–316 (ed. A. L. Notkins). Academic Press, New York.

Chantler, J. K., Ford, D. K. and Tingle, A. J. (1981). Rubella-associated arthritis: rescue of rubella virus from peripheral blood lymphocytes two years post-vaccination. *Infect. Immunity* **32**, 1274.

Chapes, S. K. and Tompkins, W. A. F. (1979). Cytotoxic macrophages induced in hamsters by vaccinia virus: selective cytotoxicity for virus-infected targets by macrophages collected late after immunization. *J. Immunol.* **123**, 303.

Charnay, P., Gervais, M., Louise, A. *et al.* (1980). Biosynthesis of hepatitis B virus surface antigen in *Escherichia coli. Nature* **286**, 893.

Chedid, L. (ed.) (1979). Immunomodulation I and II. *Springer Seminars Immunopathol.* **2**, 1.

Chedid, L. A., Parant, M. A., Audibert, F. M. *et al.* (1982). Biological activity of a new synthetic muramyl peptide adjuvant devoid of pyrogenicity. *Infect. Immunity* **35**, 417.

Chong, K. T. and Mims, C. A. (1981). Murine cytomegalovirus particle types in relation to sources of virus and pathogenicity. *J. Gen. Virol.* **57**, 415.

Chong, K. T. and Mims, C. A. (1982). Delayed hypersensitivity to murine cytomegalovirus and its depression during pregnancy. *Infect. Immunity* **37**, 54.

Chong, K. T. and Mims, C. A. (1983). Antigen-specific suppression of delayed type hypersensitivity to murine cytomegalovirus in MCMV-infected mice. *J. Gen. Virol.* **64**, 2433.

Chong, K. T. and Mims, C. A. (1984). Effects of pregnant mouse serum and pregnancy hormomes on the replication *in vitro* of murine cytomegalovirus. *Arch. Virol.* (in press).

Chong, K. T., Gould, J. J. and Mims, C. A. (1981). Neutralization of different strains of murine cytomegalovirus (MCMV)—effect of *in vitro* passage. *Arch. Virol.* **69**, 95.

Chong, K. T., Gresser, I. and Mims, C. A. (1983). Interferon as a defence mechanism in mouse cytomegalovirus infection. *J. Gen. Virol.* **64**, 461.

Choppin, P. W. and Compans, R. W. (1975). Reproduction of paramyxoviruses. *Comprehen. Virol.* **4**, 95.

Choppin, P. W. and Scheid, A. (1980). The role of viral glycoproteins in adsorption, penetration and pathogenicity of viruses. *Rev. Infect. Dis.* **2**, 40.

Choppin, P. W., Richardson, C. D., Merz, D. C. *et al.* (1981). The function and inhibition of the membrane glycoprotein of paramyxoviruses and myxoviruses and the role of the measles virus M protein in subacute sclerosing panencephalitis. *J. Infect. Dis.* **143**, 352.

Christensen, P. E., Schmidt, H., Bang, H. O. *et al.* (1953). An epidemic of measles in southern Greenland, 1951. Measles in virgin soil III Measles and tuberculosis. *Acta. Med. Scand.* **144**, 450.

Christie, A. B., Allam, A. A., Aref, M. K. *et al.* (1976). Pregnancy hepatitis in Libya. *Lancet* ii, 827.

Ciavarra, R. and Forman, J. (1982). H-2L-restricted recognition of viral antigens. *J. Exp. Med.* **156**, 778.

Cines, D. B., Lyss, A. P., Bina, M. *et al.* (1982). Fc and C3 receptors induced by herpes simplex virus on cultured human endothelial cells. *J. Clin. Invest.* **69**, 123.

Clements, J. E., Pedersen, F. S., Narayan, O. *et al.* (1980). Genomic changes associated with antigenic variation of visna virus during persistent infection. *Proc. Nat. Acad. Sci. USA* **77**, 4454.

Coffin, D. L. and Liu, C. (1957). Studies on canine distemper infection by means of fluorescein-labelled antibody. II The pathology and diagnosis of the naturally occurring disease in dogs, and the antigenic nature of the inclusion body. *Virology* **3**, 132.

Coleman, D. V., Wolfendale, M. R., Daniel, R. A. *et al.* (1980). A prospective study of human polyomavirus infection in pregnancy. *J. Infect. Dis.* **142**, 1.

Collier, L. H., Scott, Q. J. and Pani, A. (1983). Variation in resistance of cells from inbred strains of mice to herpes simplex virus Type 1. *J. Gen. Virol.* **64**, 1483.

Compans, R. W. and Klenk, H.-D. (1979). Viral membranes. *Comprehen. Virol.* **13**, 293.

Compans, R. W. and Bishop, D. H. L. (eds) (1983). *Double-stranded RNA Viruses*. Elsevier, New York.

Compans, R. W., Holmes, K. V., Dales, S. *et al.* (1966). An electron microscopic study of moderate and virulent virus-cell interactions of the parainfluenza virus, SV5. *Virology* **30**, 411.

Constantine, D. G. (1971). Bat rabies: current knowledge and future research. In *Rabies* p. 253 (eds. Y. Nagano and F. M. Davenport). University of Tokyo Press, Tokyo.

Cook, M. L., Bastone, V. B. and Stevens, J. G. (1974). Evidence that neurons harbour latent herpes simplex virus. *Infect. Immunity* **9**, 946.

Cooper, N. R. (1979). Humoral immunity to viruses. In *Comprehensive Virology* vol. 15, p. 123 (eds. H. Fraenkel-Conrat and R. R. Wagner). Plenum Press, New York.

Cooper, N. R. and Oldstone, M. B. A. (1983). Virus-infected cells, IgG and the alternative complement pathway. *Immunol. Today* **4**, 107.

Cooper, N. R. and Welsh, R. M. (1979). Antibody and complement-dependent viral neutralization. *Springer Seminars Immunopath.* **2**, 285.

Cooper, N. R., Jensen, F. C., Welsh, R. M. *et al*. (1976). Lysis of RNA tumor viruses by human serum: direct antibody independent triggering of the classical complement pathway. *J. Exp. Med.* **144**, 970.

Cooper, P. D., Agol, V. I., Bachrach, H. L. *et al*. (1978). Picornaviridae: second report. *Intervirology* **10**, 165.

Cords, C. E. and Holland, J. J. (1964). Alteration of the species and tissue specificity of poliovirus by enclosure of its RNA within the protein capsid of coxsackie B1 virus. *Virology* **24**, 492.

Corey, L., Adams, H. G., Brown, Z. A. *et al*. (1983). Genital herpes simplex virus infections: clinical manifestations, course, and complications. *Ann. Intern. Med.* **98**, 958.

Couch, R. B. (1981). The effects of influenza on host defences. *J. Infect. Dis.* **144**, 284.

Couch, R. B. and Kasel, J. A. (1983). Immunity to influenza in man. *Ann. Rev. Microbiol.* **37**, 529.

Couch, R. B., Chanock, R. M., Cate, T. R. *et al*. (1963). Immunization with types 4 and 7 adenovirus by selective infection of the intestinal tract. *Am. Rev. Resp. Dis.* **88** (Part 2), 394.

Couch, R. B., Kasel, J. A., Six, H. R. *et al*. (1981). The basis of immunity to influenza in man. In *Genetic Variation among Influenza Viruses* pp. 535–546 (ed. D. P. Nayak). Academic Press, New York.

Couch, R. D., Cate, T. R., Douglas, R. G. *et al*. (1966). Effect of route of inoculation on experimental respiratory viral disease in volunteers and evidence for airborne transmission. *Bact. Rev.* **30**, 517.

Coulon, P., Rollin, P., Aubert, M. *et al*. (1982). Molecular basis of rabies virus virulence. I. Selection of avirulent mutants of the CVS strain with anti-G monoclonal antibodies. *J. Gen. Virol.* **61**, 97.

Coulon, P., Rollin, P. E. and Flamand, A. (1983). Molecular basis of rabies virus virulence. II. Identification of a site on the CVS glycoprotein associated with virulence. *J. Gen. Virol.* **64**, 693.

Coyle, P. K. and Wolinsky, J. S. (1981). Characterization of immune complexes in progressive rubella panencephalitis. *Ann. Neurol.* **9**, 557.

Coyle, P. K., Wolinsky, J. S., Buimovici-Klein, E. *et al*. (1981). Rubella specific immune complexes following congenital infection and live virus vaccination. *Neurology* **31**, 126.

Craighead, J. E. and Steinke, J. (1971). Diabetes mellitus-like syndrome in mice infected with encephalomyocarditis virus. *Am. J. Path.* **63**, 119.

Crawford, D. H., Brickell, P., Tidman, N. *et al*. (1981). Increased numbers of cells with suppressor T cell phenotype in the peripheral blood of patients with infectious mononucleosis. *Clin. Exp. Immunol.* **43**, 291.

Crawford, T. B., Cheevers, W. P., Klevjer-Anderson, P. *et al*. (1978). Equine Infectious Anemia: virion characteristics, virus-cell interaction and host responses. In *Persistent Viruses* (eds. J. G. Stevens, G. J. Todaro and C. F. Fox). Academic Press, New York.

Crawford, T. B., Adams, D. S., Cheevers, W. P. *et al*. (1980). Chronic arthritis in goats caused by a retrovirus. *Science* **207**, 997.

Crick, F. (1979). Split genes and RNA splicing. *Science* **204**, 264.

Crick, F. H. C. and Watson, J. D. (1956). Structure of small viruses. *Nature Lond.* **177**, 473.

Cross, S. S., Parker, J. C., Rowe, W. P. *et al*. (1979). Biology of mouse thymic virus, a herpesvirus of mice, and the antigenic relationship to mouse cytomegalovirus. *Infect. Immunity* **26**, 1186.

Crowell, R. L. and Philipson, L. (1971). Specific alterations of coxsackievirus B3 eluted from HeLa cells. *J. Virol.* **8**, 509.

Cunningham, A. L. and Merigan, T. C. (1983). γ interferon production appears to predict time of recurrences of herpes labialis. *J. Immunol.* **130**, 2397.

Daemer, R. J., Feinstone, S. M., Gust, I. D. *et al*. (1981). Propagation of human hepatitis A virus in African green monkey cell culture: primary isolation and serial passage. *Infect. Immunity* **32**, 388.

Dales, S. and Pogo, B. G. T. (1981). *Biology of Poxviruses*. Virology Monographs, 18. Springer-Verlag, Wien, New York.

Dales, S., Fujinami, R. S. and Oldstone, M. B. A. (1983). Infection with vaccinia favours the selection of hybridomas synthesizing antibodies against intermediate filaments, one of them cross reacting with the viral haemaglutinin. *J. Immunol.* **131**, 1546.

Dalldorf, G. and Sickles, G. M. (1948). An unidentified, filtrable agent isolated from the feces of children with paralysis. *Science* **108**, 61.

Daniels, C. A., Le Goff, S. G. and Notkins, A. L. (1975). Shedding of infectious virus-antibody complexes from vesicular lesions of patients with recurrent herpes labialis. *Lancet* ii, 524.

Darnell, J. E. (1982). Variety in the level of gene control in eukaryotic cells. *Nature* **297**, 365.

Daughaday, C. C., Brandt, W. E., McCown, J. M. *et al*. (1981). Evidence for two mechanisms of dengue virus infection of adherent human monocytes: trypsin-sensitive virus receptors and trypsin-resistant immune complex receptors. *Infect. Immunity* **32**, 469.

Dausset, J. and Svejgaard, A. (eds.) (1977). *HLA and Disease*. Munksgaard, Copenhagen.

Davis, A. R., Bos, T., Ueda, M. *et al*. (1983). Immune response to human influenza virus hemagglutinin expressed in *Escherichia coli*. *Gene* **21**, 273.

Davis, L. E. and Johnson, R. T. (1979). An explanation for the localization of herpes simplex encephalitis. *Ann. Neurol.* **5**, 2.

Davis, L. E., Cole, L. L., Lockwood, S. J. *et al*. (1983). Experimental influenza B virus toxicity in mice: a possible model for Reye's syndrome. *Lab. Investig.* **48**, 140.

Degre, M. (1970). Synergistic effect in viral-bacterial infection II. Influence of viral infection on the phagocytic ability of alveolar macrophages. *Acta. Path. Microbiol. Scand.* B. **78**, 41.

Deinhardt, F. and Gust, I. D. (1982). Viral hepatitis. *Bull WHO* **60**, 661.

Della-Porta, A. J. and Westaway, E. G. (1978). A multihit model for the neutralization of animal viruses. *J. Gen. Virol.* **38**, 1.

Denman, A. M., Bacon, T. H. and Pelton. B. K. (1983). Viruses: Immunosuppressive effects. *Phil. Trans. R. Soc. Lond.* B. **303**, 137.

Derynck, R., Remaut, E., Saman, E. *et al*. (1980). Expression of human fibroblast interferon gene in *Escherichia coli*. *Nature* **287**, 193.

de Sena, J. and Torian, B. (1980). Studies on the *in vitro* uncoating of poliovirus.

III. Roles of membrane-modifying and stabilizing factors in the generation of subviral particles. *Virology* **104**, 149.

De Stefano, E., Friedman, R. M., Friedman-Kien, A. E. *et al*. (1982). Acid-labile human leukocyte interferon in homosexual men with Kaposi's sarcoma and lymphadenopathy. *J. Infect. Dis.* **146**, 451.

De Vries, R. R. P., Kreeftenberg, H. G., Loggen, H. G. *et al*. (1977). *In vitro* immune responsiveness to vaccinia virus and HLA. *New Engl. J. Med.* **297**, 692.

Diamond, L. S. and Mattern, C. F. T. (1976). Protozoal viruses. *Adv. Virus Res.* **20**, 87.

Dickinson, A. G. (1975). Host-pathogen interactions in scrapie. *Genetics* **79** (Suppl), 387.

Dickinson, A. G., Fraser, H. and Outram, G. W. (1975). Scrapie incubation time can exceed natural lifespan. *Nature* **256**, 732.

Diener, E. and Feldmann, M. (1972). Mechanisms at the cellular level during induction of high zone tolerances *in vitro*. *Cell Immunol.* **5**, 130.

Diener, T. O. (1982). Viroids and their interactions with host cells. *Ann. Rev. Microbiol.* **36**, 239.

Dienstag, J. L., Stevens, C. E., Bahn, A. K. *et al*. (1982). Hepatitis B vaccine administered to chronic carriers of hepatitis B surface antigen. *Ann. Intern. Med.* **96**, 575.

Dietzschold, B., Cohen, G., Eisenberg, R. *et al*. (1984). Synthesis of an antigenic determinant of the herpes simplex virus (HSV) glycoprotein D which stimulates the production of virus neutralizing antibodies and which confers protection against a lethal challenge infection of HSV. In *Modern Approaches to Vaccines* (R. A. Lerner and R. M. Chanock, eds.). Cold Spring Harbor Laboratory, New York.

Dillard, S. H., Cheatham, W. J. and Moses, H. L. (1972). Electron microscopy of zosteriform herpes simplex infection in mouse. *Lab. Investig.* **26**, 391.

Dimmock, N. J. (1982). Initial stages in infection with animal viruses. *J. Gen. Virol.* **59**, 1.

Doherty, P. C. and Zinkernagel, R. M. (1974). T cell mediated immunopathology in viral infections. *Transplant. Rev.* **19**, 89.

Doherty, P. C., Blanden, R. V. and Zinkernagel, R. M. (1976). Specificity of virus-immune effector T cells for H-2K or H-2D compatible interactions: implications for H-antigen diversity. *Transplant Rev.* **29**, 89.

Doherty, P. C., Lopes, A. D., Greenspan, N. *et al*. (1982). Therapeutic potential of monoclonal antibodies in virus-induced neurological disease. In *Viral Diseases in South-East Asia and the Western Pacific* pp. 183–90 (ed. J. S. Mackenzie). Academic Press, New York.

Doherty, R. L., Whitehead, R. H., Gorman, B. M. *et al*. (1963). The isolation of a third group A arbovirus in Australia, with preliminary observations on its relationship to epidemic polyarthritis. *Austral. J. Sci.* **26**, 183.

Dossetor, J. F. B. and Whittle, H. C. (1975). Protein-losing enteropathy and maladsorption in acute measles-enteritis. *Br. Med. J.* **2**, 592.

Dowdle, W. R. (1981). Influenza immunoprophylaxis after 30 years' experience. In *Genetic Variation among Influenza Viruses* (ed. D. Nayak). ICN-UCLA Symposium no. 21, pp. 525–34. Academic Press, New York.

Dowler, K. W. and Veltri, R. W. (1983). *In vitro* neutralization of HSV-2; inhibition by binding of normal IgG and purified Fc to virion Fc receptor (FcR). *J. Med. Microbiol.* (in press).

Downs, W. G. (1982). The Rockefeller Foundation Virus Program: 1951–1971 with update to 1981. *Ann. Rev. Med.* **33**, 1.

Doyle, L. B., Doyle, M. V. and Oldstone, M. B. (1980). Susceptibility of newborn mice with H2K backgrounds to lymphocytic choriomeningitis virus infection. *Immunology* **40**, 589.

Dreesman, G. R., Sanchez, Y., Ionescu-Matiu, I. *et al.* (1982). Antibody to hepatitis B surface antigen after a single inoculation of uncoupled synthetic HBsAg peptides. *Nature* **295**, 158.

Dubois-Dalcq, M., Hooghe-Peters, E. L. and Lazzarini, R. A. (1980). Antibody-induced modulation of rhabdovirus infection of neurones *in vitro*. *J. Neuropath. Exp. Neurol.* **39**, 507.

Dubovi, E. J., Geratz, J. D. and Tidwell, R. R. (1983). Enhancement of respiratory syncytial virus-induced cytopathology by trypsin, thrombin and plasma. *Infect. Immunity* **40**, 351.

Dudgeon, J. A. (1979). Rubella: the U.K. experience. *Develop. Biol. Stand.* **43**, 327. Karger, Basel.

Dunlop, M. B. C. and Blanden, R. V. (1977). Mechanism of suppression of cytotoxic T cell responses in murine lymphocytic choriomeningitis virus infection. *J. Exp. Med.* **145**, 1131.

Dunnick, J. K. and Galasso, G. J. (1979, 1980). Clinical trials with exogenous interferon. *J. Infect. Dis.* **139**, 109; **142**, 293.

Dutko, F. J. and Oldstone, M. B. A. (1981). Cytomegalovirus causes a latent infection in undifferentiated cells and is activated by induction of cell differentiation. *J. Exp. Med.* **154**, 1636.

Dutton, R. W. and Swain, S. L. (1982). Regulation of the immune response: T-cell interactions. *Crit. Rev. Immunol.* **3**, 209.

Easton, J. M. (1964). Cytopathic effect of Simian virus 40 on primary cell cultures of rhesus monkey kidney. *J. Immunol.* **93**, 716.

Edelman, R. (1980). Vaccine adjuvants. *Rev. Infect. Dis.* **2**, 370.

Edelman, R., Ascher, M. S., Oster, C. N. *et al.* (1979). Evaluation in humans of a new, inactivated vaccine for Venezuelan encephalitis virus (C-84). *J. Infect. Dis.* **140**, 708.

Edelman, R., Hardegree, M. C. and Chedid, L. (1980). Summary of an international symposium on potentiation of the immune response to vaccines. *J. Infect. Dis.* **141**, 103.

Editorial (1981). Immunocompromised homosexuals. *Lancet* ii, 1325.

Edman, J. C., Hallewell, R. A., Valenzuela, P. *et al.* (1981). Synthesis of hepatitis B surface and core antigens in *E. coli*. *Nature* **291**, 503.

Edmonson, W. P., Purcell, R. H., Gundelfinger, B. F. *et al.* (1966). Immunization by selective infection with type 4 adenovirus grown in human diploid tissue culture. II. Specific protection effect against epidemic disease. *J. Am. Med. Assoc.* **195**, 453.

Edy, V. G., Augenstein, D. C., Edwards, C. R. *et al.* (1982). Large-scale tissue culture for human IFN-β production. *Texas Reports Biol. Med.* **41**, 169.

Eklund, C. M., Kennedy, R. C. and Hadlow, W. J. (1967). Pathogenesis of scrapie virus infection in the mouse. *J. Infect. Dis.* **117**, 15.

Elek, S. D. and Stern, H. (1974). Development of a vaccine against mental retardation caused by cytomegalovirus infection *in utero*. *Lancet* i, 1.

Embil, J. A., Manuel, F. R., Garner, J. B. *et al.* (1982). Cytomegalovirus in the semen. *J. Can. Med. Assoc.* **126**, 391.

Emini, E. A., Jameson, B. A. and Wimmer, E. (1983). Priming for and induction of anti-poliovirus neutralizing antibodies by synthetic peptides. *Nature, Lond.* **304**, 699.

Emmons, R. W., Oshiro, L. S., Johnson, H. M. *et al.* (1972). Intraerythrocyte location of Colorado Tick Fever virus. *J. Gen. Virol.* **17**, 185.

Emtage, J. S., Tacon, W. C. A., Catlin, G. H. *et al.* (1980). Influenza antigenic determinants are expressed from haemagglutinin genes cloned in *Escherichia coli*. *Nature* **283**, 171.

Enders, J. F. and Katz, S. L. (1967). Present status of live rubeola vaccines in the United States. In *First International Conference on Vaccines against Viral and Rickettsial Diseases of Man*, p. 295. Sci. Publ. No. 147. Pan Am. Health Organ., Washington, D.C.

Enders, J. F., Weller, T. H. and Robbins, F. C. (1949). Cultivation of Lansing strain of poliomyelitis virus in cultures of various human embryonic tissues. *Science* **109**, 85.

Ennis, F. A. (1973). Host defence mechanisms against herpes simplex virus. II. Protection conferred by sensitized spleen cells. *J. Infect. Dis.* **127**, 632.

Epstein, L. B. (1981). Interferon-gamma: is it really different from other interferons? In *Interferon 3* pp. 13–44 (ed. I. Gresser). Academic Press, New York.

Epstein, L. B., Lee, S. H. and Epstein, C. J. (1980). Enhanced sensitivity of trisomy 21 monocytes to the maturation-inhibiting effect of interferon. *Cell. Immunol.* **50**, 191.

Epstein, M. A. and Achong, B. G. (1977). Pathogenesis of infectious mononucleosis. *Lancet* ii, 1270.

Epstein, M. A. and Achong, B. G. (eds.). (1979). *The Epstein-Barr Virus*. Springer-Verlag, Berlin.

Epstein, M. A. and Morgan, A. J. (1983). Clinical consequences of Epstein-Barr virus infection and possible control by an antiviral vaccine. *Clin. Exp. Immunol.* **53**, 257.

Epstein, M. A., North, J. R. and Morgan, A. J. (1983). Possibilities for antiviral vaccine intervention in nasopharyngeal carcinoma. In *Proceedings of the Third International Symposium on Nasopharyngeal Carcinoma*.

Ertl, H. C. (1981). Adoptive transfer of delayed hypersensitivity to Sendai virus. I. Induction of two different subsets of T lymphocytes which differ in H2 restriction as well as in the Lyt phenotype. *Cell. Immunol.* **62**, 38.

Essex, M., Todaro, G. and zur Hausen, H. (eds.) (1980). *Viruses in Naturally Occurring Cancers*. Cold Spring Harbor Laboratory, New York.

Estes, M. K., Palmer, E. L. and Obijeski, J. F. (1983). Rotaviruses: A review. *Curr. Topics Microbiol. Immunol.* **105**.

Evans, D. M., Minor, P. D., Schild, G. C. *et al.* (1983). Critical role of an eight-amino acid sequence of VP_1 in neutralization of poliovirus type 3. *Nature* **304**, 459.

Evans, R. and Riley, V. (1968). Circulating interferon in mice infected with the lactic dehydrogenase elevating virus. *J. Gen. Virol.* **3**, 449.

Favila, L., Howes, E. L., Taylor, W. A. *et al*. (1982). An adoptive transfer system for the evaluation of immunity to herpes simplex virus in mice. *Clin. Exp. Immunol*. **48**, 307.

Fazekas de St. Groth, S. (1950). Influenza: a study in mice. *Lancet* i, 1101.

Fazekas de St. Groth, S. (1962). The neutralization of viruses. *Adv. Virus Res.* **9**, 1.

Feldmann, M. and Kontiainen, S. (1981). The role of antigen-specific T-cell factors in the immune response. *Lymphokines* **2**, 87.

Feldmann, M. and Schreier, M. H. (eds.) (1982). *Lymphokines. 5. Monoclonal T Cells and their Products*. Academic Press, New York.

Fenner, F. (1948). The pathogenesis of the acute exanthems. *Lancet* ii, 915.

Fenner, F. (1949). Mousepox (infectious ectromelia of mice): a review. *J. Immunol*. **63**, 341.

Fenner, F. (1969). Conditional lethal mutants of animal viruses. *Curr. Topics Microbiol. Immunol*. **48**, 1.

Fenner, F. (1972). The possible use of temperature-sensitive conditional lethal mutants for immunization in viral infections. In *Immunity in Viral and Rickettsial Diseases*, p. 131 (eds. A. Kohn and M. A. Klinberg). Plenum Press, New York.

Fenner, F. (1982). A successful eradication campaign. Global eradication of smallpox. *Rev. Infect. Dis.* **4**, 916.

Fenner, F. and Woodroofe, G. M. (1953). The pathogenesis of infectious myxomatosis: The mechanism of infection and the immunological response in the European rabbit (*Oryctolagus cuniculus*). *Br. J. Exp. Pathol*. **34**, 400.

Fenner, F. and Sambrook, J. F. (1964). The genetics of animal viruses. *Ann. Rev. Microbiol*. **18**, 47.

Fenner, F. and Gibbs, A. (1983). Cryptograms—1982. *Intervirology* **19**, 121.

Fenner, F., McAuslan, B. R., Mims, C. A. *et al*. (1974). *The Biology of Animal Viruses*, 2nd edn. Academic Press, New York.

Fenner, F., Henderson, D. A., Arita, I. *et al*. (in press). *Smallpox and its Eradication*. World Health Organization, Geneva.

Fields, B. N. (1982). Molecular basis of reovirus virulence. *Arch. Virol*. **71**, 95.

Fields, B. N. and Weiner, H. L. (1977). Neutralization of reovirus: the gene responsible for the neutralization antigen. *J. Exp. Med*. **146**, 1305.

Fields, B. and Jaenisch, R. (eds.) (1980). *Animal Virus Genetics*. Academic Press, New York.

Fields, B. N. and Byers, K. (1983). The genetic basis of viral virulence. *Phil. Trans. R. Soc. Lond. B.* **303**, 209.

Fields, B. N. and Greene, M. I. (1982). Genetic and molecular mechanisms of viral pathogenesis: implications for prevention and treatment. *Nature* **300**, 19.

Fiers, W., Contreras, R., Haegeman, G. *et al*. (1978). Complete nucleotide sequence of SV40 DNA. *Nature* **273**, 113.

Finberg, R., Spriggs, D. R. and Fields, B. N. (1982). Host immune response to reovirus: CTL recognize the major neutralization domain of the viral haemagglutinin. *J. Immunol*. **129**, 2235.

Finter, N. B. (1982). Large-scale production of human interferon from lymphoblastoid cells. *Texas Reports Biol. Med.* **41**, 175.

Finter, N. B. (ed.) (1983–4). *Interferons*, 3rd edn, vols. 1–4. Elsevier North-Holland, Amsterdam.

Fishaut, M., Tubergin, D. and McIntosh, K. (1979). Prolonged fatal respiratory virus infections in children with disorders of cell-mediated immunity. *Pediat. Res.* **13**, 447.

Fleishmann, W. R. (1982). Potentiation of the direct anticellular activity of mouse interferons: mutual synergism and interferon concentration dependence. *Cancer Res.* **42**, 869.

Flewett, T. H. and Woode, G. N. (1978). The Rotaviruses. *Arch. Virol.* **57**, 1.

Flint, S. J. (1981). Splicing and the regulation of viral gene expression. In *Initiation Signals in Viral Gene Expression*, pp. 47–80 (ed. A. J. Shatkin). Springer-Verlag, Berlin.

Forghani, B. and Schmidt, N. J. (1983). Association of herpes simplex virus with platelets in experimentally infected mice. *Arch. Virol.* **76**, 269.

Fougereau, M. and Dausset, J. (eds.) (1980). *Immunology 80*. Academic Press, New York.

Fox, J. P. and Hall, C. E. (1980). *Viruses in Families*. PSG Publications, Littleton, Mass.

Fraenkel-Conrat, H. and Wagner, R. R. (eds.) (1974–83). *Comprehensive Virology*, vols 1–8. Plenum Press, New York.

Frankel-Conrat, H. and Wagner, R. R. (eds.) (1982). *The Viruses*. A series of monographs on all families of viruses. Plenum Press, New York.

Francis, T. (1955). The current status of the control of influenza. *Ann. Intern. Med.* **43**, 534.

Fraser, H. and Dickinson, A. G. (1978). Studies of the lymphoreticular system in the pathogenesis of scrapie: the role of the spleen and thymus. *J. Comp. Pathol.* **88**, 563.

Fraser, K. B. and Martin, S. J. (1978). *Measles Virus and its Biology*. Academic Press, New York.

Fridman, W. H., Gresser, I., Bandu, M. T. *et al.* (1980). Interferon enhances the expression of Fc γ receptors. *J. Immunol.* **124**, 2436.

Friedenwald, J. S. (1923). Studies on the virus of herpes simplex. *Arch. Ophthalmol.* **52**, 105.

Friedman, R. M. (1977). Antiviral activity of interferon. *Bact. Rev.* **41**, 543.

Friedman, H. M., Macarek, E. J., MacGregor, R. A. *et al.* (1981). Virus infection of endothelial cells. *J. Infect. Dis.* **143**, 266.

Fucillo, D. A., Steele, R. W., Hensen, S. A. *et al.* (1974). Impaired cellular immunity to rubella virus in congenital rubella. *Infect. Immunity* **9**, 81.

Fujinami, R. S. and Oldstone, M. B. A. (1980). Alterations in expression of measles virus polypeptides by antibody: Molecular events in antibody-induced antigenic modulation. *J. Immunol.* **125**, 78.

Fujinami, R. S. and Oldstone, M. B. A. (1981). Failure to cleave measles virus fusion protein in lymphoid cells. A possible mechanism for viral persistence in lymphoid cells. *J. Exp. Med.* **154**, 1489.

Fujinami, R. S., Oldstone, M. B. A., Wroblewska, Z. *et al.* (1983). Molecular mimicry in virus infection. Cross reaction of measles virus phosphoprotein or of herpes simplex virus protein with human intermediate filaments. *Proc. Nat. Acad. Sci. USA* **80**, 2346.

Furukawa, T., Hornberger, E., Sakuma, S. *et al.* (1975). Demonstration of immunoglobulin G receptors induced by human cytomegalovirus. *J. Clin. Microbiol.* **2**, 332.

Gajdusek, D. C. (1977). Unconventional viruses and the origin and disappearance of kuru. *Science* **197**, 943.

Galloway, D. A., Fenoglio, C. M. and McDougall, J. K. (1982). Limited transcription of the herpes simplex virus genome when latent in human sensory ganglia. *J. Virol.* **41**, 686.

Ganem, D. (1982). Persistent infection of humans with hepatitis B virus: mechanisms and consequences. *Rev. Infect. Dis.* **4**, 1026.

Gard, S. (1960). Theoretical considerations on the inactivation of viruses by chemical means. *Ann. N.Y. Acad. Sci.* **83**, 638.

Gardner, S. D. (1977). The new human papovaviruses, their nature and significance. In *Recent Advances in Clinical Virology*, p. 93 (ed. A. P. Waterson). Churchill Livingtone, Edinburgh.

Garoff, H., Kondor-Koch, C. and Riedel, H. (1982). Structure and assembly of alphaviruses. *Curr. Top. Microbiol. Immunol.* **99**, 1.

Gerhard, W. and Webster, R. G. (1978). Antigenic drift in influenza A viruses. I. Selection and characterization of antigenic variants of A/PR8/8/34 (HON1) influenza virus with monoclonal antibodies. *J. Exp. Med.* **148**, 383.

Gehrz, R. C., Christianson, W. R., Linner, K. M. *et al.* (1981). Cytomegalovirus—specific humoral and cellular immune responses in human pregnancy. *J. Infect. Dis.* **143**, 391.

Gerin, J. L., Alexander, H., Shin, J. W.-K. *et al.* (1983). Chemically synthesized peptides of hepatitis B surface antigen duplicate the *d/y* specificities and induce subtype-specific antibodies in chimpanzees. *Proc. Nat. Acad. Sci. USA* **80**, 2365.

Germain, R. N. and Benacerraf, B. (1980). Helper and suppressor T cell factors. *Springer Seminars Immunopathol.* **3**, 93.

Germain, R. N. and Benacerraf, B. (1981). A single major pathway of T-lymphocyte interactions in antigen-specific immune suppression. *Scand. J. Immunol.* **13**, 1.

Gershon, A. A. (1980). Live attenuated varicella-zoster vaccine. *Rev. Infect. Dis.* **2**, 393.

Gershon, R. K. (1974). T cell control of antibody production. *Contemp. Top. Immunobiol.* **3**, 1.

Gershon, R. K., Eardley, D. D., Durum, S. *et al.* (1981). Contrasuppression: a novel immunoregulatory activity. *J. Exp. Med.* **153**, 1533.

Gething, M-J. and Sambrook, J. (1981). Cell-surface expression of influenza haemagglutinin from a cloned DNA copy of the RNA gene. *Nature* **293**, 620.

Gibbs, A. J. (1973). *Viruses and Invertebrates*. North Holland, Amsterdam.

Gibbs, C. J., Gajdusek, D. C. and Latarjet, R. (1978). Unusual resistance to ionizing radiation of the viruses of Kuru, Creutzfeldt-Jakob disease and scrapie. *Proc. Nat. Acad. Sci. USA* **75**, 6268.

Gidlund, M., Orn, A., Wigzell, H. *et al.* (1978). Enhanced NK cell activity in mice injected with interferon and interferon inducers. *Nature* **273**, 759.

Ginsberg, H. S. (1975). Subunit viral vaccines. In *Viral Immunology and Immunopathology* pp. 317–26 (ed. A. L. Notkins). Academic Press, New York.

Ginsberg, H. S. (ed.) (1984). *The Adenoviruses*. Plenum Press, New York.

Gipson, T. G., Daniels, C. A. and Notkins, A. L. (1974). Interaction of rheumatoid factor with infectious vaccinia virus-antibody complexes. *J. Immunol.* **112**, 2087.

Gledhill, A. W. (1956). Quantitative aspects of the enhancing action of eperythrozoa on the pathogenicity of mouse hepatitis virus. *J. Gen. Microbiol.* **15**, 292.

Glenn, J. (1981). Cytomegalovirus infections following renal transplantation. *Rev. Infect. Dis.* **3**, 1151.

Gluzman, Y. (ed.) (1982). *Eukaryotic Viral Vectors*. Cold Spring Harbor Laboratory, New York.

Goeddel, D. V., Yelverton, E., Ullrich, A. *et al.* (1980). Human leukocyte interferon produced by *E. coli* is biologically active. *Nature* **287**, 411.

Goeddel, D. V., Leung, D. W., Dull, T. J. *et al.* (1981). The structure of eight distinct cloned human leukocyte interferon cDNAs. *Nature* **290**, 20.

Goldstein, M. A. and Tauraso, N. M. (1970). Effect of formalin, β-propiolactone, merthiolate, and ultraviolet light upon influenza virus infectivity, chicken cell agglutination, hemagglutination, and antigenicity. *Appl. Microbiol.* **19**, 290.

Golub, E. S. (1981). *The Cellular Basis of the Immune Response*, 2nd edn. Sinauer, Sunderland, Mass.

Goorha, R. and Granoff, A. (1979). Icosahedral cytoplasmic deoxyriboviruses. *Comprehensive Virology*, no. **14**, 347. Plenum Press, New York.

Gordon, R. M. and Lumsden, W. H. R. (1939). A study of the behaviour of the mouth parts of mosquitoes when taking up blood from living tissue, together with some observations on the ingestion of microfilariae. *Ann. Trop. Med. Parasit.* **33**, 259.

Gottlieb, M. S., Schroff, R., Schanker, H. M. *et al.* (1981). *Pneumocystis carinii* pneumonia and mucosal candidiasis in previously healthy homosexual men: evidence of a new acquired cellular immunodeficiency. *New Engl. J. Med.* **305**, 1425.

Gottlieb, M. S., Groopman, J. E., Weinstein, W. M. *et al.* (1983). The Acquired Immunodeficiency Syndrome. *Ann. Intern. Med.* **99**, 208.

Gottschalk, A., Belyavin, G. and Biddle, F. (1972). Glycoproteins as influenza virus haemagglutinin inhibitors and as cellular virus inhibitors. In *Glycoproteins: Their Composition, Structure and Function* 2nd edn, Part B, p. 1082 (ed. A. Gottschalk). Elsevier, Amsterdam.

Gould, J. J. and Mims, C. A. (1980). Murine cytomegalovirus; reactivation in pregnancy. *J. Gen. Virol.* **51**, 397.

Gray, P. W. and Goeddel, D. V. (1982). Structure of the human immune interferon gene. *Nature* **298**, 859.

Gray, P. W., Leung, D. W., Pennica, D. *et al.* (1982). Expression of human immune interferon cDNA in *E. coli* and monkey cells. *Nature* **295**, 503.

Green, D. R., Bardley, D. D., Kimura, A. *et al.* (1981). Immunoregulatory circuits which modulate responsiveness to suppressor cell signals: characterization of an effector cell in the contrasuppressor circuit. *Eur. J. Immunol.* **11**, 973.

Green, D. R., Gold, J., St. Martin, S. *et al*. (1982). Microenvironmental immuno-regulation: possible role of contrasuppressor cells in maintaining immune responses in gut-associated lymphoid tissues. *Proc. Nat. Acad. Sci. USA* **79**, 889.

Green, D. R., Flood, P. M. and Gershon, R. K. (1983). Immunoregulatory T-cell pathways. *Ann. Rev. Immunol.* **1**, 439.

Green, N., Alexander, H., Olson, A. *et al*. (1982). Immunogenic structure of the influenza virus hemagglutinin. *Cell* **28**, 477.

Greenberg, H. B., Wyatt, R. G., Kalica, A. R. *et al*. (1981). New insights in viral gastroenteritis. *Perspect. Virol.* **11**, 163.

Greene, M. I. and Weiner, H. L. (1980). Delayed hypersensitivity in mice infected with reovirus. II induction of tolerance and suppressor T cells to viral specific gene products. *J. Immunol.* **125**, 283.

Greenlee, J. E. (1979). Pathogenesis of K virus infection in newborn mice. *Infect. Immunity* **26**, 705.

Greenlee, J. E. (1981). Effect of host age on experimental K virus infection in mice. *Infect. Immunity* **33**, 297.

Gregg, N. McA. (1941). Congenital cataract following German measles in the mother. *Trans Ophthalmol. Soc. Austral.* **3**, 35.

Gregoriadis, G. (1976). The carrier potential of liposomes in biology and medicine. *New Engl. J. Med.* **295**, 704, 765.

Gresser, I. (1977). On the varied biological effects of interferon. *Cell. Immunol.* **34**, 406.

Gresser, I. (ed.) (1979, 1980, 1981, 1982). *Interferon 1, 2, 3, 4*. Academic Press, New York.

Gresser, I. (1982). Can interferon cause disease? In *Interferon 4* (ed. I. Gresser,) p. 95. Academic Press, London.

Gresser, I. and Tovey, M. G. (1978). Antitumour effects of interferon. *Biochim. Biophys. Acta* **516**, 231.

Gresser, I., Chany, C. and Enders, J. F. (1965). Persistent polioviral infection of intact human amniotic membrane without apparent cytopathic effect. *J. Bacteriol.* **89**, 470.

Gresser, I., Tovey, M. G., Maury, C. *et al*. (1976). Role of interferon in the pathogenesis of virus diseases as demonstrated by the use of anti-interferon serum. II Studies with herpes simplex, Moloney sarcoma, vesicular stomatitis, Newcastle Disease and influenza viruses. *J. Exp. Med.* **144**, 1316.

Gresser, I., de Maeyer-Guignard, J., Tovey, M. G. *et al*. (1979). Electro-phoretically pure mouse interferon exerts multiple biologic effects. *Proc. Nat. Acad. Sci. USA* **76**, 5308.

Gresser, I., Maury, C. and Chandler, R. L. (1983). Failure to modify scrapie in mice by administration of interferon or anti-interferon globulin. *J. Gen. Virol.* **64**, 1387.

Grewal, A. S., Rouse, B. T. and Babiuk, L. A. (1977). Mechanisms of resistance to herpes viruses: comparison of the effectiveness of different cell types in mediating antibody-dependent cell-mediated toxicity. *Infect. Immunity* **15**, 698.

Grewal, A. S., Rouse, B. T. and Babiuk, L. A. (1980). Mechanisms of recovery from viral infections: destruction of infected cells by neutrophils and complement. *J. Immunol.* **124**, 312.

Grinnell, B. W., Padgett, B. L. and Walker, D. L. (1983). Distribution of non-integrated DNA from JC papovavirus in organs of patients with progressive multifocal leukoencephalopathy. *J. Infect. Dis*. **147**, 669.

Grist, N. R., Bell, E. J. and Assad, F. (1978). Enteroviruses in human disease. *Progr. Med. Virol*. **24**, 114.

Grundy, (Chalmer), J. E. and Melief, C. J. M. (1982). Effect of Nu/Nu gene on genetically determined resistance to murine cytomegalovirus. *J. Gen. Virol*. **61**, 133.

Grundy (Chalmer), J. E., Mackenzie, J. S. and Stanley, N. F. (1981). Influence of H-2 and non H-2 linked genes on resistance to murine cytomegalovirus infection. *Infect. Immunity* **32**, 277.

Grundy, J. E., Trapman, J., Allan, J. E. *et al*. (1982). Evidence for a protective role of interferon in resistance to murine cytomegalovirus and its control by non-H2-linked genes. *Infect. Immunity* **37**, 143.

Gut, J. P., Schmitt, S., Bingen, A. *et al*. (1982). Protective effect of colostomy on Frog Virus 3 hepatitis of rats: possible role of endotoxin. *J. Infect. Dis*. **146**, 594.

Gutterman, J. U., Fine, S., Quesaday, J. *et al*. (1982). Recombinant human leukocyte A interferon: pharmacokinetics, single-dose tolerance, and biological effects in cancer patients. *Annals Int. Med*. **93**, 549.

Gwaltney, J. M. and Hendley, J. O. (1978). Rhinovirus transmission; one if by air, two if by hand. *Am. J. Epidemiol*. **107**, 357.

Haase, A. T. (1975). The slow infection caused by visna virus. *Curr. Top. Microb. Immunol*. **72**, 101.

Hackett, C. J., Dietzschold, B., Gerhard, W. *et al*. (1983). The influenza virus site recognized by a murine helper T cell specific for H1 strains: localization of a nine amino acid sequence in the hemagglutinin molecule. *J. Exp. Med*. **158**, 294.

Hadler, S. C., de Monzon, M., Ponzetto, A. *et al*. (1984). Delta virus infection and severe hepatitis. An epidemic in the Yucpa Indians of Venezuela. *Ann. Intern. Med*. **100**, 339.

Hadlow, W. J. and Prusiner, S. B. (eds.) (1979). *Slow Transmissible Disease of the Nervous System*, vol. 2. Academic Press, New York.

Hadlow, W. J., Kennedy, R. C. and Race, R. E. (1982). Natural infection of Suffolk sheep with scrapie virus. *J. Infect. Dis*. **146**, 657.

Hahn, E. C. and Hahn, P. S. (1983). Autoimmunity in Aleutian disease: Contribution of antiviral and anti-DNA antibody to hypergammaglobulinaemia. *Infect. Immunity* **41**, 494.

Hahon, N. (1961). Smallpox and related poxvirus infections in the simian host. *Bacteriol. Rev*. **25**, 459.

Hall, C. B. (1980). Prevention of infections with respiratory syncytial virus: the hopes and hurdles ahead. *Rev. Infect. Dis*. **2**, 384.

Haller, O. (1981). Inborn resistance of mice to orthomyxoviruses. *Curr. Top. Microbiol. Immunol*. **92**, 25.

Haller, O., Arnheiter, H., Horisberger, M. A. *et al*. (1980). Interaction between interferon and host genes in antiviral defense. *Annals N. Y. Acad. Sci*. **350**, 558.

Haller, O., Arnheiter, H., Lindenmann, J. *et al*. (1981a). Host gene influences sensitivity to interferon action selectively for influenza virus. *Nature* **283**, 660.

Haller, O., Arnheiter, H., Gresser, I. *et al*. (1981b). Virus-specific interferon action: protection of newborn Mx carriers against lethal infection with influenza virus. *J. Exp. Med.* **154**, 199.

Halpern, M. S., England, J. M., Deery, D. T. *et al.* (1983). Viral nucleic acid synthesis and antigen accumulation in pancreas and kidney of Pekin ducks infected with duck hepatitis virus. *Proc. Nat. Acad. Sci. USA* **80**, 4865.

Halstead, S. B. (1979). In vivo enhancement of dengue virus infection in rhesus monkeys by passively transferred antibody. *J. Infect. Dis.* **140**, 527.

Halstead, S. B. (1981a). The pathogenesis of dengue. Molecular epidemiology in infectious disease. *Am. J. Epidemiol.* **114**, 632.

Halstead, S. B. (1981b). Viral haemorrhagic fevers. *J. Infect. Dis.* **143**, 127.

Hammer, S. M., Richter, B. S. and Hirsch, M. S. (1981). Activation and suppression of herpes simplex virus in a human T lymphoid cell line. *J. Immunol.* **127**, 144.

Hammon, W. McD., Kitaoka, M. and Downs, W. G. (1971). *Immunization for Japanese Encephalitis.* Igaku Shoin, Tokyo.

Hanninen, P., Arstila, P., Lang, H. *et al.* (1980). Involvement of the central nervous system in acute, uncomplicated measles virus infection. *J. Clin. Microbiol.* **11**, 610.

Hansen, B., Koprowski, H., Baron, S. *et al.* (1969). Interferon-mediated natural resistance of mice to arbo B virus infection. *Microbios.* **1B**, 51.

Hanshaw, J. B. and Dudgeon, J. A. (1978). *Viral Diseases of the Fetus and Newborn*, p. 45. W. B. Saunders, Philadelphia.

Harbour, D. A., Blyth, W. A. and Hill, T. J. (1978). Prostaglandins enhance spread of herpes simplex virus in cell cultures. *J. Gen. Virol.* **41**, 87.

Harbour, D. A., Hill, T. J. and Blyth, W. A. (1983). Recurrent herpes simplex in the mouse: inflammation in the skin and activation of virus in the ganglia following peripheral stimulation. *J. Gen. Virol.* **64**, 1491.

Harfast, B., Andersson, T. and Grandien, M. (1977). Enhanced cytotoxicity of human lymphocytes against rabies-infected cells by rabies-specific antibodies. *Scand. J. Immunol.* **11**, 391.

Harnett, G. B. and Shellam, G. R. (1983). Variation in murine cytomegalovirus replication in fibroblasts from different mouse strains in vitro: correlation with in vivo resistance. *J. Gen. Virol.* **62**, 39.

Hartsough, G. R. and Burger, D. (1965). Encephalopathy of mink. I Epizootiologic and clinical observations. *J. Infect. Dis.* **115**, 387.

Härvast, B., Örvell, C., Alsheikhly, A. *et al.* (1980). The role of viral glycoproteins in mumps-virus-dependent lymphocyte-mediated cytotoxicity *in vitro. Scand. J. Immunol.* **11**, 391.

Haspel, M. V., Onodera, T., Prabhakar, B. S. *et al.* (1983). Virus-induced autoimmunity: monoclonal antibodies that react with endocrine tissues. *Science* **220**, 305.

Hawkes, R. A. and Lafferty, K. J. (1967). The enhancement of virus infectivity by antibody. *Virology* **33**, 250.

Hayashi, K., Kurata, T., Morishima, T. *et al.* (1980). Analysis of the inhibitory effect of peritoneal macrophages on the spread of herpes simplex virus. *Infect. Immunity* **28**, 350.

Hayden, G. F., Preblub, S. R., Orenstein, W. A. *et al.* (1978). The current status of mumps and mumps vaccine in the United States. *Pediatrics* **62**, 965.

Head, H. and Campbell, A. W. (1900). Pathology of herpes zoster and its bearing on sensory localization. *Brain* **23**, 353.

Heath, R. B. (1979). The pathogenesis of respiratory viral infection. *Postgrad. Med. J.* **55**, 122.

Helenius, A., Kartenbeck, J., Simons, K. *et al*. (1980). On the entry of Semliki Forest virus into BHK-21 cells. *J. Cell Biol.* **84**, 404.

Henle, W. (1963). Interferon and interference in persistent viral infection of cell cultures. *J. Immunol.* **91**, 145.

Hennessen, W. and Huygelen, C. (eds.) (1979). Immunization: Benefit versus Risk Factors. *Develop. Biol. Stand.* **43**. Karger, Basel.

Hennessen, W. and van Wezel, A. L. (eds.) (1981). Reassessment of Inactivated Poliomyelitis Vaccine. *Develop. Biol. Stand.* **47**, Karger, Basel.

Henson, J. B. and McGuire, T. C. (1974). Equine infectious anaemia. *Progr. Med. Virol.* **18**, 143.

Herberman, R. B. and Ortaldo, J. R. (1981). Natural killer cells: their role in defences against diseases. *Science* **214**, 24.

Hercend, T., Reinherz, E. L., Meuer, S. *et al*. (1983). Phenotypic and functional heterogeneity of human cloned natural killer cell lines. *Nature* **301**, 158.

Heritage, J., Chesters, P. M. and McCance, D. J. (1981). The persistence of papovavirus BK DNA sequences in normal human renal tissue. *J. Med. Microbiol.* **8**, 143.

Hers, J. F. P. and Mulder, J. (1961). Broad aspects of the pathology and pathogenesis of human influenza. *Am. Rev. Resp. Dis.* (Suppl.) **83**, 84.

Hicks, J. T., Ennis, F. A., Kim, E. *et al*. (1978). The importance of an intact complement pathway in recovery from a primary viral infection: influenza in decomplemented and C5-deficient mice. *J. Immunol.* **121**, 1437.

Higgins, P. G. (1982). Enteroviral conjunctivitis and its neurological complications. *Arch. Virol.* **73**, 91.

Hill, T. J. (1983). Herpes simplex virus latency. In *Herpesviruses*, (ed. B. Roizman). Comprehensive Virology, vol. 2. Plenum Press, New York.

Hill, T. J. and Blyth, W. A. (1976). An alternative theory of herpes simplex recurrence and a possible role for prostaglandins. *Lancet* i, 397.

Hill, T. J., Field, H. J. and Blyth, W. A. (1975). Acute and recurrent infection with herpes simplex virus in the mouse: a model for studying latency and recurrent disease. *J. Gen. Virol.* **28**, 341.

Hill, T. J., Blyth, W. A. and Harbour, D. A. (1978). Trauma to the skin causes recurrence of herpes simplex in the mouse. *J. Gen. Virol.* **39**, 21.

Hill, T. J., Harbour, D. A. and Blyth, W. A. (1980). Isolation of herpes simplex virus from the skin of clinically normal mice during latent infection. *J. Gen. Virol.* **47**, 205.

Hilleman, M. R. (1966). Critical appraisal of emulsified oil adjuvants applied to viral vaccines. *Progr. Med. Virol.* **8**, 131.

Hilleman, M. R. (1980). New developments with new vaccines. In *New Developments with Human and Veterinary Vaccines* (eds. A. Mizrahi *et al*.). *Prog. Clin. Biol. Res.* **47**, 21. Alan R. Liss, New York.

Hilleman, M. R., Buynak, E. B., McAleer, W. J. *et al*. (1981a). Newer developments with human hepatitis vaccines. *Perspect. Virol.* **11**, 219.

Hilleman, M. R., Larson, V. M., Lehman, E. D. *et al*. (1981b). Subunit herpes simplex 2 vaccine. In *The Human Herpesviruses* (eds. A. J. Nahmias, W. R. Dowdle, and R. F. Schinazi), pp. 503–6. Elsevier, New York.

Hilleman, M. R., Buynak, E. B., McAleer, W. J. *et al.* (1982). Hepatitis A and hepatitis B vaccines. In *Viral Hepatitis* (eds. W. Szmuness, H. J. Alter and J. M. Maynard), pp. 385–97. Franklin Institute Press, Philadelphia.

Hilleman, M. R., McAleer, W. J., McLean, A. A. *et al.* (1983). Stabilized measles vaccine in a novel single dose delivery system: a practical reality for world wide elimination of measles. *Rev. Infect. Dis.* **5**, 511.

Hinman, A. R., Brandling-Bennett, A. D., Bernier, R. H. *et al.* (1980). Current features of measles in the United States: feasibility of measles elimination. *Epidemiol. Rev.* **2**, 153.

Hinze, H. C. and Walker, D. L. (1971). Comparison of cytocidal and non-cytocidal strains of Shope rabbit fibroma virus. *J. Virol.* **7**, 577.

Hirsch, M. S., Zisman, B. and Allison, A. C. (1970). Macrophages and age-dependent resistance to herpes simplex virus in mice. *J. Immunol.* **104**, 1160.

Hirsch, M. S., Schooley, R. T., Cosimi, A. B. *et al.* (1983). Effects of interferon-alpha on cytomegalovirus reactivation syndromes in renal transplant recipients. *New Engl. J. Med.* **308**, 1489.

Hirsch, R. L. (1982). The complement system: its importance in the host response to viral infection. *Microbiol. Rev.* **46**, 71.

Hirsch, R. L., Griffin, D. E. and Winkelstein, J. A. (1980). The role of complement in viral infections. II. The clearance of Sindbis virus from the bloodstream and central nervous system of mice depleted of complement. *J. Infect. Dis.* **141**, 212.

Hirsch, R. L., Griffin, D. E. and Winkelstein, J. A. (1981). Host modification of Sindbis virus sialic acid content influences alternative complement pathway activation and virus clearance. *J. Immunol.* **127**, 1740.

Hirsch, R. L., Griffin, D. E. and Winkelstein, J. A. (1983). Natural immunity to Sindbis virus is influenced by host tissue sialic acid content. *Proc. Nat. Acad. Sci. USA* **80**, 548.

Ho, M. (1977). Virus infections after transplantation in man. *Arch. Virol.* **55**, 1.

Ho, M. (1982). *Cytomegalovirus: Biology and Infection*. Plenum Press, New York.

Holland, J. J., McLaren, L. C. and Syverton, J. T. (1959). The mammalian cell virus relationship. IV Infection of naturally insusceptible cells with entero-virus ribonucleic acid. *J. Exp. Med.* **110**, 65.

Holland, J. J., Grabau, E., Jones, C. L. *et al.* (1979). Evolution of multiple genome mutations during long-term persistent infections by vesicular stomatitis virus. *Cell* **16**, 495.

Holland, J. J., Kennedy, I. T., Semler, B. L. *et al.* (1980). Defective interfering RNA viruses and the host-cell response. In *Comprehensive Virology*, vol. 16, p. 137. Plenum Press, New York.

Holland, J. J., Spindler, K., Horodyski, F. *et al.* (1982). Rapid evolution of RNA genomes. *Science* **215**, 1577.

Hollinger, F. B., Adam, E., Heiberg, D. *et al.* (1982). Response to hepatitis B vaccine in a young adult population. In *Viral Hepatitis* (eds. W. Szmuness, H. J. Alter, and J. M. Maynard), pp. 361–72. Franklin Institute Press, Philadelphia.

Hollings, M. (1978). Mycoviruses: viruses that infect fungi. *Adv. Virus Res.* **22**, 1.

Holmberg, C. A., Gribble, D. H., Takemoto, K. K. *et al.* (1977). Isolation of

Simian virus 40 from rhesus monkeys (Macaca mulatta) with spontaneous progressive multifocal leukoencephalopathy. *J. Infect. Dis.* **136**, 593.

Holmes, I. H. (1979). Viral gastroenteritis. *Progr. Med. Virol.* **25**, 1.

Hoofnagle, J. H. (1981). Serological markers of hepatitis B infection. *Ann. Rev. Med.* **32**, 1.

Hooks, J. J., Burns, W., Hayashi, K. *et al*. (1976). Viral spread in the presence of neutralizing antibody: mechanisms of persistence in foamy virus infections. *Infect. Immunity* **14**, 1172.

Horne, R. W. and Wildy, P. (1979). An historical account of the development and applications of the negative staining technique to the electron microscopy of viruses. *J. Microscopy* **117**, 103.

Horstmann, D. M. (1979). Viral vaccines and their ways. *Rev. Infect. Dis.* **1**, 502.

Hoskins, T. W., Davies, J. R., Smith, A. J. *et al*. (1979). Assessment of inactivated influenza-A vaccine after three outbreaks of influenza A at Christ's Hospital. *Lancet* i, 33.

Hotchin, J. (1974). The role of transient infection in arenavirus persistence. *Progr. Med. Virol.* **18**, 81.

Hotchin, J. and Seegal, R. (1977). Virus-induced behavioural alteration of mice. *Science* **196**, 671.

Hovanessian, A. G., la Bonnardière, C. and Falcoff, E. (1980). Action of murine γ (immune) interferon on β (fibroblast)-interferon resistant L1210 and embryonal carcinoma cells. *J. Interferon Res.* **1**, 125.

Howard, R. J., Miller, J. and Najarian, J. S. (1974). Cytomegalovirus-induced immune suppression. II. Cell-mediated immunity. *Clin. Exp. Immunol.* **18**, 109.

Howes, E. L., Taylor, W., Mitchison, N. A. *et al*. (1979). MHC matching shows that at least two T cell subsets determine resistance to HSV. *Nature* **277**, 67.

Huang, A. S. (1977). Viral pathogenesis and molecular biology. *Bact. Rev.* **41**, 811.

Huang, A. S. and Baltimore, D. (1977). Defective interfering animal viruses. In *Comprehensive Virology*, vol. 10, p. 73. Plenum Press, New York.

Huddleston, J. R., Lampert, P. W. and Oldstone, M. B. A. (1980). Virus-lymphocyte interactions: Infection of TG and TM subsets by measles virus. *Clin. Immunol. Immunopathol.* **15**, 502.

Hudson, J. B. (1979). The murine cytomegalovirus as a model for the study of viral pathogenesis and persistent infections. *Arch. Virol.* **62**, 1.

Hurd, J. and Robinson, T. W. E. (1976). Herpes simplex: aspects of reactivation in a mouse model. *J. Antimicrob. Chemoth.* **3**, 99.

Hurst, E. W., Melvin, P. A. and Thorpe, J. M. (1960). The influence of cortisone, ACTH, thyroxine and thiouracil on equine encephalomyelitis in the mouse and on its treatment with mepacrine. *J. Comp. Pathol.* **70**, 361.

Husseini, R. H., Sweet, C., Collie, M. H. *et al*. (1982). Elevation of nasal viral levels by suppression of fever in ferrets infected with influenza viruses of differing virulence. *J. Infect. Dis.* **145**, 520.

Huygelen, C., Peetermans, J. and Prinzie, A. (1969). An attenuated rubella virus vaccine (Cendehill 51 strain) grown in primary rabbit kidney cells. *Progr. Med. Virol.* **11**, 107.

Huxley, E. J., Viroslav, J., Gray, W. R. *et al*. (1978). Pharyngeal aspiration in normal adults and in patients with depressed consciousness. *Am. J. Med.* **64**, 564.

Hyman, R. W., Ecker, J. R. and Tenser, R. B. (1983). Varicella-zoster virus RNA in human trigeminal ganglia. *Lancet* ii, 814.

Ichihashi, Y., Matsumoto, S. and Dales, S. (1971). Biogenesis of poxviruses: role of A type inclusions and host cell membranes in virus dissemination. *Virology* **46**, 507.

Inada, T. and Uetake, H. (1977). Virus-induced specific cell surface antigen(s) on mouse adenovirus-infected cells. *Infect. Immunity* **18**, 41.

Inada, T. and Uetake, H. (1978). Cell-mediated immunity assayed by ^{51}Cr release test in mice infected with mouse adenovirus. *Infect. Immunity* **20**, 1.

Inglot, A. D. (1983). The hormonal concept of interferon. *Arch. Virol.* **76**, 1.

Ionescu-Matiu, I., Kennedy, R. C., Sparrow, J. T. *et al.* (1983). Epitopes associated with a synthetic hepatitis B surface antigen peptide. *J. Immunol* **130**, 1947.

Isaacs, A. and Lindenmann, J. (1957). Virus interference. I The interferon, *Proc. Roy. Soc. Lond. B.* **147**, 258.

Isaacs, D., Clarke, J. R., Tyrrell, D. A. *et al.* (1981). Deficient production of leucocyte interferon (interferon α) in vitro and in vivo in children with recurrent respiratory tract infections. *Lancet* 2, 950.

Isaacs, S. T., Shen, C. J., Hearst, J. E. *et al.* (1977). Synthesis and characterization of new psoralen derivatives with superior photoreactivity with DNA and RNA. *Biochemistry* **16**, 1058.

Isaak, D. D. and Carny, J. (1983). T and B lymphocyte susceptibility to murine leukemia virus Moloney. *Infect. Immunity* **40**, 977.

Isacson, P. and Stone, A. (1971). Allergic reactions associated with viral vaccines. *Progr. Med. Virol.* **13**, 239.

Isakov, N., Segal, S. and Feldman, M. (1980). Infection of mice with lactic dehydrogenase virus (LDV) impairs the antigen-presenting capacity of macrophages but not their phagocytic activity. IVth Int. Congress Immunology, Paris. Abstract No. 11.2.09.

Isakov, N., Feldman, M. and Segal, S. (1982). The mechanism of modulation of immune responses after infection of mice with lactic dehydrogenase virus. *J. Immunol.* **128**, 969.

Israel, E., Beiss, B. and Wainberg, M. A. (1980). Viral abrogation of lymphocyte mitogenesis: induction of a soluble factor inhibitory to cellular proliferation. *Immunology* **40**, 77.

Jackson, D. C., Murray, J. M., Brown, L. E. *et al.* (1981). Immunochemical properties of influenza virus hemagglutinin and its fragments. In *Genetic Variation among Influenza Viruses* (ed. D. Nayak), ICN-UCLA Symposium **21**, pp. 355–72. Academic Press, New York.

Jackson, D. C., Murray, J. M., White, D. O. *et al.* (1982). Antigenic activity of a synthetic peptide comprising the 'loop' region of influenza virus hemagglutinin. *Virology* **120**, 273.

Jackson, D. C., Murray, J. M., Anders, E. M. *et al.* (1983). Expression of a unique antigenic determinant on influenza virus hemagglutinin at pH 5. In *The Origin of Pandemic Influenza Viruses* (ed. W. G. Laver), pp. 29–38. Elsevier, Amsterdam.

Jackson, G. G. and Muldoon, R. L. (1973). Viruses causing common respiratory infections in man. II. Enteroviruses and paramyxoviruses. *J. Infect. Dis.* **128**, 387.

Jackson, G. C. and Muldoon, R. L. (eds.) (1975). *Viruses Causing Common Respiratory Infections in Man*. University of Chicago Press, Chicago.

Jacobse-Geels, H. E. L., Daha, M. R. and Horsinek, M. C. (1982). Antibody, immune complexes, and complement activity fluctuations in kittens with experimentally induced feline infectious peritonitis. *Am. J. Vet. Res.* **43**, 666.

Jacobson, S., Friedman, R. M. and Pfau, C. J. (1981). Interferon induction by lymphocytic choriomeningitis viruses correlates with maximum virulence. *J. Gen. Virol.* **57**, 275.

Jakab, G. J. and Dick, E. C. (1973). Synergistic effect in viral-bacterial infection: combined infection of the murine respiratory tract with Sendai virus and Pasteurella pneumotropica. *Infect. Immunity* **8**, 762.

Jarrett, O. (1980). Natural occurrence of sub-groups of feline leukaemia virus. In *Viruses in Naturally Occurring Cancers* (eds. M. Essex., G. J. Todaro and H. zur Hausen), p. 603. Cold Spring Harbor Laboratory, New York.

Jenner, E. (1798). *An enquiry into the causes and effects of the variolae vaccinae, a disease discovered in some western counties of England, particularly Gloucestershire, and known by the name of cow pox*. Reprinted by Cassell, London, 1896.

Jerne, N. K. (1974). Towards a network theory of the immune system. *Ann. Immunol.* (Inst. Pasteur, Paris) **125C**, 373.

Joachim, H. L. and Sabbath, M. (1979). Redistribution and modulation of Gross murine leukemia virus antigens induced by specific antibodies. *J. Nat. Cancer Inst.* **62**, 169.

Johnson, H. M. and Baron, S. (1977). Evaluation of effects of interferon and interferon inducers on the immune response. *Pharmacol. Therap. (A)* **1**, 349.

Johnson, R. T. (1964a). The pathogenesis of herpes virus encephalitis I. Virus pathways to the nervous system of suckling mice demonstrated by fluorescent antibody staining. *J. Exp. Med.* **119**, 343.

Johnson, R. T. (1964b). The pathogenesis of herpes virus encephalitis. II A cellular basis for the development of resistance with age. *J. Exp. Med.* **120**, 359.

Johnson, R. T. (1974). Pathophysiology and epidemiology of acute viral infections of the nervous system. *Adv. Neurol.* **6**, 27.

Johnson, R. T. (1980). Selective vulnerability of neural cells to viral infection. *Brain* **103**, 447.

Johnson, R. T. (1982). *Viral Infections of the Nervous System*. Raven Press, New York.

Joklik, W. K. (1980). The Genetics of Animal Viruses. In *Zinsser Microbiology* (eds. W. K. Joklik, H. P. Willett and D. B. Amos), 17th edn, p. 1096. Appleton-Century-Croft, New York.

Joklik, W. K. (1981). Structure and function of the reovirus genome. *Microbiol. Rev.* **45**, 483.

Joklik, W. K. (ed.) (1983). *The Reoviridae*. Plenum Press, New York.

de Jong, P. J., Valderrama, G., Spigland, I. *et al.* (1983). Adenovirus isolated from urine of patients with acquired immunodeficiency syndrome. *Lancet* ii, 1293.

Jordan, M. C. (1983). Latent infection and the elusive cytomegalovirus. *Rev. Infect. Dis.* **5**, 205.

Jordan, M. C. and Mar. V. L. (1982). Spontaneous activation of latent cyto-megalovirus from murine spleen explants. Role of lymphocytes and macrophages in release and replication of virus. *J. Clin. Investig.* **70**, 762.

Joseph, B. S. and Oldstone, M. B. A. (1975). Immunologic injury in measles virus infection. II Suppression of immune injury through antigenic modulation. *J. Exp. Med.* **142**, 864.

Jubelt, J., Narayan, O. and Johnson, R. T. (1980). Pathogenesis of human polio-virus infection in mice. II Age dependency of paralysis. *J. Neuropath. Exp. Neurol.* **39**, 149.

Kadish, A. S., Tarsey, F. A., Yu, G. S. M. *et al*. (1980). Interferon as a mediator of human lymphocyte suppression. *J. Exp. Med.* **151**, 637.

Kalter, S. S., Ablashi, D., Espana, C. *et al*. (1980). Simian virus nomenclature. *Intervirol.* **13**, 317.

Kantoch, M., Warwick, A. and Bang, F. B. (1963). The cellular nature of genetic susceptibility to a virus. *J. Exp. Med.* **117**, 781.

Kapikian, A. Z., Wyatt, R. G., Greenberg, H. B. *et al*. (1980). Approaches to immunization of infants and young children against gastroenteritis due to rotaviruses. *Rev. Infect. Dis.* **2**, 459.

Kapoor, A. K., Nash, A. A. and Wildy, P. (1982a). Pathogenesis of herpes simplex virus in B cell suppressed mice: the relative roles of cell-mediated and humoral immunity. *J. Gen. Virol.* **61**, 127.

Kapoor, A. K., Nash, A. A., Wildy, P. *et al*. (1982b). Pathogenesis of herpes simplex virus in congenitally athymic mice: the relative roles of cell-mediated and humoral immunity. *J. Gen. Virol.* **60**, 225.

Kark, J. D., Lubiush, M. and Rannon, L. (1982). Cigarette smoking as a risk factor for epidemic A (H_1N_1) influenza in young men. *New Engl. J. Med.* **307**, 1042.

Kaschula, R. O. C., Druker, J. and Kipps, A. (1983). Late morphological consequences of measles: a lethal debilitating lung disease among the poor. *Rev. Infect. Dis.* **5**, 395.

Kass, E. H. and Finland, M. (1958). Corticosteroids and infections. *Adv. Intern. Med.* **9**, 45.

Kastroff, L., Long, C., Doherty, P. C. *et al*. (1981). Isolation of virus from brain after immunosuppression of mice with latent herpes simplex. *Nature* **291**, 432.

Kato, N. and Okada, A. (1961). The relation of the toxic agent to the subunits of influenza virus particles. *Br. J. Exp. Pathol.* **42**, 253.

Kato, S. *et al*. (1982). HLA-DR antigens and the rubella-specific immune response in man. *Tissue Antigen* **19**, 140.

Katz, S. L., Krugman, S. K. and Quinn, T. C. (eds.) (1983). International Symposium on Measles Immunization. *Rev. Infect. Dis*. **5**, 389.

Kaufer, I. and Weiss, E. (1980). Significance of Bursa of Fabricius as target organ in infectious bursal disease of chickens. *Infect. Immunity* **27**, 364.

Kendal, A. P., Maassab, H. F., Alexandrova, G. I. *et al*. (1982). Development of cold-adapted recombinant live attenuated influenza A vaccines in the U.S. and U.S.S.R. *Antiviral Research* **1**, 339.

Kennedy, P. G. E., Clements, G. B. and Brown, S. M. (1983). Differential susceptibility of human neural cell types in culture to infection with herpes simplex virus. *Brain* **106**, 101.

Kerr, I. M. and Brown, R. E. (1978). pppA2'p5'A2'p5'A: an inhibitor of protein synthesis synthesized with an enzyme fraction from interferon-treated cells. *Proc. Nat. Acad. Sci. USA* **75**, 256.

Kew, O. M., Nottay, B. K., Hatch, M. H. *et al*. (1981). Multiple genetic changes in the oral poliovaccines upon replication in humans. *J. Gen. Virol.* **56**, 337.

Khuroo, M. S., Teli, M. R., Skidmore, S. *et al*. (1981). Incidence and severity of viral hepatitis in pregnancy. *Am. J. Med.* **70**, 252.

Kieff, E., Dambaugh, T., Heller, M. *et al*. (1982). The biology and chemistry of Epstein-Barr virus. *J. Infect. Dis.* **146**, 506.

Kilbourne, E. D. (1968). Recombination of influenza A viruses of human and animal origin. *Science* **160**, 74.

Kilbourne, E. D. (1969). Future influenza vaccines and the use of genetic recombinants. *Bull. WHO* **41**, 643.

Kilbourne, E. D. and Horsfall, F. L. (1951). Lethal infection with Coxsackie virus of adult mice given cortisone. *Proc. Soc. Exp. Biol. Med.* **77**, 135.

Kilbourne, E. D. and Murphy, J. S. (1960). Genetic studies of influenza viruses. I. Viral morphology and growth capacity as exchangeable genetic traits. Rapid *in ovo* adaptation of early passage avian strain isolates by combination with PR8. *J. Exp. Med.* **111**, 387.

Kilbourne, E. D., Laver, W. G. and Schulman, J. L. (1968). Antiviral activity of antiserum specific for an influenza virus neuraminidase. *J. Virol.* **2**, 281.

Kiley, M. P., Bowen, E. T. W., Eddy, G. A. *et al*. (1982). Filoviridae: a taxonomic home for Marburg and Ebola viruses? *Intervirology* **18**, 24.

Kilham, L. and Margolis, G. (1966). Spontaneous hepatitis and cerebellar hypoplasia in suckling rats due to congenital infections with rat virus. *Am. J. Pathol.* **49**, 457.

Kimberlin, R. H. (1981). Scrapie as a model slow virus disease: problems, progress and diagnosis. In *Comparative Diagnosis of Viral Diseases*, vol. III A, p. 349 (eds. E. Kurstak and C. Kurstak). Academic Press, New York.

Kimberlin, R. H. and Walker, C. A. (1980). Pathogenesis of mouse scrapie; evidence for neural spread of infection to the CNS. *J. Gen. Virol.* **51**, 183.

Kimberlin, R. J. (ed.) (1976). Slow virus diseases of animals and man. North-Holland, Amsterdam.

Kimchi, A., Shure, H. and Revel, M. (1981). Anti-mitogenic function of interferon-induced (2'5') oligoadenylate and growth-related variations in enzymes that synthesize and degrade this oligonucleotide. *Europ. J. Biochem.* **114**, 5.

Kimura, Y., Ito, Y., Shimokata, K. *et al*. (1975). Temperature-sensitive virus derived from BHK cells persistently infected with HVJ (Sendai virus). *J. Virol.* **15**, 55.

Kirn, A. and Keller, F. (1983). How viruses may overcome non-specific defences in the host. *Phil. Trans. Roy. Soc. Lond. B* **303**, 115.

Kirn, A., Damron, A., Braunwald, J. *et al*. (1966). Role de la fievre dans la pneumonie vaccinale du lapin. Etude comparee du developpement viral in vivo chez les animaux febrile et apyretique. *Ann. Inst. Past.* **110**, 697.

Kishimoto, T., Suemura, M., Sugimura, K. *et al*. (1982). Characteristics of T cell-derived immunoregulatory molecules from murine or human T hybrid-omas. *Lymphokines* **5**, 129.

Kitamura, N., Semler, B. L., Rothberg, P. G. *et al*. (1981). Primary structure, gene organization and polypeptide expression of poliovirus RNA. *Nature* **291**, 547.

Kleid, D. G., Yansura, D., Small, B. *et al*. (1981). Cloned viral protein vaccine for foot-and-mouth disease: responses in cattle and swine. *Science* **214**, 1125.

Klein, G. (ed.) (1980). *Viral Oncology*. Raven Press, New York.

Klein, G. (ed.) (1982–84). *Advances in Viral Oncology*, vols. 1–4. Raven Press, New York.

Klein, G. (1983). Specific chromosomal translocations and the genesis of B-cell-derived tumours in mice and men. *Cell* **32**, 311.

Klein, J. (1981). The Histocompatibility-2 (H-2) Complex. In *The Mouse in Biomedical Research*, vol. I, p. 120 (eds. H. L. Foster, J. D. Small and J. G. Fox). Academic Press, New York.

Klein, R. J. (1982). The pathogenesis of acute, latent and recurrent herpes simplex infections. *Arch. Virol.* **72**, 143.

Klenk, H. D. and Rott, R. (1980). Cotranslational and posttranslational processing of viral glycoproteins. *Curr. Top. Microbiol. Immunol.* **90**, 19.

Klenk, H. D., Garten, W., Bosch, F. X. *et al*. (1982). Viral glycoproteins as determinants of pathogenicity. *Med. Microbiol. Immunol.* **170**, 145.

Knight, V., Fleet, W. F. and Lang, D. J. (1964). Inhibition of measles rash by chicken pox. *J.A.M.A.* **188**, 690.

Knobler, R. L., Lampert, P. W. and Oldstone, M. B. (1982). Virus persistence and recurring demyelination produced by a temperature sensitive mutant of MHV-4. *Nature* **298**, 279.

Knop, J., Stemmer, R., Neumann, C. *et al*. (1982). Interferon inhibits the suppressor T cell response of delayed-type hypersensitivity. *Nature* **296**, 757.

Knox, E. G. (1980). Strategy for rubella vaccination. *Internat. J. Epidemiol.* **9**, 13.

Kohl, S. and Loo, L. S. (1980). Ontogeny of murine cellular cytotoxicity to herpes simplex virus-infected cells. *Infect. Immunity* **30**, 847.

Kohl, S. and Loo, L. S. (1982). Protection of neonatal mice against herpes simplex virus infection: probable in vivo antibody-dependent cellular cytotoxicity. *J. Immunol.* **129**, 370.

Kohler, G. and Milstein, C. (1975). Continuous cultures of fused cells secreting antibody of predefined specificity. *Nature* **256**, 495.

Kohler, P. F., Cronin, R. E., Hammond, W. S. *et al*. (1974). Chronic membranous glomerulonephritis caused by hepatitis B antigen-antibody immune complexes. *Ann. Intern. Med.* **81**, 448.

Kono, R. (ed.) (1982). *Proceedings of the Conference on Clinical Potential of Interferon in Viral Diseases and Malignant Tumours*. Tokyo University Press, Tokyo.

Kono, Y., Kobayashi, K. and Fukunaga, Y. (1973). Antigenic drift of equine infectious anemia in chronically infected horses. *Arch. Ges. Virusforsch* **41**, 1.

Kono, R. and Vilcek, J. (eds.) (1982). *The Clinical Potential of Interferons*. Tokyo University Press, Tokyo.

Koprowski, H. (1957). Discussion of properties of attenuated poliovirus and their behaviour in human beings. In *Cellular Biology, Nucleic Acids and Viruses* (ed. T. M. Rivers), spec. publ. vol. 5, p. 128. New York Academy of Science, New York.

Koschel, K. and Halbach, M. (1979). Rabies virus infection selectively impairs membrane receptor functions in neuronal model cells. *J. Gen. Virol.* **42**, 627.

Koster, F. T., Curlin, G. C., Aziz, K. M. A. *et al*. (1981). Synergistic impact of measles and diarrhoea on nutrition and mortality in Bangladesh. *Bull. WHO* **59**, 901.

Koszinowski, U. H., Allen, H., Gething, M.-J. *et al*. (1980). Recognition of viral glycoproteins by influenza A-specific cross-reactive cytolytic T lymphocytes. *J. Exp. Med.* **151**, 945.

Kozak, M. (1981). Mechanism of mRNA recognition by eukaryotic ribosomes during initiation of protein synthesis. In *Initiation Signals in Viral Gene Expression* (ed. A. J. Shatkin). pp. 81–124. Springer-Verlag, Berlin.

Kreth, H. W., ter Meulen, V. and Eckert, G. (1979). Demonstration of HLA restricted killer cells in patients with acute measles. *Med. Microbiol. Immunol.* (Berl.) **165**, 203.

Kristensson, K., Lycke, E. and Sjostrand, J. (1971). The spread of herpes simplex in peripheral nerves. *Acta. Neuropathol.* (Berl.) **17**, 44.

Kristensson, K., Vahine, A., Persson, L. A. *et al*. (1978). Neural spread of herpes simplex virus types 1 and 2 in mice after corneal or subcutaneous (footpad) inoculation. *J. Neurol. Sci.* **35**, 331.

Krug, R. M. (1981). Priming of influenza viral RNA transcription by capped heterologous RNAs. In *Initiation Signals in Viral Gene Expression* (ed. A. J. Shatkin), pp. 124–49. Springer-Verlag, Berlin.

Krugman, S. (1977). Present status of measles and rubella immunization in the United States: a medical progress report. *J. Pediatr.* **90**, 1.

Krugman, S. (1983). Further attenuated measles vaccine: characteristics and use. *Rev. Infect. Dis.* **5**, 477.

Kumm, H. W. and Laemmert, H. W. (1950). A study of the concentration of yellow fever virus which will infect certain species of Aedes mosquitoes. *Am. J. Trop. Med.* **30**, 749.

Küpper, H., Keller, W., Kurz, C. *et al*. (1981). Cloning of cDNA of major antigen of foot and mouth disease virus and expression in *E. coli. Nature* **289**, 555.

Lachmann, P. J. and Peters, D. K. (eds.) (1982). *Clinical Aspects of Immunology*, 4th edn. Blackwell Scientific Publications, Oxford.

Lai, C-J., Markoff, L. J., Zimmerman, S. *et al*. (1980). Cloning DNA sequences from influenza viral RNA segments. *Proc. Nat. Acad. Sci. USA* **77**, 210.

Lamb, J. R., Eckels, D. D., Lake, P. *et al*. (1982). Human T cell clones recognize chemically synthesized peptides of influenza haemagglutinin. *Nature* **300**, 66.

Lamb, J. R., Skidmore, B. J., Green, N. *et al*. (1983). Induction of tolerance in influenza virus-immune T lymphocyte clones with synthetic peptides of influenza haemagglutinin. *J. Exp. Med.* **157**, 1434.

Lamb, R. A. and Choppin, P. W. (1983). The gene structure and replication of influenza virus. *Ann. Rev. Biochem.* **52**, 467.

Lancaster, W. D. and Olson, C. (1982). Animal papillomaviruses. *Microbiol. Revs.* **46**, 191.

Lando, Z., Sarin, P., Megson, M. *et al*. (1983). Association of human T-cell leukemia/lymphoma virus with the Tac antigen marker for the human T-cell growth factor receptor. *Nature* **305**, 733.

Lang, D. J. (1980). Cytomegalovirus immunization: status, prospects and problems. *Rev. Infect. Dis.* **2**, 449.

Lang, D. J. and Kummer, J. F. (1972). Demonstration of cytomegalovirus in semen. *New Engl. J. Med.* **287**, 756.

Lang, D. J. and Kummer, J. F. (1975). Cytomegalovirus in semen: observations in selected populations. *J. Infect. Dis.* **132**, 472.

Langbeheim, H., Arnon, R. and Sela, M. (1976). Antiviral effect on MS-2 coliphage obtained with a synthetic antigen. *Proc. Nat. Acad. Sci. USA* **73**, 4636.

Langford, M. P., Villarreal, A. L. and Stanton, C. J. (1983). Antibody and interferon act synergistically to inhibit enterovirus, adenovirus, and herpes simplex viral infection. *Infect. Immunity* **41**, 214.

Laufs, R. and Steinke, H. (1975). Vaccination of non-human primates against malignant lymphoma. *Nature* **253**, 71.

Laver, W. G. and Air, G. M. (eds.) (1980). *Structure and Variation in Influenza Virus*. Elsevier North-Holland, Amsterdam.

Laver, W. G., Air, G. M. and Webster, R. G. (1981). Mechanism of antigenic drift in influenza. Amino acid sequence changes in an antigenically active region of Hong Kong (H3N2) influenza virus hemagglutinin. *J. Mol. Biol.* **145**, 339.

Lazarowitz, S. G. and Choppin, R. W. (1975). Enhancement of the infectivity of influenza A and B viruses by proteolytic cleavage of the hemagglutinin polypeptide. *Virology* **48**, 440.

Lebleu, B. and Content, J. (1982). Mechanisms of interferon action: biochemical and genetic approaches. In *Interferon 4*, (ed. I. Gresser) pp. 47–94. Academic Press, London.

Lee, S. H., Weck, P. K., Moore, J. *et al*. (1982). Pharmacological comparison of two hybrid recombinant DNA-derived human leukocyte interferons. In *Interferons* (eds. T. C. Merigan and R. M. Friedman) UCLA Symposium of Molecular and Cell Biology vol. XXV, pp. 341–52. Academic Press, New York.

Lehmann-Grube, F. (1971). Lymphocytic choriomeningitis virus. *Virol. Monogr.* **10**, 1.

Lehmann-Grube, F. (1982). Lymphocytic choriomeningitis virus. In *The Mouse in Biomedical Research*, vol. II, p. 255 (eds. H. L. Foster, J. D. Small and J. G. Fox). Academic Press, New York.

Lehmann-Grube, F., Slenczka, W. and Tees, R. (1969). A persistent and inapparent infection of L-cells with the virus of lymphocytic choriomeningitis. *J. Gen. Virol.* **5**, 63.

Lehmann-Grube, F., Cihak, J., Varho, M. *et al*. (1982a). The immune response of the mouse to lymphocytic choriomeningitis virus. II Active suppression of cell-mediated immunity by infection with high virus doses. *J. Gen. Virol.* **58**, 223.

Lehmann-Grube, F., Peralta, L. M., Bruns, M. *et al*. (1982b). Persistent infection of mice with the lymphocytic choriomeningitis virus. In *Comprehensive Virology* vol. 18, p. 43 (ed. H. Fraenkel-Conrat and R. R. Wagner). Plenum Press, New York.

Lengyel, P. (1981). Mechanisms of interferon action: the (2'-5') (A)$_n$ synthetase-RNase L pathway. In *Interferon 3* (ed. I. Gresser), pp. 77–99. Academic Press, New York.

Lengyel, P. (1982). Biochemistry of interferons and their actions. *Ann. Rev. Biochem.* **51**, 251.

Lentz, T. L., Smith, A. L., Crick, J. *et al*. (1982). Is the acetylcholine receptor a rabies virus receptor? *Science* **215**, 182.

Leong, S. S. and Horoszewicz, J. S. (1981). Production and preparation of human fibroblast interferon for clinical trials. *Meth. Enzymol.* **78**, 87.

Lerner, R. A. (1982). Tapping the immunological repertoire to produce antibodies of predetermined specificity. *Nature* **299**, 592.

Lerner, R. A. and Chanock, R. M. (eds.) (1984). *Modern Approaches to Vaccines.* Cold Spring Harbor Laboratory, New York.

Lerner, R. A., Green, R. A., Alexander, H. *et al*. (1981). Chemically synthesized peptides predicted from the nucleotide sequence of the hepatitis B virus genome elicit antibodies reactive with native envelope protein of Dane particles. *Proc. Nat. Acad. Sci. USA* **78**, 3403.

Letvin, N. L., Kauffman, R. S. and Finberg, R. (1982). An adherent cell lyses virus-infected targets: characterization, activation and fine specificity of the cytotoxic cell. *J. Immunol.* **129**, 2396.

Letvin, N. L., King, N. W., Daniel, M. D. *et al*. (1983). Experimental transmission of macaque AIDS by means of inoculation of macaque lymphoma tissue. *Lancet* Sept. 10, 599.

Leung, K. N. and Ada, G. L. (1980). Cells mediating delayed hypersensitivity in the lungs of mice infected with an influenza A virus. *Scand. J. Immunol.* **12**, 393.

Leung, K. N. and Ada, G. L. (1981). Effect of helper T cells on the primary *in vitro* production of delayed-type hypersensitivity to influenza virus. *J. Exp. Med.* **153**, 1029.

Levin, S. and Hahn, T. (1982). Interferon system in acute viral hepatitis. *Lancet* i, 592.

Levine, M., Goldii, A. L. and Glorioso, J. (1980). Persistence of herpes simplex virus genes in cells of neuronals origin. *J. Virol.* **35**, 203.

Levinthal, J. D., Jakobovits, M. and Eaton, M. D. (1962). Polyoma disease and tumors in mice: the distribution of viral antigen detected by immunofluorescence. *Virology* **16**, 314.

Levy, G. A., Leibowitz, J. L. and Edgington, T. S. (1981). Induction of monocyte procoagulant activity by murine hepatitis virus type 3 parallels disease susceptibility in mice. *J. Exp. Med.* **154**, 1150.

Levy-Leblond, E. and Dupuy, J. M. (1977). Neonatal susceptibility to MHV$_3$ infection in mice. I Transfer of resistance. *J. Immunol.* **118**, 1219.

Liew, F. Y. (1982). Regulation of delayed-type hypersensitivity to pathogens and alloantigens. *Immunol. Today* **3**, 18.

Liew, F. Y. and Russell, S. M. (1980). Delayed-type hypersensitivity to influenza virus. Induction of antigen-specific suppressor T cells for delayed-type hypersensitivity to hemagglutinin during influenza virus infection in mice. *J. Exp. Med.* **151**, 799.

Liew, F. Y. and Russell, S. M. (1983). Inhibition of pathogenic effect of effector T cells by specific suppressor T cells during influenza virus infection in mice. *Nature* **304**, 541.

Lin, Y. L. and Askonas, B. A. (1980). Cross-reactivity for different type A influenza viruses of a cloned T-killer cell line. *Nature* **288**, 164.

Lin, Y. L. and Askonas, B. A. (1981). Biological properties of an influenza A virus-specific killer T cell clone. *J. Exp. Med.* **154**, 225.

Lindahl, P., Leary, P. and Gresser, I. (1972). Enhancement by interferon of the specific toxicity of sensitized lymphocytes. *Proc. Nat. Acad. Sci. USA* **69**, 721.

Linde, G. A., Hammarstrom, L., Persson, M. A. A. *et al*. (1983). Virus specific antibody activity of different subclasses of immunoglobulin G and A in cytomegalovirus infections. *Infect. Immunity* **42**, 237.

Lindenmann, J. and Klein, P. A. (1967). Viral oncolysis: increased immunogenicity of host cell antigen associated with influenza virus. *J. Exp. Med.* **126**, 93.

Lipton, H. L. (1975). Theilers virus infection in mice: an unusual biphasic disease process leading to demyelination. *Infect. Immunity* **11**, 1147.

Lipton, H. L. and Johnson, R. T. (1972). The pathogenesis of rat virus infections in the newborn hamster. *Lab. Invest.* **27**, 508.

Little, L. M. and Shadduck, J. A. (1982). Pathogenesis of rotavirus infection of mice. *Infect. Immunity* **38**, 755.

Lodish, H. F. and Potter, M. (1980). Specific incorporation of host cell surface proteins into budding vesicular stomatitis virus particles. *Cell* **19**, 161.

Lodmell, D. L. (1983). Genetic control of resistance to street rabies virus in mice. *J. Exp. Med.* **157**, 451.

LoGrippo, G. A. (1960). Investigations of the use of beta-propiolactone in virus inactivation. *Annals N.Y. Acad. Sci.* **83**, 578.

Loh, L. and Hudson, J. B. (1982). Murine cytomegalovirus-induced immunosuppression. *Infect. Immunity* **36**, 89.

Lonberg-Holm, K. and Philipson, L. (1981). *Animal Virus Receptors. Series B: Receptors and Recognition*. Chapman and Hall, London.

London, W. T. (1977). Epizootiology, transmission and approach to prevention of fatal simian haemorrhagic fever in rhesus monkeys. *Nature* **268**, 344.

London, W. T., Drew, J. S., Lustbader, E. D. *et al*. (1977). Host responses to hepatitis B infection in patients in chronic haemodialysis unit. *Kidney Internat.* **12**, 51.

Loosli, C. G., Stinson, S. F., Ryan, D. P. *et al*. (1975). The destruction of Type 2 pneumocytes by airborne influenza PR8-A virus: its effect of surfactant and lecithin content of the pneumonic lesions of mice. *Chest* **67** (Suppl.), 7s.

Lopez, C. (1980). Resistance to HSV-1 in the mouse is governed by two major, independently segregating, non H-2 loci. *Immunogenetics* **11**, 87.

Lopez, C. (1981). Resistance to herpes simplex virus—type I (HSV-1). *Curr. Top. Microbiol. Immunol.* **92**, 15.

Lopez, C., Ryslike, R. and Bennett, M. (1980). Marrow-dependent cells depleted by ^{89}Sr mediated genetic resistance to herpes simplex virus type I infection in mice. *Infect. Immunity* **28**, 1028.

Lubeck, M. D. and Gerhard, W. (1981). Topological mapping of antigenic sites on the influenza A/PR8/8/34 virus haemagglutinin using monoclonal antibodies **113**, 64.

Lucas, C. J., Ubeis-Postma, J. C., Rezee, A. *et al*. (1978). Activation of measles virus from silently infected human lymphocytes. *J. Exp. Med.* **148**, 940.

Luria, S. E., Darnell, J. E., Baltimore, D. *et al*. (1978). *General Virology*, 3rd edn. Wiley, New York.

Lustbader, E. D., Hann, H. W. L. and Blumberg, B. (1983). Serum ferritin as a predictor of host response to hepatitis B virus infection. *Science* **220**, 423.

Lutley, R., Petursson, G., Palsson, P. A. *et al*. (1983). Antigenic drift in visna: virus variation during long-term infection of Icelandic sheep. *J. Gen. Virol.* **64**, 1433.

Lwoff, A. (1959). Factors influencing the evolution of viral diseases at the cellular level and in the organism. *Bact. Rev.* **23**, 109.

Lwoff, A. (1969). Death and transfiguration of a problem. *Bact. Rev.* **33**, 390.

Lwoff, A., Tournier, P. and Cartreaud, J. P. (1959). L'influence de l'hyperthermie provoquée sur l'infection poliomyélitique de la souris. *CR Acad. Sci.* (Paris) **248**, 1876.

Lyons, M. J., Faust, I. M., Hemmes, R. B. *et al.* (1982). A virally induced obesity syndrome in mice. *Science* **216**, 82.

Maassab, H. F., Monto, A. S., deBorde, D. C. *et al.* (1981). Development of cold recombinants of influenza virus as live virus vaccines. In *Genetic Variation among Influenza Viruses* (ed. D. Nayak), ICN-UCLA Symp. 21, pp. 617–37. Academic Press, New York.

McAleer, W. J., Markus, H. Z., McLean, A. A. *et al.* (1980). Stability on storage at various temperatures of live measles, mumps and rubella virus vaccines in new stabilizer. *J. Biol. Stand.* **8**, 281.

McAleer, W. J., Buynak, E. B., Maigetter, R. Z. *et al.* (1984). Human hepatitis B vaccine from recombinant yeast. *Nature* **307**, 178.

McAllister, P. E. (1979). Fish viruses and viral infections. In *Comprehensive Virology*, vol. 14, 401. Plenum Press, New York.

McCance, D. J. and Mims, C. A. (1979). Reactivation of polyoma virus in kidneys of persistently infected mice during pregnancy. *Infect. Immunity* **25**, 998.

McCance, D. J., Sebesteny, A., Griffin, B. E. *et al.* (1983). A paralytic disease in nude mice associated with polyma virus infection. *J. Gen. Virol.* **64**, 57.

McClintock, P. R., Billups, L. C. and Notkins, A. L. (1980). Receptors for encephalomyocarditis virus on murine and human cells. *Virology* **106**, 261.

McConnell, I., Munro, A. and Waldman, H. (1981). *The Immune System: A Course on the Molecular and Cellular Basis of Immunology*. Blackwell Scientific Publications, Oxford.

McCormick, J. B. and Johnson, K. M. (1984). Viral hemorrhagic fevers. In *Tropical and Geographic Medicine* (eds K. S. Warren and A. D. F. Mahmoud). McGraw-Hill, Maidenhead, Berkshire.

Macfarlan, R. I. and White, D. O. (1983). Macrophages bind directly to Semliki Forest virus-infected cells and mediate antibody-dependent cell-mediated cytotoxicity. *Aust. J. Exp. Biol. Med. Sci.* **62**.

Macfarlan, R. I., Burns, W. H. and White, D. O. (1977). Two cytotoxic cells in peritoneal cavity of virus-infected mice: antibody-dependent macrophages and non-specific killer cells. *J. Immunol.* **119**, 1569.

McGeogh, D. J. (1981). Structural analysis of animal virus genomes. *J. Gen. Virol.* **55**, 1.

McIntosh, K. and Fishaut, J. M. (1980). Immunopathic mechanisms in lower respiratory tract disease of infants due to respiratory syncytial virus. *Progr. Med. Virol.* **26**, 94.

Mackay, P., Pasek, M., Magazin, M. *et al.* (1981). Production of immunologically active surface antigens of hepatitis B virus by *Escherichia coli*. *Proc. Nat. Acad. Sci. USA* **78**, 4510.

McKenzie, I. F. C. and Potter, T. (1979). Murine lymphocyte surface antigens. *Adv. Immunol.* **27**, 179.

Mackenzie, J. S. (1969). Virulence of temperature-sensitive mutants of influenza virus. *Br. Med. J.* **3**, 757.

McKinnon, K. P., Hale, A. H. and Ruebush, M. J. (1981). Elicitation of natural killer cells in beige mice by infection with vesicular stomatitis virus. *Infect. Immunity* **32**, 204.

McLaren, L. C., Holland, J. J. and Syverton, J. T. (1959). The mammalian cell-virus relationship. I. Attachment of poliovirus to cultivated cells of primate and non-primate origin. *J. Exp. Med.* **109**, 475.

McLennan, J. L. and Darby, G. (1980). Herpes simplex virus latency: the cellular location of virus in dorsal root ganglia and the fate of the infected cell following virus activation. *J. Gen. Virol.* **51**, 233.

McMichael, A. J., Gotch, F. M., Noble, G. R. *et al.* (1983). Cytotoxic T cell immunity to influenza. *New Engl. J. Med.* **309**, 13.

McNabb, P. C. and Tomasi, T. B. (1981). Host defence mechanisms at mucosal surfaces. *Ann. Rev. Microbiol.* **35**, 477.

Macnaughton, M. R. (1982). The structure and replication of rhinoviruses. *Curr. Top. Microbiol. Immunol.* **97**, 1.

de Maeyer, E. and de Maeyer-Guignard, J. (1979). Interferons. In *Comprehensive Virology*, vol. 15, 205. Plenum Press, New York.

de Maeyer, E. and de Maeyer-Guignard, J. (1980). Immunoregulatory action of type I interferon in the mouse. *Annals. NY Acad. Sci.* **350**, 1.

de Maeyer, E., Galasso, G. and Schellekens, H. (eds.) (1981). *The Biology of the Interferon System*. Elsevier North-Holland, Amsterdam.

de Maeyer, E. and Schellekens, H. (eds.) (1983). *The Biology of the Interferon System 1983*. Elsevier, Amsterdam.

Maiztegui, J. I., Fernandez, N. J. and de Damilano, A. J. (1979). Efficacy of immune plasma in treatment of Argentine haemorrhagic fever and association between treatment and a late neurological syndrome. *Lancet* ii, 1216.

Mak, N. K., Leung, K. N. and Ada, G. L. (1982). The generation of 'cytotoxic' macrophages in mice during infection with influenza A or Sendai virus. *Scand. J. Immunol.* **15**, 553.

Makinodan, T. and Kay, M. M. B. (1980). Age influence on the immune response. *Adv. Immunol.* **29**, 287.

Mandel, B. (1967). The interaction of neutralized poliovirus with HeLa cells. II. Elution, penetration, uncoating. *Virology* **31**, 248.

Mandel, B. (1979). Interaction of viruses with neutralizing antibodies. In *Comprehensive Virology*, vol. 15, p. 37 (eds. H. Fraenkel-Conrat and R. R. Wagner). Plenum Press, New York.

Mandel, T. E., Phipps, R. P., Abbot, A. *et al.* (1980). The follicular dendritic cell: long term antigen retention during immunity. *Immunol. Rev.* **53**, 29.

Maniatis, T., Fritsch, E. F. and Sambrook, J. (1982). *Molecular Cloning: a Laboratory Manual*. Cold Spring Harbor Laboratory, New York.

Mantei, N. and Weissmann, C. (1982). Controlled transcription of a human α-interferon gene introduced into mouse L cells. *Nature* **297**, 128.

Marcus, P. I. (1982). The interferon inducer moiety of viruses: a single molecule of dsRNA. *Texas Reports Biol. Med.* **41**, 70.

Margolis, G. and Kilham, L. (1968). Virus-induced cerebellar hypoplasia. *Res. Publ. Assoc. Nerv. Mental Dis.* **44**, 113.

Margolis, G., Jacobs, L. R. and Kilham, L. (1976). Oxygen tension and the selective tropism of K-virus for mouse pulmonary endothelium. *Am. Rev. Respir. Dis.* **114**, 45.

Marion, P. L. and Robinson, W. S. (1983). Hepadna viruses: hepatitis B and related viruses. *Curr. Top. Microbiol. Immunol.* **105**, 99.

Marker, S. C. and Jahrling, P. B. (1979). Correlation between virus-cell receptor properties of alphaviruses in vitro and virulence in vivo. *Arch. Virol.* **62**, 53.

Markwell, M. A. K., Svennerholm, L. and Paulson, J. C. (1981). Specific gangliosides function as host cell receptors for Sendai virus. *Proc. Nat. Acad. Sci. USA* **78**, 5406.

Marshall, I. D. (1959). The influence of ambient temperature on the course of myxomatosis in rabbits. *J. Hyg.* **57**, 484.

Massey, R. J. and Schochetman, G. (1981). Viral epitopes and monoclonal antibodies: isolation of blocking antibodies that inhibit virus neutralization. *Science* **213**, 447.

Masters, C. L., Harris, J. O., Gajdusek, D. C. *et al.* (1980). Creutzfeld-Jakob disease: patterns of worldwide occurrence and the significance of familial and sporadic clustering. *Ann. Neurol.* **5**, 177.

Masur, H., Michelis, M. A., Greene, J. B. *et al.* (1981). An outbreak of community-acquired *Pneumocystis carinii* pneumonia, initial manifestation of cellular immune dysfunction. *New Engl. J. Med.* **305**, 1431.

Mata, L. J. (1975). Malnutrition-infection interactions in the tropics. *Am. J. Trop. Med. Hyg.* **24**, 564.

Mathur, A., Arora, K. K. and Chaturvedi, U. C. (1982). Transplacental Japanese encephalitis virus (JEV) infection in mice during consecutive pregnancies. *J. Gen. Virol.* **59**, 213.

Mathur, A., Rawat, S. and Chaturvedi, U. C. (1983). Induction of suppressor cells in Japanese encephalitis virus infected mice. *Br. J. Exp. Pathol.* **64**, 336.

Matthews, R. E. F. (1981). *Plant Virology*, 2nd edn. Academic Press, New York.

Matthews, R. E. F. (1982). Classification and Nomenclature of Viruses. Fourth Report of the International Committee on Taxonomy of Viruses. *Intervirology* **17**, 1–200.

Matthews, R. E. F. (1983). The history of virus taxonomy. In *A Critical Appraisal of Viral Taxonomy* (ed. R. E. F. Matthews). CRC Press, Florida.

Maupas, P. and Guesry, P. (eds.) (1981). *Hepatitis B Vaccine*. INSERM Symposium 18. Elsevier North-Holland, Amsterdam.

Maupas, P., Goudeau, A., Coursaget, P. *et al.* (1976). Immunization against hepatitis B in man. *Lancet* i, 1367.

Melnick, J. L. (1977). Viral vaccines. *Progr. Med. Virol.* **23**, 158.

Melnick, J. L. (1978). Advantages and disadvantages of killed and live poliomyelitis vaccines. *Bull. WHO* **56**, 21.

Melnick, J. L. (1980). Poliomyelitis vaccines: an appraisal after 25 years. *Compr. Ther.* **6**, 6.

Melnick, J. L. and Riordan, J. T. (1947). Latent mouse encephalomyelitis. *J. Immunol.* **57**, 331.

Menser, M. A., Forrest, J. M. and Bransby, R. D. (1978). Rubella infection and diabetes mellitus. *Lancet* i, 57.

Merigan, T. C. (1981). Present appraisal of and future hopes for clinical utilization of human interferons. In *Interferon 3* (ed. I. Gresser), pp. 135–54. Academic Press, New York.

Merigan, T. C. and Friedman, R. M. (eds.) (1982). *Interferons*. UCLA Symposium of Molecular Cell Biology, vol. XXV. Academic Press, New York.

Merz, D. C., Scheid, A. and Choppin, P. W. (1980). Importance of antibodies to the fusion glycoprotein of paramyxoviruses in the prevention of spread of infection. *J. Exp. Med.* **151**, 275.

ter Meulen, V. and Carter, M. J. (1982). Morbillivirus persistent infections in animals and man. In *Virus Persistence*, p. 97 33rd Symposium Soc. Gen. Microbiol, (eds. B. W. J. Mahy, A. C. Minson and G. K. Darby). Cambridge University Press, Cambridge.

Meyer, H. M., Hopps, H. E. and Parkman, P. D. (1980). Appraisal and reappraisal of viral vaccines. *Adv. Intern. Med.* **25**, 533.

Miller, A. E. (1980). Selective decline in cellular immune response to varicella-zoster in the elderly. *Neurology* **30**, 582.

Miller, C. A. and Carrigan, D. R. (1982). Reversible repression and activation of measles virus infection in neural cells. *Proc. Nat. Acad. Sci. USA* **79**, 1629.

Miller, D. A., Miller, O. J., Dev, V. G. *et al.* (1974). Human chromosome 19 carries a poliovirus receptor gene. *Cell* **1**, 167.

Mims, C. A. (1957). Rift Valley Fever virus in mice VI. Histological changes in the liver in relation to virus multiplication. *Aust. J. Exp. Biol. Med. Sci.* **35**, 595.

Mims, C. A. (1959). The response of mice to large intravenous injections of ectromelia virus. II The growth of virus in the liver. *Br. J. Exp. Pathol.* **40**, 543.

Mims, C. A. (1960). An analysis of the toxicity for mice of influenza virus. I. Intracerebral toxicity. *Br. J. Exp. Pathol.* **41**, 586.

Mims, C. A. (1960b). An analysis of the toxicity for mice of influenza virus. II Intravenous toxicity. *Br. J. Exp. Pathol.* **41**, 593.

Mims, C. A. (1964). Aspects of the pathogenesis of virus diseases. *Bact. Rev.* **28**, 30.

Mims, C. A. (1966). Immunofluorescence study of the carrier state and mechanism of vertical transmission in lymphocytic choriomeningitis virus infection in mice. *J. Pathol. Bacteriol.* **91**, 395.

Mims, C. A. (1968a). The response of mice to the intravenous injection of cowpox virus. *Br. J. Exp. Pathol.* **49**, 24.

Mims, C. A. (1968b). Pathogenesis of viral infections of the fetus. *Progr. Med. Virol.* **10**, 194.

Mims, C. A. (1969). Effect on the fetus of maternal infection with lymphocytic choriomeningitis (LCM) virus. *J. Infect. Dis.* **120**, 582.

Mims, C. A. (1970). Observations on mice infected congenitally or neonatally with lymphocytic choriomeningitis (LCM) virus. *Arch. Ges. Virusforsch.* **30**, 67.

Mims, C. A. (1974). Factors in the mechanism of persistent viral infections. *Progr. Med. Virol.* **18**, 1.

Mims, C. A. (1978). General features of persistent virus infections. *Postgrad. Med. J.* **54**, 581.

Mims, C. A. (1981). Vertical transmission of viruses. *Microbiol. Rev.* **45**, 267.

Mims, C. A. (1982a). *The Pathogenesis of Infectious Disease*, 2nd edn. Academic Press, New York.

Mims, C. A. (1982b). Immunopathology of Viral Infection. In *Viral Diseases in South-East Asia and the Western Pacific*. (ed. J. S. Mackenzie), pp. 46–55. Academic Press, New York.

Mims, C. A. (1982c). Role of persistence in viral pathogenesis. In *Virus*

Persistence, (eds. B. W. J. Mahy, A. C. Minson and G. K. Darby). Cambridge University Press, Cambridge.

Mims, C. A. and Blanden, R. V. (1972). Antiviral activity of immune lymphocytes in lymphocytic choriomeningitis virus infection of mice. *Infect. Immunity* **6**, 695.

Mims, C. A. and Gould, J. (1978). Infection of salivary glands, kidneys, adrenals, ovaries and epithelia by murine cytomegalovirus. *J. Med. Microbiol.* **12**, 113.

Mims, C. A. and Murphy, F. A. (1973). Parainfluenza virus Sendai infection in macrophages, ependyma, choroid plexus, vascular endothelium and respiratory tract of mice. *Am. J. Pathol.* **70**, 315.

Mims, C. A. and Subrahmanyan, T. P. (1966). Immunofluorescent study of the mechanism of resistance to superinfection in mice carrying the lymphocytic choriomeningitis virus. *J. Pathol. Bact.* **91**, 403.

Mims, C. A. and Tosolini, F. A. (1969). Pathogenesis of lesions in lymphoid tissue of mice infected with lymphocytic choriomeningitis (LCM) virus. *Br. J. Exp. Pathol.* **50**, 584.

Mims, C. A. and Wainwright, S. (1968). The immunodepressive action of lymphocytic choriomeningitis virus in mice. *J. Immunol.* **101**, 717.

Miyanohara, A., Toh-e, A., Nozaki, C. *et al.* (1983). Expression of hepatitis B surface antigen in yeast. *Proc. Nat. Acad. Sci. USA* **80**, 1.

Mogensen, S. G. (1979). Role of macrophages in natural resistance to virus infection. *Microbiol. Rev.* **43**. 1.

Mok, C. H. (1971). Zoster-like disease in infants and young children. *New Engl. J. Med.* **285**, 294.

Möller, G. (ed.) (1974). The Immune Response to Infectious Diseases. *Transplant. Rev.* **19**.

Möller, G. (ed.) (1981a). T cell Clones. *Immunol. Rev.* **54**.

Möller, G. (ed.) (1981b). MHC Restriction of Anti-Viral Immunity. *Immunol. Rev.* **58**.

Möller, G. (ed.) (1981c). Accessory Cells in the Immune Response. *Immunol. Rev.* **53**.

Möller, G. (ed.) (1982). Interleukins and Lymphocyte Activation. *Immunol. Rev.* **63**.

Monath, T. P., Kinney, R. M., Schlesinger, J. J. *et al.* (1983). Ontogeny of yellow fever 17D vaccine: RNA oligonucleotide fingerprint and monoclonal antibody analysis of vaccines produced worldwide. *J. Gen. Virol.* **64**, 627.

Montagnon, B. J., Janget, B., and Nicolas, A. J. (1981). The large scale cultivation of VERO cells in microcarrier culture for virus vaccine production. Preliminary results for killed poliovirus vaccine. *Develop. Biol. Stand.* **47**, 55.

Moore, M. (1983). Interferon and the immune system. 2: Effect of IFN on the immune system. In *Interferons* (eds. D. C. Burke and A. G. Morris), Symposium of the Society of General Microbiology, vol. 35, pp. 181–209. Cambridge University Press, Cambridge.

Moore, M., Katona, P., Kaplan, J. E. *et al.* (1982). Poliomyelitis in the United States, 1969–1981. *J. Infect. Dis.* **146**, 558.

Morahan, P. S. (1980). Macrophage nomenclature: where are we going? *J. Reticuloendothel. Soc.* **27**, 223.

Morgan, D. G., Niederman, J. C., Miller, G. *et al.* (1979). Site of Epstein-Barr replication in the oropharynx. *Lancet* ii, 1154.

Morgan, D. O., Moore, D. M. and McKercher, P. D. (1980). Vaccination against foot-and-mouth disease. In *New Developments with Human and Veterinary Vaccines* (eds. A. Mizrahi *et al.*). *Progr. Clin. Biol. Res.* **47**, 169. Alan R. Liss, New York.

Morishima, T., McClintock, P. R., Billups, L. C. *et al.* (1982). Expression and modulation of virus receptors on lymphoid and myeloid cells; relation to infectivity. *Virology* **116**, 605.

Morley, D. C. (1967). Measles and measles vaccine in preindustrial countries. *Mod. Trends. Med. Virol.* **1**, 141.

Morley, D. C. (1969). The severe measles of West Africa. *Proc. Roy. Soc. Med.* **57**, 846.

Morley, D. C. (1980). Severe measles: a barometer of childhood nutrition. In *Potency and Efficacy of Vaccines* (ed. F. E. Andre), pp. 143–56. Smith Kline-RIT, U.S.A.

Morris, A. G., Lin, Y. L. and Askonas, B. A. (1982). Immune interferon release when a cloned cytotoxic T-cell line meets its correct influenza-infected target cell. *Nature* **295**, 150.

Morse, S. S. and Morahan, P.S. (1981). Activated macrophages mediate interferon-independent inhibition of herpes simplex virus. *Cell. Immunol.* **58**, 72.

Mozes, L. W., Schultz, J., Scott, W. A. *et al.* (eds.) (1981). *Cellular Responses to Molecular Modulators*. Miami Winter Symp. no. 18. Academic Press, New York.

Müller, G. M., Shapira, M. and Arnon, R. (1982). Anti-influenza response achieved by immunization with a synthetic conjugate. *Proc. Nat. Acad. Sci. USA* **79**, 569.

Münk, K. and Kirchner, H. (1982). *Interferons: Properties, Mode of Action, Production, Clinical Application*. Karger, Basel.

Murphy, B. R. and Chanock, R. M. (1981). Genetic approaches to the prevention of influenza A virus infection. In *Genetic Variation among Influenza Viruses* (ed. D. Nayak), ICN-UCLA Symp. no. 21, pp. 601–15. Academic Press, New York.

Murphy, B. R., Tolpin, M. D., Massicot, J. *et al.* (1980). Escape of a highly defective influenza A virus mutant from its *ts* phenotype by extragenic suppression and other types of mutation. *Ann. N. Y. Acad. Sci.* **354**, 142.

Murphy, B. R., Sly, D. L., Tierney, E. L. *et al.* (1982). Reassortant virus derived from avian and human influenza A virus is attenuated and immunogenic in monkeys. *Science* **218**, 1330.

Murphy, F. A. (1977). Rabies pathogenesis—brief review. *Arch. Virol.* **54**, 279.

Murphy, F. A., Taylor, W. P., Mims, C. A. *et al.* (1973). Pathogenesis of Ross River virus infection in mice. II Muscle, heart and brown fat lesions. *J. Infect. Dis.* **127**, 129.

Murray, K. (1980). Genetic engineering: possibilities and prospects for its application in industrial microbiology. *Phil. Trans. Roy. Soc. Lond. B* **290**, 369.

Naeye, R. L. and Blanc, W. (1965). Pathogenesis of congenital rubella. *J. Am. Med. Assoc.* **194**, 1277.

Nagai, Y., Klenk, H. D. and Roth, R. (1976). Proteolytic cleavage of the viral glycoproteins and its significance for the virulence of Newcastle Disease virus. *Virology* **68**, 494.

Nagata, S., Taira, H., Hall, A. *et al*. (1980). Synthesis in *E. coli* of a polypeptide with human leukocyte interferon activity. *Nature* **284**, 316.

Nahmias, A. J. and O'Reilly, R. J. (1982). Immunology of Human Infection, Part 2. Viruses. In *Comprehensive Immunology*, vol. 9. Plenum Press, New York.

Nahmias, A. J., Griffith, D., Salsbury, C. *et al*. (1967). Thymic aplasia with lymphopenia, plasma cells and normal immunoglobulins: relation to measles virus infection. *J.A.M.A.* **201**, 792.

Nahmias, A. J., Dowdle, W. R. and Schinazi, R. F. (eds.) (1981). *The Human Herpesviruses: An Interdisciplinary Perspective*. Elsevier, New York.

Nakamura, M., Manser, T., Pearson, G. D. N. *et al*. (1984). Effect of IFN-γ on the immune response in vivo and on gene expression in vitro. *Nature* **307**, 381.

Nakano, J. H., Hatch, M. H., Thieme, M. L. *et al*. (1978). Parameters for differentiating vaccine-derived and wild poliovirus strains. *Progr. Med. Virol.* **24**, 178.

Narayan, O., Griffin, D. E. and Chase, J. (1977). Antigenic shift of visna virus in persistently infected sheep. *Science* **197**, 376.

Narayan, O., Griffin, D. E. and Clements, J. E. (1978). Virus mutation during 'slow infection': temporal development and characterization of mutants of visna virus recovered from sheep. *J. Gen. Virol.* **41**, 343.

Narayan, O., Clements, J. E., Strandberg, J. D. *et al*. (1980). Biological characterization of the virus causing leukoencephalitis and arthritis in goats. *J. Gen. Virol.* **50**, 69.

Narayan, O., Wolinsky, J. S., Clements, J. E. *et al*. (1982). Slow virus replication: the role of macrophages in the persistence and expression of visna viruses of sheep and goats. *J. Gen. Virol.* **59**, 345.

Narayan, O., Kennedy-Stoskopf, S., Sheffer, D. *et al*. (1983a). Activation of caprine arthritis-encephalitis virus expression during maturation of monocytes to macrophages. *Infect. Immunity* **41**, 67.

Narayan, O., Strandberg, J. D., Griffin, D. E. *et al*. (1983b). Aspects of the pathogenesis of visna in sheep. In *Viruses and Demyelinating Diseases*, (eds. C. A. Mims, M. L. Cuzner and R. E. Kelly). Academic Press, New York.

Nash, A. A. and Ashford, N. P. N. (1982). Split T cell tolerance in herpes simplex virus infected mice and its implication for antiviral immunity. *Immunology* **45**, 761.

Nash, A. A., Field, H. J. and Quartey-Papafio, R. (1980). Cell-mediated immunity in herpes simplex virus infected mice: induction, characterization and antiviral effects of delayed type hypersensitivity. *J. Gen. Virol.* **48**, 351.

Nash, A. A., Phelan, J., Gell, P. G. *et al*. (1981). Tolerance and immunity in mice infected with herpes simplex virus: studies on the mechanism of tolerance to delayed type hypersensitivity. *Immunology* **43**, 363.

Nash, A. A., Phelan, J. and Wildy, P. (1981). Cell-mediated immunity in herpes simplex virus infected mice: H_2 mapping of the delayed type hypersensitivity response and the antiviral T cell response. *J. Immunol.* **126**, 1260.

Nathanson, N. and Martin, J. R. (1979). The epidemiology of poliomyelitis: enigmas surrounding its appearance, epidemicity, and disappearance. *Am. J. Epidemiol.* **110**, 672.

Nathanson, N., Georgsson, G., Lutley, R. *et al*. (1983). Pathogenesis of visna in Icelandic sheep. Demyelinating lesions and antigenic drift. In *Viruses and*

Demyelinating Diseases (eds. C. A. Mims, M. L. Cuzner, and R. E. Kelly). Academic Press, New York.

Nawrocki, J. F., Pease, L. R. and Murphy, W. H. (1980). Etiologic role of lactic dehydrogenase virus infection in an age-dependent neuroparalytic disease in C_{58} mice. *Virology* **103**, 259.

Nayak, D. (ed.) (1981). *Genetic Variation among Influenza Viruses*. ICN-UCLA Symposium no. 21. Academic Press, New York.

Naylor, P. T., Larsen, H. S., Huang, L. *et al*. (1982). *In vivo* induction of anti-herpes simplex virus immune response by type 1 antigens and lipid A incorporated into liposomes. *Infect. Immunity* **36**, 1209.

Naylor, S. L., Sakaguchi, A. Y., Shows, T. B. *et al*. (1983). Human immune interferon gene is located on chromosome 12. *J. Exp. Med.* **157**, 1020.

Nazarian, K. and Witter, R. L. (1970). Cell-free transmission and in vivo replication of Marek's disease virus. *J. Virol.* **5**, 388.

Neff, B. J., Weibel, R. E., Buynak, E. B. *et al*. (1979). Clinical and laboratory studies of live cytomegalovirus vaccine Ad-169(40382). *Proc. Soc. Exp. Biol. Med.* **160**, 32.

Neff, B. J., Weibel, R. E., Villarejos, V. M. *et al*. (1981). Clinical and laboratory studies of KMcC strain of live attenuated varicella virus (41071). *Proc. Soc. Exp. Biol. Med.* **166**, 339.

O'Neill, H. C. and Blanden, R. V. (1983). Mechanisms determining innate resistance to ectromelia virus infection in C57 BL mice. *Infect. Immunity* **41**, 1391.

Nemazee, D. A. and Sato, V. L. (1982). Enhancing antibody: a novel component of the immune response. *Proc. Nat. Acad. Sci. USA* **79**, 3828.

Nepom, J. T., Weiner, J. L., Dichter, M. A. *et al*. (1982). Identification of a hemagglutinin-specific idiotype associated with reovirus recognition shared by lymphoid and neural cells. *J. Exp. Med.* **155**, 155.

Newby, T. J., Stokes, C. R. and Bourne, F. J. (1982). Immunological activities of milk. *Vet. Immunol. Immunopathol.* **3**, 67.

Newhouse, M., Sanchis, J. and Bienenstock, J. (1976). Lung defence mechanisms. *New Engl. J. Med.* **295**, 990.

Ng, A. B., Reagen, J. W. and Yen, S. S. (1970). Herpes genitalis; clinical and cytopathologic experience with 256 patients. *Obstet. Gynaecol.* **36**, 645.

Nichols, W. W. (1970). Virus-induced chromosome abnormalities. *Ann. Rev. Microbiol.* **24**, 479.

Nightingale, E. O. (1977). Recommendations for a national policy on poliomyelitis vaccination. *New Engl. J. Med.* **297**, 249.

Nishiyama, Y. (1977). Studies of L cells persistently infected with VSV: factors involved in the regulation of persistent infections. *J. Gen. Virol* **35**, 265.

Nomoto, A., Omata, T., Toyoda, H. *et al*. (1982). Complete nucleotide sequence of the attenuated poliovirus Sabin 1 strain genome. *Proc. Nat. Acad. Sci. USA* **79**, 5793.

Norkin, L. C. (1982). Papovaviral persistent infections. *Microbiol. Rev.* **46**, 384.

Norrby, E., Enders-Ruckle, G. and ter Meulen, V. (1975). Differences in the appearance of antibodies to structural components of measles virus after immunization with inactivated and live virus. *J. Infect. Dis.* **132**, 262.

North, J. R., Morgan, A. J., Thompson, J. L. *et al*. (1982). Purified EB virus gp 340 induces potent virus-neutralizing antibodies when incorporated in liposomes. *Proc. Nat. Acad. Sci. USA* **79**, 7504.

Noseworthy, J. H., Fields, B. N., Dichter, M. A. *et al.* (1983). Cell receptors for the mammalian reovirus I. Syngeneic monoclonal anti-idiotypic antibody identifies a cell surface receptor for reovirus. *J. Immunol.* **131**, 2533.

Notkins, A. L. (1974). Immune mechanisms by which the spread of viral infections is stopped. *Cell. Immunol.* **11**, 478.

Notkins, A. L. (ed.) (1975). *Viral Immunology and Immunopathology*. Academic Press, New York.

Notkins, A. L. (1977). Virus-induced diabetes mellitus. *Arch. Virol.* **54**, 1.

Notkins, A. L., Mahar, S., Scheele, C. *et al.* (1966). Infectious virus-antibody complex in the blood of chronically infected mice. *J. Exp. Med.* **124**, 81.

Notkins, A. L., Mergenhagen, S. E. and Howard, R. J. (1970). Effect of virus infections on the function of the immune system. *Ann. Rev. Microbiol.* **24**, 525.

Noyes, W. F. and Mellors, R. C. (1957). Fluorescent antibody detection of the antigens of the Shope papilloma virus in papillomas of the wild and domestic rabbit. *J. Exp. Med.* **106**, 552.

O'Connell, A. P., Urban, M. K. and London, W. T. (1983). Naturally occurring infection of Pekin duck embryos by duck hepatitis B virus. *Proc. Nat. Acad. Sci. USA* **80**, 1703.

Ofosu-Amah, S., Kratzer, J. H. and Nicholas, D. D. (1977). Is Poliomyelitis a serious problem in developing countries?—lameness in Ghanian schools. *Br. Med. J.* i, 1012.

Ogata, M. and Shigeta, S. (1979). Appearance of immunoglobulin G Fc receptor in cultured human cells infected with varicella-zoster virus. *Infect. Immunity* **26**, 770.

Ogra, P. L. (1971). The secretory immunoglobulin system of the gastrointestinal tract. In *The Secretory Immunologic System* (eds. D. H. Dayton, P. A. Small, R. M. Chanock *et al.*). p. 259. National Inst. Child Health and Human Development, National Institutes of Health, Bethesda, Maryland.

Ogra, P. L. and Herd, J. K. (1971). Arthritis associated with induced rubella infection. *J. Immunol.* **107**, 810.

Ogra, P. L., Fishaut, M. and Gallagher, M. R. (1980). Viral vaccination via the mucosal routes. *Rev. Infect. Dis.* **2**, 352.

Ohkuma, S. and Poole, B. (1978). Fluorescent probe measurement of the intra-lysosomal pH in living cells and the perturbation of pH by various agents. *Proc. Nat. Acad. Sci. USA* **75**, 3327.

Oldstone, M. B. A. and Dixon, F. J. (1967). Lymphocytic choriomeningitis: production of antibody by 'tolerant' infected mice. *Science* **158**, 1193.

Oldstone, M. B. A. and Dixon, F. J. (1969). Pathogenesis of chronic disease associated with persistent lymphocytic choriomeningitis viral infection. I Relationship of antibody production to disease in neonatally infected mice. *J. Exp. Med.* **129**, 483.

Oldstone, M. B. A. and Dixon, F. J. (1971). Immune complex disease in chronic viral infections. *J. Exp. Med.* **134**, 32s.

Oldstone, M. B. A. and Tishon, A. (1978). Immunologic injury in measles virus infection. IV Antigenic modulation and abrogation of lymphocyte lysis of virus-infected cells. *Clin. Immunol. Immunopathol.* **9**, 55.

Oldstone, M. B. A. and Fujinami, R. S. (1982). Virus persistence and avoidance of immune surveillance: how measles viruses can be induced to persist in cells, escape immune assault and injure tissues. In *Virus Persistence*, (eds. B. W. J. Mahy, A. C. Minson and G. K. Derby), 33rd Symp. Soc. Gen. Microbiol. Cambridge University Press, Cambridge.

Oldstone, M. B. A., Dixon, F. J., Mitchell, G. F. *et al.* (1973). Histocompatibility-linked genetic control of disease susceptibility. Murine lymphocytic choriomeningitis virus infection. *J. Exp. Med.* **137**, 1201.

Oldstone, M. B. A., Cooper, N. R. and Larson, D. L. (1974). Formation and biologic role of polyoma virus-antibody complexes: a critical role for complement. *J. Exp. Med.* **140**, 549.

Oldstone, M. B. A., Holmstoen, J. and Welsh, R. M. (1977). Alterations of acetylcholine enzymes in neuroblastoma cells persistently infected with lymphocytic choriomeningitis virus. *J. Cell. Physiol.* **91**, 459.

Oldstone, M. B. A., Fujinami, R. S. and Lampert, P. W. (1980). Membrane and cytoplasmic changes in virus-infected cells induced by interaction of antiviral antibody with surface viral antigen. *Progr. Med. Virol.* **26**, 45.

Oldstone, M. B. A., Sinha, Y. M., Bhount, P. *et al.* (1982). Virus-induced alterations in homeostasis leading to disease: alterations in differentiated but not vital functions of infected cells in vivo. *Science* **218**, 1125.

Oldstone, M. B. A., Tishon, A. and Buchmeier, M. J. (1983). Virus-induced immune complex disease: genetic control of C1q binding complexes in the circulation of mice persistently infected with lymphocytic choriomeningitis virus. *J. Immunol.* **130**, 912.

Onodera, T., Toniolo, T., Ray, U. R. *et al.* (1981). Virus-induced diabetes mellitus XX. Polyendocrinopathy and autoimmunity. *J. Exp. Med.* **153**, 1457.

Openshaw, H., Puga, A. and Notkins, A. L. (1979). Latency and reactivation of herpes simplex virus in sensory ganglia of mice. *Devel. Immunol.* **7**, 301.

Osborn, J. E. (1979). Viral vaccines under development: a third generation. *Adv. Exp. Biol. Med. Biol.* **118**, 61.

Osborn, J. E. (1981). Cytomegalovirus: pathogenicity, immunology, and vaccine initiatives. *J. Infect. Dis.* **143**, 618.

Osborn, J. E. and Walker, D. L. (1971). Virulence and attenuation of murine cytomegalovirus. *Infect. Immunity* **3**, 228.

Osborn, J. E., Blazkovec, A. A. and Walker, D. L. (1968). Immunosuppression during acute murine cytomegalovirus infection. *J. Immunol.* **100**, 835.

Oshiro, L. S., Dondero, D. V., Emmons, R. W. *et al.* (1978). The development of Colorado Tick Fever virus within cells of the haemopoetic system. *J. Gen. Virol.* **39**, 73.

Owens, S. L., Osebold, J. W. and Zee, Y. C. (1981). Dynamics of B lymphocytes in the lungs of mice exposed to aerosolized influenza virus. *Infect. Immunity* **33**, 231.

Owerbach, D., Rutter, W. J., Shows, T. B. *et al.* (1981). Leukocyte and fibroblast interferon genes are located on human chromosome 9. *Proc. Nat. Acad. Sci. USA* **78**, 3123.

Palese, P. and Roizman, B. (eds.) (1980). Genetic Variation of Viruses. *Annals N.Y. Acad. Sci.* **354**.

Pancic, F., Carpenter, D. C. and Caine, P. E. (1980). Role of infectious secretions in the transmission of rhinoviruses. *J. Clin. Microbiol.* **12**, 567.

Panem, S., Check, I. J., Henriksen, D. *et al.* (1982). Alpha interferon and antibody to alpha interferon in systemic lupus erythematosus. In *Interferons* (eds. T. C. Merigan and R. M. Friedman), UCLA Symposium of Molecular and Cell Biology, vol. XXV, pp. 233–40. Academic Press, New York.

Pang, T. (1983). Delayed-type hypersensitivity: probable role in the pathogenesis of dengue hemorrhagic fever/dengue shock syndrome. *Rev. Infect. Dis.* **5**, 346.

Pang, T. and Lam, K. S. K. (1983). The immunopathogenesis of dengue hemorrhagic fever. *Immunology Today* **4**, 46.

Panicali, D., Davis, S. W., Weinberg, R. L. *et al.* (1983). Construction of live vaccines by using genetically engineered poxviruses: biological activity of recombinant vaccinia virus expressing influenza virus hemagglutinin. *Proc. Nat. Acad. Sci. USA* **80**, 5364.

Para, M. F., Zezulak, K. M., Conley, A. J. *et al.* (1983). Use of monoclonal antibodies against two 75,000 – molecular weight glycoproteins specified by herpes simplex virus type 2 in glycoprotein identification and gene mapping. *J. Virol.* **45**, 1223.

Park, M. M., Griffin, D. E. and Johnson. R. T. (1981). Studies of immune responses during recovery from Sindbis virus encephalitis in selectively reconstituted thymectomized, lethally irradiated mice. *Infect. Immunity* **34**, 306.

Parker, R. F. and Thompson, R. L. (1942). The effect of external temperature on the course of infectious myxomatosis of rabbits. *J. Exp. Med.* **75**, 567.

Parkman, P. D. and Meyer, H. M. (1969). Prospects for a rubella virus vaccine. *Progr. Med. Virol.* **11**, 80.

Parks, W. P. and Rapp, F. (1975). Prospects for herpesvirus vaccination—safety and efficacy considerations. *Progr. Med. Virol.* **21**, 188.

Pasteur, L. (1885). Methode pour prévenir la rage après morsure. *C.R. Acad. Sci.* **101**, 765.

Paterson, P. Y., Day, E. D. and Whitacre, C. C. (1981). Neuroimmunologic disease: effector cell responses and immunoregulatory mechanisms. *Immunol. Rev.* **55**, 90.

Paucker, K., Cantell, K., and Henle, W. (1962). Quantitative studies of viral interference in suspended L cells. Effect of interfering viruses and interferon on the growth rate of cells. *Virology* **17**, 324.

Payne, L. N., Frazier, J. A. and Powell, P. C. (1976). Pathogenesis of Marek's disease. *Internat. Rev. Pathol.* **16**, 59.

Pazin, G. J., Ho, M. and Jannetta, P. J. (1978). Reactivation of herpes simplex virus after decompression of the trigeminal nerve root. *J. Infect. Dis.* **138**, 405.

Pearse, B. M. F. and Bretscher, M. S. (1981). Membrane recycling by coated vesicles. *Ann. Rev. Biochem.* **50**, 85.

Peiris, J. S. M. and Porterfield, J. S. (1981). Antibody-dependent enhancement of plaque formation on cell lines of macrophage origin—a sensitive assay for antiviral antibody. *J. Gen. Virol.* **57**, 119.

Peiris, J. S. M., Porterfield, J. S. and Roehrig, J. T. (1982). Monoclonal antibodies against the flavivirus West Nile. *J. Gen. Virol.* **58**, 283.

Pepose, J. S., Stevens, J. G., Cook, M. L. *et al.* (1981). Marek's disease as a model for the Landry-Guillain-Barre syndrome; latent viral infection in non-neuronal cells accompanied by specific immune responses to peripheral nerve and myelin. *Am. J. Pathol.* **103**, 309.

Pereira, R. S., James, D. C. O. and Stern, H. (1978). Correlation between cytomegalovirus infection and HLA-BW15. *Br. Med. J.* ii, 126.

Perez-Bercoff, R. (ed.) (1979). *The Molecular Biology of Picornaviruses*. Plenum Press. New York.

Perkins, F. T. and Regamey, R. H. (eds.) (1977). International Symposium on Influenza Immunization. *Dev. Biol. Stand.* **39**. Karger, Basel.

Perrault, J. (1981). Origin and replication of defective interfering particles. In *Initiation Signals in Viral Gene Expression* (ed. A. J. Shatkin), pp. 151–207. Springer-Verlag, Berlin.

Pestka, S. (ed.) (1981). Interferons, Parts A & B. *Meth. Enzymol.* **78** & **79**.

Pestka, S. (1983). The human interferons—from protein purification and sequence to cloning and expression in bacteria: before, between, and beyond. *Arch. Biochim. Biophys.* **221**, 1.

Pestka, S., Maeda, S., Hobbs, D. S. *et al.* (1981). The human interferons. In *Cellular Responses to Molecular Modulators* (eds. L. W. Mozes *et al.*), pp. 455–93. Academic Press, New York.

Pestka, S., Evinger, M., Maeda, S. *et al.* (1982). Biological properties of natural and recombinant interferons. *Texas Repts. Biol. Med.* **41**, 31.

Petchclai, B. and Saelim, P. (1978). Circulating immune complexes in dengue haemorrhagic fever. *Lancet* ii, 638.

Petricciani, J. C., Hopps, H. E. and Chapple, P. J. (eds.) (1979). Cell Substrates: Their Use in the Production of Vaccines and other Biologicals. *Adv. Exp. Med. Biol.* **118**. Plenum Press, New York.

Pfau, C. J., Valenti, J. K., Pevear, D. C. *et al.* (1982). Lymphocytic chorio-meningitis virus killer T cells are lethal only in weekly disseminated murine infections. *J. Exp. Med.* **156**, 79.

Pfeffer, L. M., Wang, E. and Tamm, I. (1980). Interferon effects on microfilament organization, cellular fibronectin distribution, and cell motility in human fibroblasts. *J. Cell Biol.* **85**, 9.

Pfizenmaier, K., Jung, H., Starzinski-Powitz, A. *et al.* (1977). The role of T cells in anti-herpes simplex virus immunity. I Induction of antigen-specific cytotoxic T lymphocytes. *J. Immunol.* **119**, 939.

Philipson, L., Lonberg-Holm, K. and Pettersson, U. (1968). Virus-receptor interaction in an adenovirus system. *J. Virol.* **2**, 1064.

Pincus, W. B. and Flick, J. A. (1963). Inhibition of the primary vaccinial lesion and of delayed hypersensitivity by an antimononuclear cell serum. *J. Infect. Dis.* **113**, 15.

Pitha, P. M., Rowe, W. P. and Oxman, M. N. (1976). Effect of interferon on exogenous, endogenous, and chronic murine leukemia virus infection. *Virology* **70**, 324.

Plotkin, S. A. (1975). Routes of fetal infection and mechanisms of fetal damage. *Am. J. Dis. Child.* **129**, 444.

Plotkin, S. A. (1980). Rabies vaccine prepared in human cell cultures: progress and perspectives. *Rev. Infect. Dis.* **2**, 433.

Plotkin, S. A., Farquhar, J. D., Katz, M. *et al.* (1969). Attenuation of RA 27/3 rubella virus in WI-38 human diploid cells. *Am. J. Dis. Child.* **118**, 178.

Plowright, W. (1965). Malignant catarrhal fever in East Africa. I Behaviour of the virus in free-living populations of Blue Wildebeeste (Corgon taurinus taurinus, Burchell). *Res. Vet. Sci.* **6**, 56.

Pollard, R. B. (1982). Interferons and interferon inducers: development of clinical usefulness and therapeutic promise. *Drugs* **23**, 37.

Pollard, R. B. and Merigan, T. C. (1978). Experience with clinical applications of interferon and interferon inducers. *Pharmacol. Therap. (A)* **2**, 783.

Pope, J. H., Horne, M. K. and Scott, W. (1968). Transformation of foetal human leukocytes *in vitro* by filtrates of a human leukemic cell line containing herpes-like virus. *Internat. J. Cancer* **3**, 857.

Popescu, M., Lohler, J. and Lehmann-Grube, F. (1979). Infectious lymphocytes in lymphocytic choriomeningitis virus carrier mice. *J. Gen. Virol.* **42**, 481.

Porter, D. D. and Larsen, A. E. (1974). Aleutian disease of mink. *Progr. Med. Virol.* **18**, 32.

Porter, D. D. and Cho, H. J. (1980). Aleutian disease of mink: a model for persistent infection. In *Comprehensive Virology* (eds. H. Fraenkel-Conrat and R. R. Wagner), vol. 16. Plenum Press, New York.

Porter, D. D., Porter, H. G. and Deerhake, B. B. (1969). Immunofluorescence assay for antigen and antibody in lactic dehydrogenase virus infection of mice. *J. Immunol.* **102**, 431.

Porter, D. D., Larsen, A. E. and Porter H. G. (1980). Aleutian disease of mink. *Adv. Immunol.* **29**, 261.

Porterfield, J. S. (1982). Immunological enhancement and the pathogenesis of dengue haemorrhagic fever. *J. Hyg.* **89**, 355.

Porterfield, J. S., Casals, J., Chumakov, M. P. *et al*. (1978). Togaviridae. *Intervirology* **9**, 129.

Possee, R. D., Schild, G. C. and Dimmock, N. J. (1982). Studies on the mechanisms of neutralization of influenza virus by antibody. Evidence that neutralizing antibody (anti-haemagglutinin) inactivates influenza virus *in vivo* by inhibiting virion transcriptase activity. *J. Gen. Virol.* **58**, 373.

Poste, G and Nicolson, G. L. (eds.) (1977). *Virus Infection and the Cell Surface*. Elsevier North-Holland, Amsterdam.

Potter, C. W. (1982). Inactivated influenza virus vaccine. In *Basic and Applied Influenza Research* (ed. A. S. Beare). CRC Press, Florida.

Pourcel, C., Sobzack, E., Dubois, M.-F. *et al*. (1982). Antigenicity and immunogenicity of hepatitis B virus particles produced by mouse cells transfected with cloned viral DNA. *Virology* **121**, 175.

Prabhakar, B. S. and Nathanson, N. (1981). Acute rabies death mediated by antibody. *Nature* **290**, 590.

Preble, O. T., Black, R. J., Klippel, J. H. *et al*. (1982). Interferon in systemic lupus erythematosus. In *Interferons* (eds. T. C. Merigan and R. M. Friedman), UCLA Symposium of Molecular and Cell Biology, vol. XXV, pp. 219–31. Academic Press, New York.

Preblud, S. R., Serdula, M. K., Frank, J. A. *et al*. (1980). Rubella vaccination in the United States: a ten-year review. *Epidemiol. Rev.* **2**, 171.

Preblud, S. R., Stetler, H. C., Frank, J. A. *et al*. (1981). Fetal risk associated with rubella vaccine. *J. Am. Med. Assoc.* **246**, 1413.

Prince, A. M., Ikram, H. and Hopp, T. P. (1982). Hepatitis B virus vaccine: Identification of HB_sAg/a and HB_sAg/d but not HB_sAg/y subtype antigenic determinants on a synthetic immunogenic peptide. *Proc. Nat. Acad. Sci. USA* **79**, 579.

Provost, P. J., Banker, F. S., Giesa, P. A. *et al*. (1982). Progress towards a live, attenuated human hepatitis A vaccine (41387). *Proc. Soc. Exp. Biol. Med.* **170**, 8.

Provost, P. J. and Hilleman, M. R. (1978). An inactivated hepatitis A virus vaccine prepared from infected marmoset liver. *Proc. Soc. Exp. Biol. Med.* **159**, 201.

Provost, P. J., Giesa, P. A., McAleer, W. J. *et al.* (1981). Isolation of hepatitis A virus *in vitro* in cell culture directly from human specimens. *Proc. Soc. Exp. Biol. Med.* **167**, 201.

Prusiner, S. B. (1982). Novel proteinaceous infectious particles cause scrapie. *Science* **216**, 136.

Puga, A., Rosenthal, J. D., Openshaw, H. *et al.* (1978). Herpes simplex virus DNA and mRNA sequences in acutely and chronically infected trigeminal ganglia of mice. *Virology* **89**, 102.

Purcell, R. H. and Gerin, J. L. (1978). Hepatitis B vaccines: a status report. In *Viral Hepatitis* (eds. G. Vyas, S. N. Cohen and R. Schmid), p. 491. Franklin Institute Press, Philadelphia.

Purchase, H. G., Okazaki, W. and Burmester, B. R. (1972). Long-term field trials with the herpesvirus of turkeys vaccine against Marek's disease. *Avian Dis.* **16**, 57.

Purchase, H. G. (1976). Prevention of Marek's disease: a review. *Cancer Res.* **36**, 696.

Purchase, H. G., Chubb, R. C. and Biggs, P. M. (1968). Effect of lymphoid leukosis and Marek's disease on the immunological responsiveness of the chicken. *J. Nat. Canc. Inst.* **40**, 583.

Quinnan, G. V., Manischewitz, J. F. and Ennis, F. A. (1978). Cytotoxic T lymphocyte response to murine cytomegalovirus infection. *Nature* **273**, 514.

Quinnan, G. V., Manischewitz, J. F. and Kirmani, N. (1982). Involvement of natural killer cells in the pathogenesis of murine cytomegalovirus interstitial pneumonitis and the immune response to infection. *J. Gen. Virol.* **58**, 173.

Racaniello, V. R. and Baltimore, D. (1981). Cloned poliovirus complementary DNA is infectious in mammalian cells. *Science* **214**, 916.

Radwan, A. I. and Crawford, T. B. (1974). The mechanism of neutralization of sensitized equine arteritis virus by complement components. *J. Gen. Virol.* **25**, 229.

Rager-Zisman, B. and Allison, A. C. (1976). Mechanisms of immunological resistance to herpes simplex virus I (HSV-1) infection. *J. Immunol.* **116**, 35.

Rager-Zisman, B. and Bloom, B. R. (1974). Immunological destruction of herpes simplex virus I infected cells. *Nature* **251**, 542.

Rager-Zisman, B., Kunkell, M., Taneka, Y. *et al.* (1982). Role of macrophage oxidative metabolism in resistance to vesicular stomatitis virus infection. *Infect. Immunity* **36**, 1229.

Rajewsky, K. and Brenig, C. (1974). Tolerance to serum albumin in T and B lymphocytes in mice. Dose dependence, specificity and kinetics of escape. *Eur. J. Immunol.* **4**, 120.

Rapp, F. (ed.) (1980). *Oncogenic Herpesviruses*, vols. 1 & 2. CRC Press, Florida.

Rapp, F., Melnick J. L., Butel, J. S. *et al.* (1964). The incorporation of SV40 genetic material into adenovirus 7 as measured by intranuclear synthesis of SV40 tumor antigen. *Proc. Nat. Acad. Sci. USA* **52**, 1348.

Rawls, W. E. (1968). Congenital rubella: the significance of virus persistence. *Progr. Med. Virol.* **10**, 238.

Rawls, W. E. and Leung, W.-C. (1979). Arenaviruses. Comprehensive Virology, no. 14, p. 157. Plenum Press, New York.

Rawls, W. E. and Melnick, J. L. (1966). Rubella virus carrier cultures derived from congenitally infected infants. *J. Exp. Med.* **123**, 795.

Reagen, K. J., Wunner, W. H., Wiktor, T. J. *et al.* (1983). Anti-idiotypic antibodies induce neutralizing antibodies to rabies virus glycoprotein. *J. Virol.* **48**, 660.

Redfield, D. C., Richman, D. D., Oxman, M. N. *et al.* (1981). Psoralen inactivation of influenza and herpes simplex viruses and of virus-infected cells. *Infect. Immunity* **32**, 1216.

Reed, S. E. (1975). An investigation of the possible transmission of rhinovirus colds through indirect contact. *J. Hyg.* **75**, 249.

Reed, S. E. and Boyle, A. (1972). Organ cultures of respiratory epithelium infected with rhinovirus or parainfluenza virus studied in a scanning electron microscope. *Infect. Immunity* **6**, 68.

Reid, L. M., Minato, N., Gresser, I. *et al.* (1981). Influence of anti-mouse interferon serum on the growth and metastasis of tumor cells persistently infected with virus and of human prostatic tumors in athymic nude mice. *Proc. Nat. Acad. Sci. USA* **78**, 1171.

Reinicke, V. (1965). The influence of steroid hormones and growth hormones on the production of influenza virus and interferon in tissue culture. II The influence of metandienonum, d-aldosterone, testosterone, oestradiol and growth hormones. *Acta. Pathol Microbiol. Scand.* **64**, 553.

Reitz, M. S., Kalyanaraman, V. S., Robert-Guroff, M. *et al.* (1983). Human T cell leukemia/lymphoma virus: the retrovirus of adult T-cell leukemia/lymphoma. *J. Infect. Dis.* **147**, 399.

Repaske, R., O'Neill, R. R., Steele, P. E. *et al.* (1983). Characterization and partial nucleotide sequencing of endogenous type C retrovirus segments in human chromosomal DNA. *Proc. Nat. Acad. Sci. USA* **80**, 678.

Revel, M. (1979). Molecular mechanisms involved in the antiviral effects of interferon. In *Interferon 1* (ed. I. Gresser), pp. 102–163. Academic Press, New York.

Richman, D. D. and Murphy, B. R. (1979). The association of the temperature-sensitive phenotype with viral attenuation in animals and humans: implications for the development and use of live virus vaccines. *Rev. Infect. Dis.* **1**, 413.

Rickinson, A. B., Moss, D. J., Wallace, L. E. *et al.* (1981). Long term T cell-mediated immunity to Epstein-Barr virus. *Cancer Research* **41**, 4216.

Riley, V. (1974). Persistence and other characteristics of the lactate dehydrogenase-elevating virus (LDH-virus). *Progr. Med. Virol.* **18**, 198.

Rima, B. K. (1983). The proteins of morbilliviruses. *J. Gen. Virol.* **64**, 1205.

Ringold, G. M., Yamamoto, K. R., Tomkins, G. M. *et al.* (1975). Dexamethazone-mediated induction of mouse mammary tumor virus RNA: a system for studying glucocorticoid action. *Cell* **6**, 299.

Rivière, Y., Gresser, I., Guillon, J. C. *et al.* (1977). Inhibition by anti-interferon serum of lymphocytic choriomeningitis disease in suckling mice. *Proc. Nat. Acad. Sci. USA* **74**, 2135.

Rivière, Y., Gresser, I., Guillon, J. C. *et al.* (1980). Severity of lymphocytic choriomeningitis virus disease in different strains of suckling mice correlates with increasing amounts of endogenous interferon. *J. Exp. Med.* **152**, 633.

Robbins, K. B., Brandling-Bennett, A. D. and Hinman, A. R. (1981). Low measles incidence: association with enforcement of school immunization laws. *Am. J. Publ. Health.* **71**, 270.

Roberts, J. A. (1962a). Histopathogenesis of mousepox I. Respiratory infection. *Br. J. Exp. Pathol.* **43**, 451.

Roberts, J. A. (1962b). Histopathogenesis of mousepox II. Cutaneous infection. *Br. J. Exp. Pathol.* **43**, 462.

Roberts, J. A. (1964a). Growth of virulent and attenuated ectromelia virus in cultured macrophages from normal and ectromelia-immune mice. *J. Immunol.* **92**, 837.

Roberts, J. A. (1964b). Histopathogenesis of mousepox. III. Ectromelia virulence. *Br. J. Exp. Pathol.* **44**, 42.

Roberts, J. A. (1964c). Enhancement of the virulence of attenuated ectromelia virus in mice maintained in a cold environment. *Austral. J. Exp. Biol. Med. Sci.* **42**, 657.

Roberts, N. J. (1979). Temperature and host defence. *Microbiol. Rev.* **43**, 241.

Robinson, J. E., Smith, D. and Niederman, J. (1981). Plasmacytic differentiation of circulating Epstein-Barr virus-infected B lymphocytes during acute infectious mononucleosis. *J. Exp. Med.* **153**, 235.

Robinson, W. S. (1982). The enigma of non-A, non-B hepatitis. *J. Infect. Dis.* **145**, 387.

Rocchi, G., de Feleci, A., Ragona, G. *et al.* (1977). Quantitative evaluation of Epstein-Barr virus infected mononuclear peripheral blood leukocytes in infectious mononucleosis. *New Engl. J. Med.* **296**, 132.

Rock, D. L. and Fraser, N. W. (1983). Detection of HSV-1 genome in central nervous system of latently infected mice. *Nature* **302**, 523.

Rodgers, B. and Mims, C. A. (1981). Interaction of influenza virus with mouse macrophages. *Infect. Immunity* **31**, 751.

Rodgers, B. and Mims, C. A. (1982). Influenza virus replication in human alveolar macrophages. *J. Med. Virol.* **9**, 177.

Rodriguez-Boulan, E. J. and Sabatini, D. D. (1978). Asymmetric budding of viruses in epithelial monolayers: a model system for study of epithelial polarity. *Proc. Nat. Acad. Sci. USA* **75**, 5071.

Rodriguez, M., Buchmeier, M. J., Oldstone, M. B. A. *et al.* (1983a). Ultrastructural localization of viral antigens in the CNS of mice persistently infected with lymphocytic choriomeningitis virus (LCMV). *Am. J. Pathol.* **110**, 95.

Rodriguez, M., Leibowitz, J. L. and Lampert, P. W. (1983b). Persistent infection of oligodendrocytes in Theiler's virus-induced encephalomyelitis. *Ann. Neurol.* **13**, 426.

Rodriguez, M., von Wedel, R. J., Garrett, R. S. *et al.* (1983c). Pituitary dwarfism in mice persistently infected with lymphocytic choriomeningitis virus. *Lab. Invest.* **49**, 48.

Roehrig, J. T., Brawner, T. A. and Riggs, H. G. (1979). Effects of 17 beta-estradiol on the replication of rubella virus in an estrogen-responsive continuous cell line. *J. Virol.* **29**, 417.

Rohatiner, A. Z. S., Prior, P. F., Burton, A. C. *et al.* (1983). Central nervous system toxicity of interferon. *Br. J. Canc.* **47**, 419.

Roitt, I. M. (1980). *Essential Immunology*, 4th edn. Blackwell Scientific Publications, Oxford.

Roizman, B. (ed.) (1982–84). *Herpesviruses*. Plenum Press, New York.

Roizman, B., Carmichael, L. E., Deinhardt, F. *et al.* (1981). Herpesviridae. *Intervirology* **16**, 201.

Roizman, B., Warren, J., Thuning, C. A. *et al.* (1982). Application of molecular genetics to the design of live herpes simplex virus vaccines. *Develop. Biol. Stand.* **52**, 287–304. Karger, Basel.

Rola-Pleszczynski, M. and Lieu, H. (1983). Natural cytotoxic cell activity linked to time of recurrence of herpes liabialis. *Clin. Exp. Immunol.* **55**, 224.

Romet-Lemonne, J. L., McLane, M. F., Elfrassi, E. *et al.* (1983). Hepatitis B virus infection in cultured human lymphoblastoid cells. *Science* **221**, 667.

Rosen, L. (1982). Dengue—an overview. In *Viral Diseases in South-East Asia and the Western Pacific* (ed. J. S. Mackenzie), p. 484. Academic Press, New York.

Rossen, R. D., Kasel, J. A. and Couch, R. B. (1971). The secretory immune system: its relation to respiratory viral infection. *Progr. Med. Virol.* **13**, 194.

Roth, M. G., Srinivas, R. V. and Compans, R. W. (1983). Basolateral maturation of retroviruses in polarized epithelial cells. *J. Virol.* **45**, 1065.

Rothman, J. E. and Fine, R. E. (1980). Coated vesicles transport newly synthesized membrane glycoproteins from endoplasmic reticulum to plasma membrane in two successive stages. *Proc. Nat. Acad. Sci. USA* **77**, 780.

Rothman, J. E. and Lodish, H. F. (1977). Synchronised transmembrane insertion and glycosylation of a nascent membrane protein. *Nature* **269**, 775.

Rott, R. (1979). Molecular basis of infectivity and pathogenicity of myxovirus. *Arch. Virol.* **59**, 285.

Rott, R., Reinacher, M., Orlich, M. *et al.* (1980). Cleavability of haemagglutinin determines spread of avian influenza viruses in the chorioallantoic membrane of chicken embryo. *Arch. Virol.* **65**, 123.

Rouse, B. T., Grewal, A. S., and Babiuk, L. A. (1977). Complement enhances antiviral antibody-dependent cell cytotoxicity. *Nature* **266**, 456.

Rowe, W. P. (1961). The epidemiology of mouse polyoma virus infection. *Bact. Rev.* **25**, 18.

Rowe, W. P. (1967). Some interactions of defective animal viruses. *Perspect. Virol.* **5**, 123.

Rowe, W. P. (1983). Deformed whiskers in mice infected with certain exogenous murine leukemia viruses. *Science* **221**, 562.

Rowe, W. P. and Baum, S. G. (1964). Evidence for a possible genetic hybrid between adenovirus type 7 and SV40 viruses. *Proc. Nat. Acad. Sci. USA* **52**, 1340.

Rowlands, D., Grabau, E., Spindler, K. *et al.* (1980). Virus protein changes and RNA termini alterations evolving during persistent infection. *Cell* **19**, 871.

Rubin, B. Y. and Gupta, S. L. (1980). Differential efficacies of human type I and type II interferons as antiviral and antiproliferative agents. *Proc. Nat. Acad. Sci. USA* **77**, 5928.

Rubin, D. and Fields, B. N. (1980). The molecular basis of reovirus virulence: the role of the M2 gene. *J. Exp. Med.* **152**, 853.

Rueckert, R. R. (1976). On the structure and morphogenesis of picornaviruses. In *Comprehensive Virology*, vol. 6, p. 131. Plenum Press, New York.

Ruff, R. L. and Secrist, D. (1982). Viral studies on benign acute childhood myositis. *Arch. Neurol.* **39**, 261.

Rundell, B. B. and Betts, R. F. (1981). Interaction of cytomegalovirus immune complexes with host cells. *Infect. Immunity* **33**, 658.

Rustigian, R., Smulow. K. B., Tye, M. *et al.* (1966). Studies on latent infection of skin and oral mucosa in individuals with recurrent herpes simplex. *J. Investig. Dermatol.* **47**, 218.

Rytel, M. W. and Kilbourne, E. D. (1966). The influence of cortisone on experimental viral infection VIII. Suppression by cortisone of interferon production in mice injected with Newcastle Disease virus. *J. Exp. Med.* **123**, 767.

Sabin, A. B. (1954). Genetic factors affecting susceptibility and resistance to virus disease of the nervous system. *Res. Publ. Assoc. Res. Nerv. Mental Dis.* **33**, 57.

Sabin, A. B. (1957). Properties of attenuated polioviruses and their behaviour in human beings. In *Cellular Biology, Nucleic Acids and Viruses* (ed. T. M. Rivers), Spec. publ. vol. 5, p. 113. N.Y. Acad. Sci., New York.

Sabin, A. B. (1980). Vaccination against poliomyelitis in economically underdeveloped countries. *Bull WHO* **58**, 141.

Sabin, A. B. (1981a). Immunization: evaluation of some currently available and prospective vaccines. *J. Am. Med. Assoc.* **246**, 236.

Sabin, A. B. (1981b). Paralytic poliomyelitis: old dogmas and new perspectives. *Rev. Infect. Dis.* **3**, 543.

Sabin, A. B., Arechiga, A. F., de Castro, J. F. *et al.* (1983). Successful immunization of children with and without maternal antibody by aerosolized measles vaccine. *J. Am. Med. Assoc.* **249**, 2651.

Sagar, A. D., Pickering, L. A., Sussman-Berger, P. *et al.* (1981). Heterogeneity of interferon mRNA species from Sendai virus-induced human lymphoblastoid (Namalva) cells and Newcastle disease virus-induced murine fibroblastoid (L) cells. *Nucleic Acids Res.* **9**, 149.

Sagar, A. D., Sehgal, P. B., Slate, D. L. *et al.* (1982). Multiple human β interferon genes. *J. Exp. Med.* **156**, 744.

Salk, D. (1980). Eradiation of poliomyelitis in the United States, I, II, III. *Rev. Infect. Dis.* **2**, 228.

Salk, J. E. (1958). Basic principles underlying immunization against poliomyelitis with a noninfectious vaccine. In *Poliomyelitis: Papers and Discussions Presented at the Fourth International Poliomyelitis Conference*. Lippincott, Philadelphia.

Salk, J. and Salk, D. (1977). Control of influenza and poliomyelitis with killed virus vaccines. *Science* **195**, 834.

Salonen, E. M., Vaheri, A., Suni, J. *et al.* (1980). Rheumatoid factor in acute viral infections: interference with determination of IgM, IgG and IgA antibodies in an enzyme immunoassay. *J. Infect. Dis.* **142**, 250.

Sambrook, J. (1981). Papovaviruses. In *DNA Tumor Viruses* (ed. J. Tooze), Cold Spring Harbor Laboratory, New York.

Sambrook, J. (1983). Biochemistry of animal viruses. In *Biochemistry* (ed. G. Zubay). Chap. 28. Addison-Wesley, New York.

Sanchez, Y., Ionescu-Matiu, I., Dreesman, G. R. *et al.* (1980). Humoral and cellular immunity to hepatitis B virus-derived antigens: comparative activity of Freund complete adjuvant, alum and liposomes. *Infect. Immunity* **30**, 728.

Sanford, B. A., Skelokov, A. and Ramsay, M. A. (1978). Bacterial adherence to virus-infected cells: a cell culture model of bacterial superinfection. *J. Infect. Dis.* **137**, 176.

Santisteran, G. A., Riley, V. and Fitzmaurice, M. A. (1972). Thymolytic and adrenal cortical responses to LDH-elevating virus. *Proc. Soc. Exp. Biol. Med.* **139**, 202.

Santoro, M. G., Jaffe, B. M., Garaci, E. *et al.* (1982). Antiviral effect of prostaglandins of the A series: Inhibition of vaccinia virus replication in cultured cells. *J. Gen. Virol.* **63**, 435.

Saron, M. F., Riviere, Y., Hovanessian, A. G. *et al.* (1982). Chronic production of interferon in carrier mice congenitally infected with lymphocytic choriomeningitis virus. *Virology* **117**, 253.

Sato, K., Inaba, Y., Shinozaki, T. *et al.* (1981). Isolation of human rotavirus in cell cultures. *Arch. Virol.* **69**, 155.

Sawyer, W. A. (1931). Persistence of yellow fever immunity. *J. Prevent. Med.* **5**, 413.

Sawyer, W. A. and Lloyd, W. (1931). Use of mice in tests of immunity against yellow fever. *J. Exp. Med.* **54**, 533.

Sawyer, W. A., Meyer, K. F., Eaton, M. D. *et al.* (1944). Jaundice in army personnel in the Western Region of the United States and its relation to vaccination against yellow fever. *Am. J. Hyg.* **39**, 337.

Schaffer, F. L. (1979). Caliciviruses. Comprehensive Virology no. 14, 249. Plenum Press, New York.

Schattner, A., Wallach, D., Merlin, G. *et al.* (1981). Assay of an interferon-induced enzyme in white blood cells as a diagnostic aid in viral diseases. *Lancet* ii, 497.

Schell, K. (1960). Studies in the innate resistance of mice to infection with mousepox. I Resistance and antibody production. *Austral. J. Exp. Biol. Med. Sci.* **38**, 271.

Schlesinger, R. W. (1980). *The Togaviruses*. Academic Press, New York.

Schluederberg, A., Ajello, C. and Evans, B. (1976). Fate of rubella genome ribonucleic acid after immune and non-immune virolysis in the presence of ribonuclease. *Infect. Immunity* **14**, 1097.

Schmaljohn, A. L., Johnson, E. D., Dalrymple, J. M. *et al.* (1982). Non-neutralizing monoclonal antibodies can prevent lethal alpha-virus encephalitis. *Nature* **297**, 70.

Schmidt, M. F. G. (1982). Acylation of viral spike glycoproteins: a feature of enveloped RNA viruses. *Virology* **116**, 327.

Schmidt, N. J. (1979). Laboratory diagnosis of viral infections. In *Antiviral Agents and Viral Diseases* (eds. G. J. Galasso *et al.*), pp. 209–52. Raven Press, New York.

Schonberger, L. B., Bregman, D. J., Sullivan-Bolyai, J. Z. *et al.* (1979). Guillain-Barré syndrome following vaccination in the National Influenza Immunization Program, United States, 1976–1977. *Am. J. Epidemiol.* **110**, 105.

Schulman, J. L. (1967). Experimental transmission of influenza virus infection in mice. IV Relationship of transmissibility of different strains of virus and recovery of airborne virus in the environment of effector mice. *J. Exp. Med.* **125**, 479.

Schultz, R. M., Chirigos, M. A. and Heine, U. I. (1978). Functional and morphologic characteristics of interferon-treated macrophages. *Cell. Immunol.* **35**, 84.

Schwartz, A. J. F. (1964). Immunization against measles: development and evaluation of a highly attenuated live measles vaccine. *Ann. Paediat.* **202**, 241.

Scott, G. M. and Tyrrell, D. A. J. (1980). Interferon: therapeutic fact or fiction for the 80's? *Br. Med. J.* i, 1558.

Scott, G. M., Secher, D. S., Flowers, D. *et al.* (1981). Toxicity of interferon. *Br. Med. J.* **282**, 1345.

Sehgal, P. B., Sagar, A. D. and Braude, I. A. (1981). Further heterogeneity of human α interferon mRNA species. *Science* **214**, 803.

Sehgal, P. B., Pfeffer, L. M. and Tamm, I. (1982). Interferon and its inducers. In *Chemotherapy of Viral Infections* (eds. P. E. Came and L. A. Caliguiri), pp. 205–311. Springer-Verlag, Berlin.

Sekizawa, T., Openshaw, H., Wohlenberg, C. *et al.* (1980). Latency of herpes simplex virus in absence of neutralizing antibody: model of reactivation. *Science* **210**, 1026.

Sela, M. (1975). Synthetic vaccines of the future. *Perspect. Virol.* **9**, 91.

Sela, M. and Arnon, R. (1980). Antiviral antibodies obtained with aqueous solution of a synthetic antigen. In *New Developments with Human and Veterinary Vaccines* (eds. A. Mizrahi *et al.*). *Progr. Clin. Biol. Res.* **47**, 315. Alan R. Liss, New York.

Sequera, L. W., Jennings, L. C., Carrasso, L. H. *et al.* (1979). Detection of herpes simplex viral genome in brain tissues. *Lancet* ii, 609.

Sethi, K. K., Omata, Y. and Schnewels, K. E. (1983). Protection of mice from fatal herpes simplex virus type I infection by adoptive transfer of cloned virus-specific and H_2-restricted cytotoxic T lymphocytes. *J. Gen. Virol.* **64**, 443.

Sever, J. and White, L. R. (1968). Intrauterine viral infections. *Ann. Rev. Med.* **19**, 471.

Shapiro, I. M. and Volsky, D. J. (1983). Infection of normal epithelial cells by Epstein-Barr virus. *Science* **219**, 1225.

Sharp, P. A. (1984). Adenovirus transcription. In *Adenoviruses* (ed. H. S. Ginsberg). Plenum Press, New York.

Shatkin, A. J. (ed.) (1981). *Initiation Signals in Viral Gene Expression*. Springer-Verlag, Berlin.

Shatkin, A. J. (1983). Molecular mechanisms of virus-mediated cytopathology. *Phil. Trans. R. Soc. Lond. B* **303**, 167.

Sheffield, W. D., Narayan, O., Strandberg, J. D. *et al.* (1980). Visna-maedi-like disease associated with an ovine retrovirus infection in a Corriedale sheep. *Vet. Pathol.* **17**, 544.

Shellam, G. R., Allan, J. E., Papadimitriou, J. M. *et al.* (1980). Increased susceptibility to cytomegalovirus infection in beige mutant mice. *Proc. Nat. Acad. Sci. USA* **78**, 5104.

Sherman, L. A. and Brown, R. M. Jr. (1978). Cyanophages and viruses of eukaryotic algae. In *Comprehensive Virology* (eds. H. Fraenkel-Conrat and R. R. Wagner), vol. 3, p. 145. Plenum Press, New York.

Shillitoe, E. J., Wilton, J. M. A. and Lehner, T. (1977). Sequential changes in cell-mediated immune responses to herpes simplex virus after recurrent herpetic infection in humans. *Infect. Immunity* **18**, 130.

Shimoda, T., Shikita, T., Karasawa, T. *et al.* (1981). Light microscope localization of hepatitis B virus antigens in the human pancreas. *Gastroenterology* **81**, 998.

Shore, S. L., Nahmias, A. J., Starr, S. E. *et al.* (1974). Detection of cell-dependent cytotoxic antibody to cells infected with herpes simplex virus. *Nature* **251**, 350.

Shore, S. L., Cromeans, T. L. and Romano, T. J. (1976). Immune destruction of virus infected cells early in the infectious cycle. *Nature* **262**, 695.

Shortman, K., Wilson, A., Scollay, R. *et al.* (1983). Development of large granular lymphocytes with anomalous non-specific cytotoxicity in clones derived from Ly-2+ T cells. *Proc. Nat. Acad. Sci. USA* **80**, 2728.

Shwartzman, G. and Aronson, S. M. (1953). Poliomyelitis infection by parenteral routes made possible by cortisone. *Ann. N. Y. Acad. Sci.* **56**, 793.

Shyamala, G. and Dickson, C. (1976). Relationship between receptor and mammary tumor virus production after stimulation by glucocorticoid. *Nature* **262**, 107.

Siddell, S., Wege, H. and ter Meulen, V. (1983). The biology of coronaviruses. *J. Gen. Virol.* **64**, 761.

Sigurdsson, B. (1954). Rida: a chronic encephalitis of sheep. With general remarks on infections which develop slowly and some of their special characteristics. *Br. Vet. J.* **110**, 341.

Silverstein, S. C., Astell, C., Levin, D. *et al.* (1974). The role of lysosomes in the uncoating and activation of the reovirus genome. *Adv. Biosciences* **11**, 3.

Simons, K. and Garoff, H. (1980). The budding mechanisms of enveloped animal viruses. *J. Gen. Virol.* **50**, 1.

Simons, K., Helenius, A., Leonard, K. *et al.* (1978). Formation of protein micelles from amphiphilic membrane proteins. *Proc. Nat. Acad. Sci. USA* **75**, 5306.

Simons, K., Helenius, A., Morein, B. *et al.* (1980). Development of effective subunit vaccines against enveloped viruses. In *New Developments with Human and Veterinary Vaccines* (eds. A. Mizrahi *et al.*). *Progr. Clin. Biol. Res.* **47**, 217. Alan R. Liss, New York.

Simons, K., Garoff, H. and Helenius, A. (1982). How an animal virus gets into and out of its host cell. *Sci. Am.* **246**, 46.

Sissons, J. G. and Oldstone, M. B. A. (1980). Antibody-mediated destruction of virus infected cells. *Adv. Immunol.* **29**, 209.

Skehel, J. J., Bayley, P. M., Brown, E. B. *et al.* (1982). Changes in the conformation of influenza virus hemagglutinin at the pH optimum of virus-mediated membrane fusion. *Proc. Nat. Acad. Sci. USA* **79**, 968.

Skelly, J., Howard, C. R. and Zuckerman, A. J. (1981). Hepatitis B polypeptide vaccine preparation in micelle form. *Nature* **290**, 51.

Skinner, G. R. B., Woodman, C. B. J., Hartley, C. E. *et al.* (1982). The preparation and immunogenicity of a vaccine Ac NFU$_1$ (S$^-$) MRC towards prevention of herpes genitalis in human subjects. *Br. J. Venereal. Dis.* **58**, 381.

Skup, D. and Millward, S. (1980). Reovirus-induced modification of cap-dependent translation in infected L cells. *Proc. Nat. Acad. Sci. USA* **77**. 152.

Smith, G. L., Mackett, M. and Moss, B. (1983). Infectious vaccinia virus recombinants that express hepatitis B surface antigen. *Nature* **302**, 490.

Smith, J. W. and Sheppard, A. M. (1982). Activity of rabbit monocytes, macrophages and neutrophils in antibody-dependent cellular cytotoxicity of herpes simplex virus-infected corneal cells. *Infect. Immunity* **36**, 685.

Smith, T. F., McIntosh, K., Fishaut, M. *et al.* (1981). Activation of complement by cells infected with respiratory syncytial virus. *Infect. Immunity* **33**, 43.

Sonnenfeld, G. and Merigan, T. C. (1979). The role of interferon in viral infections. *Springer Seminars Immunopathol.* **2**, 311.

Sonnenfeld, G., Mandel, A. D., and Merigan, T. C. (1978). Time and dosage dependence of immuno-enhancement by murine type II interferon preparations. *Cell. Immunol.* **40**, 285.

Spruance, S. L., Overall, J. C., Kern, E. R. *et al.* (1977). The natural history of recurrent herpes simplex labialis. *New Engl. J. Med.* **297**, 69.

Spruance, S. L., Green, J. A., Chiu, G. *et al.* (1982). Pathogenesis of herpes simplex labialis: correlation of vesicle fluid interferon with lesion age and virus titre. *Infect. Immunity* **36**, 907.

Stagno, S., Reynolds, D., Tsiantos, A. *et al.* (1975). Cervical cytomegalovirus excretion in pregnant and non-pregnant women; suppression in early gestation. *J. Infect. Dis.* **132**, 522.

Stagno, S., Reynolds, D. W., Huang, E. S. *et al.* (1977). Congenital cytomegalovirus infection: occurrence in an immune population. *New Engl. J. Med.* **296**, 1254.

Stagno, S., Reynolds, D. W., Pass, R. F. *et al.* (1980). Breast milk and the risk of cytomegalovirus infection. *New Engl. J. Med.* **302**, 1073.

Stagno, S., Pass, R. F., Dworsky, M. F. *et al.* (1982). Congenital cytomegalovirus infection. *New Engl. J. Med.* **306**, 945.

Stalder, H. and Ehrensberger, A. (1980). Microneutralization of cytomegalovirus. *J. Infect. Dis.* **142**, 102.

Starr, S. and Berkovich, S. (1964). Effects of measles, gammaglobulin modified measles and vaccine measles on the tuberculin test. *New Engl. J. Med.* **270**, 386.

Starr, S. E. and Allison, A. C. (1977). Role of T lymphocytes in recovery from murine cytomegalovirus infection. *Infect. Immunity* **17**, 458.

Starr, S. E., Glazer, J. P., Friedman, H. M. *et al.* (1981). Specific cellular and humoral immunity after immunization with live Towne strain cytomegalovirus vaccine. *J. Infect. Dis.* **143**, 585.

Steck, A. J., Tschannen, R. and Schaefer, R. (1981). Induction of antimyelin and antioligodendrocyte antibodies by vaccinia virus. *J. Neuroimmunol.* **1**, 117.

Stevens, J. G. and Cook, M. L. (1973). Latent herpes simplex virus in sensory ganglia. *Perspect. Virol.* **8**, 171.

Stiehm, E. R., Kronenberg, L. H., Rosenblatt, H. M. *et al.* (1982). UCLA conference. Interferon: immunobiology and clinical significance. *Ann. Intern. Med.* **96**, 80.

Stohlmann, S. A., Woodward, J. G. and Frelinger, J. A. (1982). Macrophage antiviral activity: extrinsic versus intrinsic activity. *Infect. Immunity* **36**, 672.

Stokes, J., Weibel, R. E., Villarejos, V. M. *et al.* (1971). Trivalent combined measles-mumps-rubella vaccine. *J. Am. Med. Assoc.* **218**, 57.

Stone, J. D. (1948). Prevention of virus infection with enzyme of V. cholerae II Studies with influenza virus in mice. *Austral. J. Exp. Biol. Med. Sci.* **26**, 287.

Strauss, E. G. and Strauss, J. H. (1983). Replication strategies of the single-stranded RNA viruses of eukaryotes. *Curr. Top. Microbiol. Immunol.* **105**, 1.

Strober, W., Hanson, L. A. and Sell, K. W. (eds.) (1982). *Recent Advances in Mucosal Immunity*. Raven Press, New York.

Stroop, W. G. and Baringer, J. R. (1982). Persistent, slow and latent viral infections. *Progr. Med. Virol.* **28**, 1.

Stueckemann, J. A., Ritzi, D. M. and Plagemann, P. G. W. (1981). Replication of lactate dehydrogenase-elevating virus in macrophages. I Evidence for cytocidal replication. *J. Gen. Virol.* **59**, 245.

Stueckemann, J. A., Holth, M., Swart, W. J. *et al.* (1982). Replication of lactate dehydrogenase-elevating enzyme in macrophages. 2 Mechanism of persistent infection in mice and in cell cultures. *J. Gen. Virol.* **59**, 263.

Sugden, B. (1982). Epstein-Barr virus: a human pathogen inducing lympho-proliferation in vivo and in vitro. *Rev. Infect. Dis.* **4**, 1048.

Sullivan, J. L., Mayner, R. E., Barry, D. W. *et al.* (1976). Influenza virus infections in nude mice. *J. Infect. Dis.* **133**, 91.

Summers, B. A., Griesen, H. A. and Appel, M. J. G. (1978). Possible initiation of viral encephalitis in dogs by migrating lymphocytes infected with distemper. *Lancet* i, 187.

Sundquist, V. A., Linde, A. and Wahren, B. (1983). Virus-specific IgG sub-classes in herpes simplex and varicella-zoster infections.

Suter, E. R. and Majno, G. (1965). Passage of lipid across vesicular endothelium in newborn rats. *J. Cell Biol.* **27**, 163.

Sveda, M. M. and Lai, C.-J. (1981). Functional expression in primate cells of cloned DNA coding for the hemagglutinin surface glycoprotein of influenza virus. *Proc. Nat. Acad. Sci. USA* **78**, 5488.

Sveda, M. M., Markoff, L. J. and Lai, C.-J. (1982). Cell surface expression of the influenza virus hemagglutinin requires the hydrophobic carboxyterminal sequences. *Cell* **30**, 649.

Swarz, J. R., Brooks, B. R. and Johnson, R. T. (1981). Spongiform polio-encephalomyelopathy caused by a murine retrovirus. II Ultrastructural localization of virus replication and spongiform changes in the central nervous system. *Neuropathol. Applied Neurobiol.* **7**, 365.

Sweet, B. H. and Hilleman, M. R. (1960). The vacuolating virus, SV40. *Proc. Soc. Exp. Biol. Med.* **105**, 420.

Sweet, C. and Smith, H. (1980). Pathogenicity of influenza virus. *Microbiol. Revs.* **44**, 303.

Symington, J., McCann, A. K. and Schlesinger, M. J. (1977). Infectious virus-antibody complexes of Sindbis virus. *Infect. Immunity* **15**, 720.

Szmuness, W., Stevens, C. E., Harley, E. J. *et al.* (1980). Hepatitis B vaccine: demonstration of efficacy in a controlled clinical trial in a high-risk population in the United States. *New Engl. J. Med.* **303**, 833.

Szmuness, W., Stevens, C. E., Harley, E. J. *et al.* (1981a). The immune response of healthy adults to a reduced dose of hepatitis B vaccine. *J. Med. Virol.* **8**, 123.

Szmuness, W., Stevens, C. E., Oleszko, W. R. *et al.* (1981b). Passive-active immunization against hepatitis B: immunogenicity studies in adult Americans. *Lancet* i, 575.

Szmuness, W., Alter, H. J. and Maynard, J. E. (eds.) (1982). *Viral Hepatitis*. Franklin Institute Press, Philadelphia.

Tada, T. and Okamura, K. (1979). The role of antigen-specific T cell factors in the immune response. *Adv. Immunol.* **28**, 1.

Taguchi, F., Yamada, A. and Fujiwara, F. (1979). Factors involved in the age-dependent resistance of mice infected with low virulence mouse hepatitis virus. *Arch. Virol.* **62**, 333.

Taguchi, F., Yamaguchi, R., Makino, S. *et al.* (1981). Correlation between growth potential of mouse hepatitis viruses in macrophages and their virulence for mice. *Infect. Immunity* **34**, 1059.

Takahashi, M., Asano, Y., Kamiya, H. *et al.* (1981). Active immunization for varicella-zoster virus. In *The Human Herpesviruses* (eds. A. J. Nahmias, W. R. Dowdle and R. F. Schinazi), pp. 414–31. Elsevier, Amsterdam.

Takemoto, K. K. and Habel, K. (1959). Virus-cell relationship in a carrier culture of HeLa cells and Coxsackie A9 virus. *Virology* **7**, 28.

Talal, N. and Steinberg, A. D. (1974). The pathogenesis of auto-immunity in New Zealand Black mice. *Curr. Topics Microbiol. Immunol.* **64**, 79.

Tamm, I. (1975). Cell injury with viruses. *Am. J. Pathol.* **81**, 163.

Tan, Y. H. (1977). Genetics of the human interferon system. In *Interferons and their Actions* (ed. W. E. Stewart), pp. 73–90. CRC Press, Florida.

Taniguchi, T., Guarente, L., Roberts, T. M. *et al.* (1980). Expression of the human fibroblast interferon gene in *Escherichia coli. Proc. Nat. Acad. Sci. USA* **77**, 5230.

Tashiro, M. and Homma, M. (1983). Pneumotropism of Sendai virus in relation to protease-mediated activation in mouse lungs. *Infect. Immunity* **39**, 879.

Tattersall, P. and Bratton, J. (1983). Reciprocal productive and restrictive virus-cell interactions of immunosuppressive and prototype strains of minute virus of mice. *J. Virol.* **46**, 944.

Taylor-Papadimitriou, J. (1980). Effects of interferons on cell growth and function. In *Interferon 2* (ed. I. Gresser), pp. 13–46. Academic Press, New York.

Tesh, R. B. (1982). Arthritides caused by mosquito-borne viruses. *Ann. Rev. Med.* **33**, 31.

Theiler, M. and Downs, W. G. (1973). *The Arthropod-Borne Viruses of Vertebrates*. Yale University Press, New Haven.

Theiler, M. and Smith, H. H. (1937). The use of yellow fever virus modified by *in vitro* cultivation for human immunization. *J. Exp. Med.* **65**, 787.

Thompson, R. L. (1938). The influence of temperature upon proliferation of infectious fibroma and infectious myxoma *in vivo. J. Infect. Dis.* **62**, 307.

Thomsen, A. R., Bro-Jorgensen, K. and Jensen, B. L. (1982). Lymphocytic choriomeningitis virus-induced immunosuppression: evidence for viral interference with T cell maturation. *Infect Immunity* **37**, 981.

Thomsen, A. R., Bro-Jorgensen, K. and Volkert, M. (1983). Fatal meningitis following lymphocytic choriomeningitis virus infection reflects delayed-type hypersensitivity rather than cytotoxicity. *Scand. J. Immunol.* **17**, 139.

Thormar, H., Barshatsky, M. R., Arnesen, K. *et al.* (1983). Emergence of antigenic variants is a rare event in long-term visna virus infection in vivo. *J. Gen. Virol.* **64**, 1427.

Tinsley, T. W. and Harrap, K. A. (1978). Viruses of invertebrates. In *Comprehensive Virology*, vol. 12, p. 1. Plenum Press, New York.

Tiollais, P., Charney, P. and Vyas, G. N. (1981). Biology of hepatitis B virus. *Science* **213**, 406.

Todaro, C. J., Callahan, R., Sherr, C. J. *et al.* (1978). Genetically transmitted viral genes of rodents and primates. In *Persistent Viruses* (eds. J. G. Stevens, G. J. Todaro and C. F. Fox), pp. 133–45. Academic Press, New York.

Toms, G. L., Rosztoczy, I. and Smith, H. (1974). The localization of influenza virus, minimal infectious dose determination and single cycle kinetic studies on organ cultures of respiratory and other ferret tissues. *Br. J. Exp. Pathol.* **55**, 116.

Tooze, J. (1980). *The Molecular Biology of Tumor Viruses. DNA Tumor Viruses.* Cold Spring Harbor Laboratory, New York.

Top, F. H., Grossman, R. A., Bartelloni, P. J. *et al.* (1971). Immunization with live types 7 and 4 adenovirus vaccines. I Safety, infectivity, antigenicity, and potency of adenovirus type 7 vaccine in humans. *J. Infect. Dis.* **124**, 148.

Tosolini, F. A. and Mims, C. A. (1971). Effect of murine strain and viral strain on the pathogenesis of lymphocytic choriomeningitis virus infection and a study of footpad responses. *J. Infect. Dis.* **123**, 134.

Trachsel, H., Sonenberg, N., Shatkin, A. J. *et al.* (1980). Purification of a factor that restores translation of vesicular stomatitis virus mRNA in extracts from poliovirus-infected HeLa cells. *Proc. Nat. Acad. Sci. USA* **77**, 770.

Trinchieri, G. and Santoli, D. (1978). Antiviral activity induced by cultured lymphocytes with tumor-derived or virus-transformed cells: enhancement of human natural killer cell activity by interferon and antagonistic inhibition of susceptibility of target cells to lysis. *J. Exp. Med.* **147**, 1314.

Tsai, K. and Karstad, L. (1973). The pathogenesis of epizootic haemorrhagic disease of deer. *Am. J. Pathol.* **70**, 379.

Tsiang, H. (1982). Neuronal function impairment in rabies-infected rat brain. *J. Gen. Virol.* **61**, 277.

Tyeryar, F. J., Richardson, L. S. and Belshe, R. B. (1978). Report of a workshop on respiratory syncytial virus and parainfluenza viruses. *J. Infect. Dis.* **137**, 835.

Tyrrell, D. A. J. and Burke, D. C. (eds.) (1982). Interferon: 25 years on. *Phil. Trans. Roy. Soc. Lond.* **299**, 1–144.

Tyrrell, D. A. J. and Smith, J. W. G. (1979). Vaccination against influenza A. *Br. Med. Bull.* **35**, 77.

Tyrrell, D. A. J., Schild, G. C., Dowdle, W. R. *et al.* (1981). Development and use of influenza vaccines. *Bull. WHO* **59**, 165.

Unanue, E. R. (1981). The regulatory role of macrophages in antigenic stimulation. *Adv. Immunol.* **31**, 1.

Urasawa, T., Urasawa, S. and Taniguchi, K. (1981). Sequential passages of human rotavirus in MA-104 cells. *Microbiol. Immunol.* **25**, 1025.

Vainio, T. (1963a). Virus and hereditary resistance in vitro I. Behaviour of West Nile (E-101) virus in the cultures prepared from genetically resistant and susceptible strains of mice. *Ann. Med. Exp. Biol. Fenniae* **41** (suppl.), 1.

Vainio, T. (1963b). Virus and hereditary resistance in vitro II. Behaviour of West Nile (E-101) virus in cultures prepared from challenged backcross and non-challenged susceptible mice. *Ann. Med. Exp. Biol. Fenniae* **41** (suppl.), 25.

Valentine, R. C. and Pereira, H. G. (1965). Antigens and the structure of the adenovirus. *J. Mol. Biol.* **13**, 13.

Valenzuela, P., Medina, A., Rutter, W. J. *et al.* (1982). Synthesis and assembly of hepatitis B virus surface antigen particles in yeast. *Nature* **298**, 347.

van Damme, J. and Billiau, A. (1981). Large scale production of human fibroblast interferon. *Meth. Enzymol.* **78**, 101.

Vandenbussche, P., Divizia, M., Verhaegen-Lewalle, M. *et al.* (1981). Enzymatic activities induced by interferon in human fibroblast cell lines differing in their sensitivity to the anticellular activity of interferon. *Virology* **111**, 11.

Van Wezel, A. L. (1981). Present state and developments in the production of inactivated poliomyelitis vaccine. *Develop. Biol. Stand.* **47**, 7.

Van Wezel, A. L., van Steenis, G., Hannik, Ch. A. *et al.* (1978). New approach to the production of concentrated and purified inactivated polio and rabies tissue culture vaccines. *Develop. Biol. Stand.* **41**, 159.

Varho, M., Lehmann-Grube, F. and Simon, M. M. (1981). Effector T lymphocytes in lymphocytic choriomeningitis virus infected mice. *J. Exp. Med.* **153**, 992.

Varmus, H. E. (1982). Form and function of retroviral proviruses. *Science* **216**, 812.

Verwoerd, D. W., Huismans, H. and Erasmus, B. J. (1979). Orbiviruses. In *Comprehensive Virology*, vol. 14, p. 285. Plenum Press, New York.

Vilček, J., Gresser, I. and Merigan, T. C. (eds.) (1980). Regulatory Functions of Interferons. *Annals N.Y. Acad. Sci.* **350**, 1.

Vilček, J., Yip, Y. K., Pang, R. H. L. *et al.* (1981). How many interferons are there? In *Cellular Responses to Molecular Modulators* (eds. L. W. Mozes *et al.*), pp. 331–45. Academic Press, New York.

Virelizier, J.-L. and Gresser, I. (1978). Role of interferon in the pathogenesis of viral diseases of mice as demonstrated by the use of anti-interferon serum. V. Protective role in mouse hepatitis virus type 3 infection of susceptible and resistant strains of mice. *J. Immunol.* **120**, 1616.

Virelizier, J. L., Postlethwaite, R., Schild, G. C. *et al.* (1974). Antibody responses to antigenic determinants of influenza virus haemagglutinin. I Thymus dependence of antibody formation and thymus independence of immunological memory. *J. Exp. Med.* **140**, 1559.

Vodinelich, L., Sutherland, R., Schneider, C. *et al.* (1983). Receptor for transferrin may be 'target' structure for natural killer cells. *Proc. Nat. Acad. Sci. USA* **80**, 835.

Vyas, G., Cohen, S. N. and Schmid, R. (eds.) (1978). *Viral Hepatitis*. Franklin Institute Press, Philadelphia.

Wachendorfer, G. and Frost, J. W. (1978). Epizootiological aspects of rabies in central Europe. Proceedings of 3rd Munich Symposium on Microbiology. Who Collaborating Centre, Munich.

Wagner, R. R. (1955). A pantropic strain of influenza virus: Generalized infection and viraemia in the infant mouse. *Virology* **1**, 497.

Walker, D. H., Murphy, F. A., Whitfield, S. G. *et al.* (1975). Lymphocytic choriomeningitis: Ultrastructural pathology. *Exp. Molec. Pathol.* **23**, 245.

Walker, D. H., McCormick, J. B., Johnson, K. M. *et al.* (1982). Pathologic and virologic study of fatal Lassa fever in man. *Am. J. Pathol.* **107**, 349.

Wallach, D., Fellous, M. and Revel, M. (1982). Preferential effect of γ interferon on the synthesis of HLA antigens and their mRNAs in human cells. *Nature* **299**, 833.

Wallnerova, Z. and Mims, C. A. (1970). Thoracic duct cannulation and hemal node formation in mice infected with cowpox virus. *Br. J. Exp. Pathol.* **51**, 118.

Wallnerova, A. and Mims, C. A. (1971). Thoracic lymph duct cannulation of mice infected with lymphocytic choriomeningitis (LCM) and ectromelia viruses. *Arch. Ges. Virusforsch.* **35**, 152.

Walsh, J. A. and Warren, K. S. (1979). Selective primary health care. An interim strategy for disease control in developing countries. *New Engl. J. Med.* **301**, 967.

Ward, D. C. and Tattersall, P. (eds.) (1978). *Replication of Mammalian Parvoviruses*. Cold Spring Harbor Laboratory, New York.

Watanabe, R., Wege, H. and ter Meulen, V. (1983). Adoptive transfer of EAE-like lesions from rats with coronavirus-induced demyelinating encephalomyelitis. *Nature* **305**, 150.

Watson, H. D., Tignor, G. H. and Smith, A. L. (1981). Entry of rabies virus into the peripheral nerves of mice. *J. Gen. Virol.* **56**, 371.

Watson, R. J., Weis, J. H., Salstrom, J. S. *et al.* (1982). Herpes simplex type-1 glycoprotein D gene: nucleotide sequence and expression in *Escherichia coli*. *Science* **218**, 381.

Watt, R. G., Plowright, W., Sabo, A. *et al.* (1973). A sensitive cell culture for the virus of porcine inclusion body rhinitis (cytomegalic inclusion disease). *Res. Vet. Sci.* **14**, 119.

Weber, C., Martinez-Peralta, L. and Lehmann-Grube, F. (1983). Persistent infection of cultivated cells with lymphocytic choriomeningitis virus: regulation of virus replication. *Arch. Virology* **77**, 271.

Webster, L. T. (1937). Inheritance of resistance of mice to enteric bacterial and neurotropic virus infections. *J. Exp. Med.* **65**, 261.

Webster, R. G. and Laver, W. G. (1975). Antigenic variation of influenza viruses. In *The Influenza Viruses and Influenza* (ed. E. D. Kilbourne), pp. 269–314. Academic Press, New York.

Webster, R. G., Yakhno, M., Hinshaw, V. S. *et al.* (1978). Intestinal influenza; replication and characterization of influenza viruses in ducks. *Virology* **84**, 268.

Webster, R. G., Laver, W. G., Air, G. M. *et al.* (1982). Molecular mechanisms of variation in influenza viruses. *Nature* **296**, 115.

Webster, R. G., Laver, W. G. and Air, G. M. (1984). Antigenic variation among type A influenza viruses. *Virology Monographs*, in press.

de Weck, A., Kristensen, F. and Landy, M. (eds.) (1980). *Biochemical Characterization of Lymphokines*. Academic Press, New York.

Weck, P. K., Apperson, S., May, L. *et al.* (1981). Comparison of the antiviral activities of various cloned human interferons in mammalian cell culture. *J. Gen. Virol.* **57**, 233.

Weibel, R. E., Buynak, E. B., McLean, A. A. *et al.* (1979). Follow-up surveillance for antibody in human subjects following live attenuated measles, mumps and rubella virus vaccines. *Proc. Soc. Exp. Biol. Med.* **162**, 328.

Weinberg, R. A. (1982). Oncogenes of spontaneous and chemically induced tumors. *Adv. Canc. Res.* **36**, 149.

Weiner, H. L., Powers, M. L. and Fields, B. N. (1980). Absolute linkage of virulence and central nervous system cell tropism of reoviruses to viral haemagglutinin. *J. Infect. Dis.* **141**, 609.

Weinstein, L. (1957). Influence of age and sex on susceptibility and clinical manifestations in poliomyelitis. *New Engl. J. Med.* **257**, 47.

Weis, J. H., Enquist, L. W., Salstrom, J. S. *et al.* (1983). An immunologically active chimaeric protein containing herpes simplex virus type 1 glycoprotein D. *Nature* **302**, 72.

Weiss, R. A. (1982). The persistence of retroviruses. In *Virus Persistence*, Symposium 33, Soc. Gen. Microbiol. (eds. B. W. J. Mahy, A. C. Minson and G. K. Darby). Cambridge University Press, Cambridge.

Weiss, R. A., Teich, N., Varmus, H. E. *et al.* (eds.) (1982). *RNA Tumor Viruses.* Cold Spring Harbor Laboratory, New York.

Weiss, R. C. and Scott, F. W. (1981). Antibody-mediated enhancement of disease in feline infectious peritonitis: comparisons with dengue hemorrhagic fever. *Comp. Immunol. Microbiol. Infect. Dis.* **4**, 175.

Weiss, R. C., Dodds, W. J. and Scott, F. W. (1980). Disseminated intravascular coagulation in experimentally induced feline infectious peritonitis. *Am. J. Vet. Res.* **41**, 663.

Weissenbach, J., Chernajovsky, Y., Zeevi, M. *et al.* (1980). Two interferon mRNAs in human fibroblasts: *in vitro* translation and *Escherichia coli* cloning studies. *Proc. Nat. Acad. Sci. USA* **77**, 7152.

Weissmann, C. (1981). The cloning of interferon and other mistakes. In *Interferon 3* (ed. I. Gresser), pp. 101–34. Academic Press, New York.

Weissmann, C., Nagata, S., Boll, W. *et al.* (1982). Structure and expression of human alpha-interferon genes. In *Interferons* UCLA Symposium of Molecular and Cell Biology, vol. XXV, pp. 295–326. (eds. T. C. Merigan and R. M. Friedman). Academic Press, New York.

Welliver, R. C., Wong, D. T., Sun, M. *et al.* (1981). The development of respiratory syncytial virus-specific IgE and the release of histamine in nasopharyngeal secretions after infection. *New Engl. J. Med.* **305**, 841.

Wells, A., Koide, N., Stein, H. *et al.* (1983). The Epstein-Barr virus receptor is distinct from the C3 receptor. *J. Gen. Virol.* **64**, 449.

Wells, M. A., Daniels, S., Djeu, J. Y. *et al.* (1983). Recovery from a viral respiratory tract infection. IV Specificity of protection by cytotoxic T lymphocytes. *J. Immunol.* **130**, 2908.

Welsh, J. K., Skurrie, I. J. and May, J. T. (1978). Use of Semliki Forst virus to identify lipid-mediated antiviral activity and anti-alphavirus immunoglobulin A in human milk. *Infect. Immunity* **19**, 395.

Welsh, R. M. (1978). Mouse natural killer cells: induction, specificity and function. *J. Immunol.* **121**, 1631.

Welsh, R. M. and Hallenbeck, L. A. (1980). Effect of virus infections on target cell susceptibility to natural killer cell mediated lysis. *J. Immunol.* **124**, 2491.

Welsh, R. M., Zinkernagel, R. M. and Hallenbeck, L. A. (1979). Cytotoxic cells induced during lymphocytic choriomeningitis virus infection of mice. II Specificities of the natural killer cells. *J. Immunol.* **122**, 475.

Westmoreland, D. and Watkins, J. F. (1974). The IgG receptors induced by herpes simplex virus: studies using radioiodinated IgG. *J. Gen. Virol.* **24**, 167.

Wheeler, C. E. (1960). Further studies on the effect of neutralizing antibody upon the course of herpes simplex infections in tissue culture. *J. Immunol.* **84**, 394.

White, D. O. (1984). *Antiviral Chemotherapy, Interferons and Vaccines*. Monographs in Virology, vol. 16. Karger, Basel.

Whitley, R., Lakeman, A. D., Nahmias, A. *et al.* (1982). DNA restriction-enzyme analysis of herpes simplex virus isolates obtained from patients with encephalitis. *New Engl. J. Med.* **307**, 1060.

Whittle, H. C., Mee, J., Werblinska, J. *et al.* (1980). Immunity to measles in malnourished children. *Clin. Exp. Immunol.* **42**, 144.

Wigand, R., Bartha, A., Dreizin, R. S. *et al.* (1982). Adenoviridae: second report. *Intervirology* **18**, 169.

Wigdahl, B. L., Scheck, A. C., De Clercq, E. *et al.* (1982). High efficiency latency and activation of herpes simplex virus in human cells. *Science* **217**, 1145.

Wigdahl, B. L., Ziegler, R. J., Sneve, M. *et al.* (1983). Herpes simplex virus latency and reactivation in isolated rat sensory neurones. *Virology* **127**, 159.

Wiktor, T. J. and Koprowski, H. (1982). Does the existence of rabies antigenic variants warrant re-evaluation of rabies vaccines? Proceedings of the First International Conference on the Impact of Viral Diseases on the Development of Latin American Countries and the Caribbean Region.

Wiktor, T. J., Plotkin, S. A. and Koprowski, H. (1978). Development and clinical trials of the new human rabies vaccine of tissue culture (human diploid cell) origin. *Dev. Biol. Stand.* **40**, 3.

Wildy, P., Cell, P. G. H., Rhodes, J. *et al.* (1982a). Inhibition of herpes virus multiplication by activated macrophages: a role for arginase. *Infect. Immunity* **37**, 40.

Wildy, P., Field, H. J. and Nash, A. A. (1982b). *Classical herpes latency revisited*. Soc. Gen. Microbiol. Symposium 33 (eds. B. W. J. Mahy, A. C. Minson and G. K. Darby). Cambridge University Press, Cambridge.

Wiley, D. C., Wilson, I. A. and Skehel, J. J. (1981). Structural identification of the antibody binding sites of Hong Kong influenza haemagglutinin and their involvement in antigenic variation. *Nature* **289**, 373.

Wolfe, J., Rubin, D. H., Finberg, R. *et al.* (1981). Intestinal M cells: a pathway for entry of reovirus into the host. *Science* **212**, 471.

Wolfe, L. G. (1979). Primate herpes virus infections of B (Epstein-Barr virus) and T (Herpes virus Saimiri) lymphocytes. Review of biological characteristics. In *Mechanisms of Viral Pathogenesis and Virulence*, 4th Munich Symposium on Microbiology, (ed. P. A. Bachman).

Wolinsky, J. S., Klassen, T. and Baringer, J. R. (1976). Persistence of neuro-adapted mumps virus in brains of newborn hamsters after intraperitoneal inoculation. *J. Infect. Dis.* **133**, 260.

Wong, C. Y., Woodruff, J. J. and Woodruff, J. F. (1977). Generation of cytotoxic T lymphocytes during coxsackievirus B_3 infection. III Role of sex. *J. Immunol.* **119**, 591.

Wood, J. N., Hudson, L., Jessell, T. M. *et al.* (1982). A monoclonal antibody defining antigenic determinants on sub-populations of mammalian neurones and Trypanosoma cruzi parasites. *Nature* **296**, 34.

Woodruff, J. F. (1970). The influence of quantitated post-weaning under-nutrition or coxsackievirus B_3 infection of adult mice. II Alterations of host defence mechanisms. *J. Infect. Dis.* **121**, 164.

Woodruff, J. F. (1979). Lack of correlation between neutralizing antibody production and suppression of Coxsackie virus B₃ replication in target organs. Evidence for involvement of mononuclear inflammatory cells in host defence. *J. Immunol.* **123**, 31.

Woodruff, J. F. (1980). Viral myocarditis. *Am. J. Pathol.* **101**, 425.

Woods, W. A., Johnson, R. T., Hostetler, P. D. *et al.* (1966). Immunofluorescent studies on rubella-infected tissue cultures and human tissues. *J. Immunol.* **96**, 253.

Workshop (1976). Current understanding of persistent viral infections and their implications in human disease—summary of a workshop. *J. Infect Dis.* **133**, 707.

WHO (1966). The use of human immunoglobulin. WHO Technical Report Series 327. WHO, Geneva.

WHO (1971). WHO Expert Committee on Yellow Fever, Third Report. WHO Technical Report Series 479. WHO, Geneva.

WHO (1976). Immunological adjuvants. WHO Technical Report Series 595. WHO, Geneva.

WHO (1982). Interferon therapy. WHO Technical Report Series 676. WHO, Geneva.

WHO (1983a). Prevention of liver cancer. WHO Technical Report Series 691. WHO, Geneva.

WHO (1983b). *Viral Vaccines and Antiviral Drugs*. WHO, Geneva.

WHO Consultative Group (1982). The relation between persisting spinal paralysis and poliomyelitis vaccine—results of a ten-year enquiry. *Bull. WHO* **60**, 231.

Williams, A. F. (1984). The T-lymphocyte antigen receptor-elusive no more. *Nature* **308**, 108.

Worthington, B. B. and Graney, D. O. (1973). Uptake of adenovirus by intestinal absorptive cells of the suckling rat. I The neonatal ileum. *Anat. Rec.* **175**, 37.

Worthington, M., Conliffe, M. A. and Baron, S. (1980). Mechanism of recovery from systemic herpes simplex virus infection. I Comparative effectiveness of antibody and reconstitution with immune spleen cells. *J. Infect. Dis.* **142**, 163.

Wright, P. F., Okabe, N., McKee, K. T. *et al.* (1982). Cold-adapted recombinant influenza A virus vaccines in seronegative young children. *J. Infect. Dis.* **146**, 71.

Wu, B. C. and Ho, M. (1979). Characterization of infection of B and T lymphocytes from mice after inoculation with cytomegalovirus. *Infect Immunity* **24**, 856.

Wunner, W. H., Dietzschold, B., Curtis, P. J. *et al.* (1983). Rabies subunit vaccines. *J. Gen. Virol.* **64**, 1649.

Wyatt, H. V. (1973). Poliomyelitis in hypogammaglobulinaemics. *J. Infect. Dis.* **128**, 802.

Wyde, P. R. and Cate, T. R. (1978). Cellular changes in lungs of mice infected with influenza virus: characterization of the cytotoxic responses. *Infect. Immunity* **22**, 423.

Wylie, D. E., Sherman, L. A. and Klinman, N. R. (1982). Participation of the major histocompatibility complex in antibody recognition of viral antigens expressed on infected cells. *J. Exp. Med.* **155**, 403.

Yap, K. L., Ada, G. L. and McKenzie, I. F. C. (1978). Transfer of specific cytotoxic T lymphocytes protects mice inoculated with influenza virus. *Nature* **273**, 238.

Yarchoan, R., Tosato, G., Blaese, R. M. *et al.* (1983). Limiting dilution analysis of Epstein-Barr virus-induced immunoglobulin production by human B cells. *J. Exp. Med.* **157**, 1.

Yefenof, E. and Klein, G. (1977). Membrane receptor stripping confirms the association between EBV receptors and complement receptors on the surface of human B lymphoma lines. *Internat. J. Canc.* **20**, 347.

Yelverton, E., Norton, S., Obijeski, J. F. *et al.* (1983). Rabies virus glycoprotein analogs: biosynthesis in *Escherichia coli. Science* **219**, 614.

Yewdell, J. W., Webster, R. G. and Gerhard, W. U. (1979). Antigenic variation in three distinct determinants of an influenza type A haemagglutinin molecule. *Nature* **279**, 246.

Yip, Y. K., Barrowclough, B., Urban, C. *et al.* (1982). Purification of two sub-species of human gamma (immune) interferon. *Proc. Nat. Acad. Sci. USA* **79**, 1820.

Yoon, J. W., Austin, M., Onodera, T. *et al.* (1979). Virus induced diabetes mellitus: isolation of a virus from the pancreas of a child with diabetic ketoacidosis. *New Engl. J. Med.* **300**, 1173.

Yoshimura, A., Kuroda, K., Kawasaki, K. *et al.* (1982). Infectious cell entry mechanism of influenza virus. *J. Virol.* **43**, 284.

Yoshino, K. and Isono, N. (1978). Studies on the neutralization of herpes simplex virus. IX Variance in complement requirement among IgG and IgM from early and late sera under different sensitization conditions. *Microbiol. Immunol.* **22**, 403.

Young, E. J. and Gomez, C. I. (1979). Enhancement of herpes virus type 2 infection in pregnant mice. *Proc. Soc. Exp. Biol. Med.* **160**, 416.

Young, E. J., Killam, A. P. and Greene, J. F. (1976). Disseminated herpes virus infection. *J.A.M.A.* **235**, 2731.

Youngner, J. S., Preble, O. T. and Jones, E. V. (1978). Persistent infection of L cells with vesicular stomatitis: evolution of virus populations. *J. Virol.* **28**, 6.

Youssoufian, H., Hammer, S. M., Hirsch, M. S. *et al.* (1982). Methylation of the viral genome in an in vitro model of herpes simplex latency. *Proc. Nat. Acad. Sci. USA* **79**, 2207.

Zawatsky, R., Hilfenaus, J. and Kirchner, H. (1979). Resistance of nude mice to herpes simplex virus and correlation with *in vitro* production of interferon. *Cell. Immunol.* **47**, 424.

Zawatsky, R., Hilfenaus, J., Marcucci, F. *et al.* (1981). Experimental infection of susceptible and resistant mice with herpes simplex virus. I Investigation of humoral and cellular immunity and interferon production. *J. Gen. Virol.* **60**, 25.

Zawatsky, R., Gresser, I., de Maeyer, E. *et al.* (1982). The role of interferon in the resistance of C57 BL/6 mice to various doses of herpes simplex virus type I. *J. Infect. Dis.* **146**, 405.

Zinkernagel, R. M. (1976). H-2 restriction of virus-specific T cell-mediated effector functions in vivo. II Adoptive transfer of delayed hypersensitivity to murine lymphocytic choriomeningitis virus is restricted by the K and D region of H-2. *J. Exp. Med.* **144**, 776.

Zinkernagel, R. M. (1979). Associations between major histocompatibility antigens and susceptibility to disease. *Ann. Rev. Microbiol.* **33**, 201.

Zinkernagel, R. M. and Doherty, P. C. (1973). Cytotoxic thymus-derived lymphocytes in cerebrospinal fluid of mice with lymphocytic choriomeningitis. *J. Exp. Med.* **138**, 1266.

Zinkernagel, R. M. and Doherty, P. C. (1974). Restriction of *in vitro* T cell mediated cytotoxicity in lymphocytic choriomeningitis within a syngeneic or semiallogeneic system. *Nature* **248**, 701.

Zinkernagel, R. M. and Doherty, P. C. (1979). MHC-restricted cytotoxic T cells: studies on the biological role of polymorphic major transplantation antigens determining T-cell restriction—specificity, function and responsiveness. *Adv. Immunol.* **27**, 51.

Zisman, B., Hirsch, M. S. and Allison, A. C. (1970). Selective effects of anti-macrophage serum, silica and anti-lymphocyte serum on pathogenesis of herpes virus infection of young adult mice. *J. Immunol.* **104**, 1155.

Zisman, B., Wheelock, E. F. and Allison, A. C. (1971). Role of macrophages and antibody in resistance of mice against yellow fever virus. *J. Immunol.* **107**, 236.

Zuckerman, A. J. (1982). Persistence of hepatitis B virus in the population. In *Virus Persistence*, Symposium 33, Soc. Gen. Microbiol. (eds. B. W. J. Mahy, A. C. Minson and G. K. Darby). Cambridge University Press, Cambridge.

zur Hausen, H. (1980). The role of viruses in human tumors. *Adv. Canc. Res.* **33**, 77.

Index

Note: Page numbers in **bold** refer to those pages on which illustration/tables appear.

Abbreviations used are as follows:

H2 restrictions on response 120–1
inclusion bodies **134**, 135
monoclonal antibodies 149
primary infection 9, 206, **208**
recurrent infections 9, 185, 206–11
  immunology 210–11, 243
  models 207–8, 209
  reactivation 185, 207, **208**,
    210–12, 235
  site, neurone 207, 208, 212
  viral state in neurone 209, 243
spread of,
  via nerves 68, 206–7, 210
  prevention, macrophage 115
  via saliva 73
susceptibility to infections by 167
  age-dependence 180
  macrophage 178, 180
type I 9
  progesterone effect 194
  vaccine 259, 301–2
  virulence, genome region in
    161–2
type 2 9, 207
  vaccine 301–2
Herpesviruses 9
  lymphotropic persistent 215
  multiplication **19**, **24**, 32, 206–7
  properties 7, 9
  spread of 68
  structure 4, 7
  vaccines 300–2
  see also Cytomegalovirus;
    Epstein-Barr virus; Herpes
    simplex; Varicella-zoster
Herpesvirus saimiri 216
Herpesvirus simiae 273
Herpesvirus of turkeys 261
Heterokaryons 135
Heteroploid cell lines 273–4
Histamine release **111**, 141
HLA and susceptibility 181
  see also Major histocompatibility
    complex
Hormones,
  pathogenic effects 151–2
  in susceptibility to infections
    193–5, 213
Host, of viruses 2, 5
  body surface **40**
  cellular synthesis inhibition 32–3,
    133, 136
  damage, *see* Disease production
  defence, *see* Immune response

resistance, determinants 158, 160,
  163–97
  age, *see* Age
  cellular enzymes, mitotic state
    167
  cellular receptors for virus 165–7
  dual infections 195–7
  fever 184–5
  genes 164, 166
  hormones 193–5, 213
  immune responses 181–4
  inflammation 185–6
  interferon, *see* Interferons
  lactation 193–5
  macrophage 178–80
  nutrition 186–8
  pregnancy 193–5
  sex 193
  sialic acid 166–7
  susceptibility to infection 163, 197
  genetic differences 163–4, 167
Host range mutants 256
Human diploid cell vaccine (HDCV)
  280
Human T-cell leukaemia/lymphoma
  virus 36
Hybridisation, molecular 5
Hybridoma technology 96, 135
  IgE suppression 102
  LCM infection 226
Hyperalimentation 188
Hypercholesterolaemia 188
Hypersensitivity 139–48
  summary **140**
  type I (anaphylactic) 139–41, 155
  type 2 (cytotoxic) **140**, 141, 155
  type 3 (immune complex) **140**,
    141–5, 156
    see also Immune complex(es);
      Inflammation
  type 4 (cell-mediated, delayed)
    140, 146–8, 156
    see also Delayed hypersensitivity
Hypogammaglobulinaemia 123

Ia antigens 88, **91**, 97
  in antigen presentation 97, 114,
    128, 269, 270
  on dendritic cells 114
Icosahedron 3
Idiotypic receptors 98
Immune complex(es) 108, 141
  in acute infections 143
  antigen excess 143

Lactation 193–5
see also Breast milk
Lactic dehydrogenase (LDH) virus
   58, 60, 138, 227–8
   acute infection 227
   functional change of infected cell
      138, 227
   immune complexes **145**, 227
   immunological effects 227
   interferon not produced 247
   in vivo assay 227
   macrophage, infection of 138,
      227–8, 244–5
   persistent infection 227–8, 243, 247
Lactose 153–4
Lamina propria 105
Langerhan, islets of 150, 152
Langerhans cells 89, 114
Laryngitis **44**
Lassa fever 14, 153, 278
Late genes 18, 23, 25
   proteins 27
Latency 201
Latent period 18
Latent virus infections 200, **203**
   reactivation 191, 200–1
   see also individual infections;
      Persistent infections
LCM virus, *see* Lymphocytic
   choriomeningitis virus
Lectins 173, 174
Lentivirinae 15, 201, 216–17
Lethal dose (LD$_{50}$) **159**, 163
Leukaemias 205, 206
Leukaemia virus 236
   feline 206
   mouse **145**, 206, 238, 244
Leukovirus, avian 165
Lipids, anti-viral 188
Liposomes 267, 292
   MHC restriction, T$_c$ cells 100
Liver,
   destruction in yellow fever 152
   necrosis,
      antibody-mediated 141
      influenza virus 133
      Rift Valley fever virus 139
   virus behaviour in, types **55**
Lung,
   immunopathology 147, 190
   in infants, infection severity 190
   oedema in, vulnerability 132, 147
'Luxury functions' 138, 225
Lymphatic spread 49–51, 76, 84

Lymphatic system 49–50, 76
Lymph node 49, 104
   swelling, immunopathology 139
Lymphoblasts (blasts) 90
Lymphocytes 89
   in brain 248
   infections of, persistence
      mechanism **234**, 239, **240**
      measles, VSV 235–6
   in infections, role 49–50
   large granular, NK cells 116
   recirculation 50, 89–**90**
   virus carriage in **53**
   virus receptors 239, 241
   see also B lymphocytes; T
      lymphocytes
Lymphocytic choriomeningitis (LCM)
      virus 223–6
   depressed antibody response 119,
      197, 241
   electromelia virus susceptibility
      197
   germline transmission 64, 75
   host susceptibility, genetics 225,
      238
   immunopathology 118, 120, 138,
      139, 146–7, 225
      cell-mediated 120, 146–7, 181
      interferon in 154, 173
      weak CMI, disease resistance
         181–2
   interferon action 226, 247
   persistent infections 204, 223–6
      clonal depletion 226
      growth hormone 138, 152, 225
      immune complexes 144, **145**,
         223, 225
      immune response 224, 226, 238,
         244, 247
      luxury functions 138, 225
      mechanism 226
      in newborn, *in utero* 193, 223
      T cell responses 120, 146, 181,
         226
      virology 226, 244
   platelet infection 53
Lymphocytotrophic hormones 98
Lymphoid tissues,
   in EB virus infection 215
   infections of 239, **240**–1
   see also Macrophage
   submucosal 104, 105
Lymphokines 90, 98
   interferons as 174–5

Multiplication of viruses (*contd*)
  temperature, fever, effect of 184–5
  transcription, *see* Transcription
  transformation, *see* Transformation
  translation 26–7
  uncoating 22–3
  uptake, penetration 21–2
  viral genome expression 19–20, **24**
Multiplicity reactivation 261–2
Mumps virus 67
  vaccine **276**, **279**, 290
Muramyl dipeptide (MDP) 266
Muscle, invasion 59, 67
Mutants, vaccines 256–60, 272, 293–4
Mutations, viral 217, 248, 250
  see also Temperature-sensitive
    mutants
Myositis 67
Myxomatosis 77
Myxoma virus 164, 184–5

Nairovirus 14
Nasopharyngeal carcinoma (NPC)
  215
Nasopharyngeal secretion 81
Natural killer (NK) cells 92, 115–16,
  129
  antiviral role 122–3
  in CMV infection 122, 123
  cytotoxicity 116, 129
  in herpes simplex infection 121
  interferon, activation by 77, 116,
    123, 175
  interferon secretion 175
  origin, cell type 116
  surface markers **95**, 116
Negri bodies **134**, 135
Neoantigenic determinants 100, 109,
  127
Nerves,
  latent herpes simplex 207–9
  latent varicella-zoster 211–12
  measles virus in 217
  spread of virus 61, 68, **69**, 206–7,
    210
Neural cell infection 60, 61
Neuraminidase (NA) 12, 43
  antibody to 109
  in influenza vaccines 292, 293
  in protection from virus 165
Neuritis, acute demyelinating
  peripheral 151
Neutralisation of virus 107–9
  classical, mechanism 108–9, 245

low level, persistent infection
  242
enhancement 127
  by complement 109, **111**, 112
  by enhancing antibody 109, 244
  opsonisation, agglutination 109
Neutralising tests 243
Newborn, susceptibility of 188–9
  experimental animals 191–3
Newcastle disease virus 161
Nodaviruses 16–17
Non-neutralising antibody, *see*
  Antibody
Non-permissive host cells 33
Norwalk virus 11
Nucleic acid in viruses 2, 18, 28–9
  see also DNA; RNA
Nucleo-capsid 3, 4, 29, 218
Nutrition 79, 186–8, 287

Obesity syndrome 152
Oedema, cellular, tissue 132
  cerebral 133, 146
  'cloudy swelling' 134
  in inflammation 142
  in lung 132, 147
  role in host defence 185, 186
Okazaki fragments 28
OKT antigens 95
Olfactory nerve, invasion via 68
Oligodendrocytes 228–9, 241
Oligosaccharide core trimming 30
Oligosaccharide
  pyrophosphoryldolichol 30
Oncogenes 35, 258
Oncoviruses 15
  transformation 19, 35–6, 135, 205,
    252
O'nyong-nyong 144
Opsonization 109, 112
Orbivirus **4**, 16
Organs, virus localisation in 53, 65–8
Original antigenic sin 126–7, 270, 291
Oropharynx 45, **48**
Orthomyxoviruses 12–13
  multiplication **19**, **24**
  properties, structure **4**, **8**, 12–13
Otitis media 196, 295

Pancencephalitis **145**
  see also Subacute sclerosing
    panencephalitis